What Develops
in Emotional Development?

EMOTIONS, PERSONALITY, AND PSYCHOTHERAPY

Series Editors:

Carroll E. Izard, *University of Delaware, Newark, Delaware*
and
Jerome L. Singer, *Yale University, New Haven, Connecticut*

Current volumes in the series

THE COGNITIVE FOUNDATIONS OF PERSONALITY TRAITS
Shulamith Kreitler and Hans Kreitler

FINDING MEANING IN DREAMS: A Quantitative Approach
G. William Domhoff

FROM MEMORIES TO MENTAL ILLNESS: A Conceptual Journey
William M. Hall

IMAGERY AND VISUAL EXPRESSION IN THERAPY
Vija Bergs Lusebrink

THE PSYCHOLOGY OF EMOTIONS
Carroll E. Izard

QUANTIFYING CONSCIOUSNESS: An Empirical Approach
Ronald J. Pekala

THE ROLE OF EMOTIONS IN SOCIAL AND PERSONALITY
DEVELOPMENT: History, Theory, and Research
Carol Magai and Susan H. McFadden

SAMPLING INNER EXPERIENCE IN DISTURBED AFFECT
Russell T. Hurlburt

SAMPLING NORMAL AND SCHIZOPHRENIC INNER EXPERIENCE
Russell T. Hurlburt

WHAT DEVELOPS IN EMOTIONAL DEVELOPMENT?
Edited by Michael F. Mascolo and Sharon Griffin

A Continuation Order Plan is available for this series. A continuation order will bring delivery of each new volume immediately upon publication. Volumes are billed only upon actual shipment. For further information please contact the publisher. ·

What Develops in Emotional Development?

Edited by

Michael F. Mascolo
Merrimack College
North Andover, Massachusetts

and

Sharon Griffin
Clark University
Worcester, Massachusetts

Plenum Press • New York and London

Library of Congress Cataloging-in-Publication Data

On file

ISBN 0-306-45722-9

© 1998 Plenum Press, New York
A Division of Plenum Publishing Corporation
233 Spring Street, New York, N.Y. 10013

http://www.plenum.com

10 9 8 7 6 5 4 3 2 1

Printed in the United States of America

To Bonnie and Paul

and to Dennis McLaughlin
who inspires through his compassionate style of guidance,
support, and good humor.

Contributors

Jo Ann A. Abe • Department of Psychology, 220 Wolf Hall, University of Delaware, Newark, Delaware 19716

Brian P. Ackerman • Department of Psychology, 220 Wolf Hall, University of Delaware, Newark, Delaware 19716

Karen Caplovitz Barrett • Department of Human Development and Family Studies, Colorado State University, Fort Collins, Colorado 80523

Terrance Brown • 3530 North Lake Shore Drive, 12-A, Chicago, Illinois 60657

K. Laurie Dickson • Department of Psychology, Northern Arizona University, Flagstaff, Arizona 86011

Lori Douglas • Ontario Institute for Educational Studies, 252 Bloor Street West, Toronto Ontario, Canada M5S 1V6

Alan Fogel • Department of Psychology, University of Utah, Salt Lake City, Utah 84112

Nico H. Frijda • University of Amsterdam, Roeterstraat 15, 1018 WB Amsterdam, The Netherlands

Sharon Griffin • Frances L. Hiatt School of Psychology, Clark University, 950 Main Street, Worcester, Massachusetts 01610

Debra Harkins • Department of Psychology, Suffolk University, Boston, Massachussets 02114

Carrol E. Izard • Department of Psychology, 220 Wolf Hall, University of Delaware, Newark, Delarware 19716

Brian Knutson • Department of Psychology, Bowling Green State University, Bowling Green, Ohio 43402

Arnold Kozak • RR1, Box 1276, Cambridge, Vermont 05444

Marc D. Lewis • Ontario Institute for Educational Studies, 252 Bloor Street West, Toronto, Ontario, Canada M5S 1V6

Michael Lewis • Institute for the Study of Child Development, Robert Wood Johnson Medical School, 97 Paterson Street, New Brunswick, New Jersey 08903

James C. Mancuso • Department of Psychology, State University of New York at Albany, 1400 Washington Avenue, Albany, New York 12222

Michael F. Mascolo • Department of Psychology, Merimack College, 315 Turnpike Street, North Andover, Massachusetts 01845

Batja Mesquita • Department of Psychology, Wake Forest University, Winston-Salem, North Carolina 27101

Daniel Messinger • Departments of Pediatrics and Psychology, University of Miami, Miami, Florida 33101

Jaak Panksepp • Department of Psychology, Bowling Green State University, Bowling Green, Ohio 43402

Douglas L. Pruitt • Department of Psychology, Bowling Green State University, Bowling Green, Ohio 43402

Theodore R. Sarbin • University of California, 25515 Hatton Road, Carmel, California 93923

Foreword

The problem of development is central in the study of emotional life for two basic reasons. First, emotional life so clearly changes (dramatically in the early years) with new emotional reactions emerging against the backdrop of an increasing sensitivity to context and with self-regulation of emotion emerging from a striking dependence on regulatory assistance from caregivers. Such changes demand developmental analysis. At the same time, understanding such profound changes will surely inform our understanding of the nature of development more generally. The complexity of emotional change, when grasped, will reveal the elusive nature of development itself.

At the outset, we know that development is complex. We must take seriously what is present at any given phase, including the newborn period, because a developmental analysis disallows something emerging from nothing. Still, it is equally nondevelopmental to posit that new forms of new processes were simply present in their precursors. Rather, development is characterized by transformations in which more complex structures and organization "emerge" from new integration of prior components and new capacities. These new forms and organizations cannot be specified from prior conditions but are due to transactions of the evolving organism with its environment over time. They are not simply in the genome, and they are not simply conditioned by the environment. They are the result of the developmental process. Thus, positing a simple differentiation mechanism, in which mature forms simply "come out of" earlier forms, without specifying the nature of the interactive process is not adequate; nor is a position in which mature forms are assumed to have always been present.

Development, then, implies increasing complexity and organization, often accompanied by a more precise coordination of components and a more precise coordination between organism and environment. There are distinctive patterns of infant–environment transaction, even in the newborn. These set the stage for later processes involving subjective engagement, evaluation, and (ultimately) represented subjectivity. It is differentiation in this sense, not in the sense of more differentiated components only, that defines a developmental analysis. Yet understanding and specifying this type of developmental change is extraordinarily challenging.

The authors in this volume grapple with this complexity from many points of view, with varying emphases that sometimes seem difficult to integrate; yet integration remains the goal of all. Emotional development includes the emergence of specific affects, the growth of emotional regulation, and the increasing integration of emotion with social and cognitive development. It also includes changes in experience and changes in the narratives children and others construct of these experiences. It is all of this and more. Each of these aspects of emotional development is taken up by one contributor or another, in the knowledge that greater understanding of these various features of emotional life will contribute to the integration we seek. Some explicitly move toward an overarching integration. In their view, as in mine, what develops are not just components or facets of emotions, but changes in systemic organization of emotional life itself. This is the challenge confronted in this volume.

L. ALAN SROUFE
Institute of Child Development
University of Minnesota

Preface

The idea for this volume developed from several sources. The first involved a discussion that occurred one evening among members of a Harvard discussion group about the nature of emotional development. In that discussion, one participant expressed puzzlement over the very idea of "emotional development." He said something like "I never really understand what people mean when they talk about emotional development. Does this mean that emotions develop? I know what it means to say that thinking develops. But what does it mean to say that emotions develop?" This comment sparked much debate. One individual expressed the position that emotions, as feeling states, were largely impervious to a developmental analysis. How can something as basic as a sensory experience undergo developmental change? Another individual, with passion to match the first, said something like "but everything about emotion develops—our perceptions of the situations that elicit emotion, emotional expressions, what we do when we have an emotion, the experience of emotion, our understanding of emotion. How can we say that everything about emotion develops except the emotion? *All* psychological processes undergo development." It was clear that debaters advocated very different positions on the nature of emotion and emotional development.

This book also had its origins in our own work as emotion researchers attempting to make sense of the burgeoning literature on emotional development, and in our experiences with students who have struggled with this same literature. Even a casual perusal of the literature on emotions and emotional development indicates a lack of consensus or even clarity about the meaning of such concepts. Some researchers have provided clear definitions of what they have in mind when they speak of emotion; others, in failing to define it at all, have written as if the concept were clear and transparent. In our courses, we have led students through discussions of theoretical and empirical treatments of the nature of emotion and emotional development. In particular, for any given set of readings, we have asked students to infer how the theorist defined emotion and whether emotions could be said to develop over any period of the life span. Constructing answers to these questions has provided a considerable challenge to several groups of students over a period of several years. Although students and their professors have been able to construct answers for each theorist that were reasonably consistent from year to year, the amount of inference involved always raised questions about the faithfulness of our answers to the theorists' own conceptions. Would they agree with our renditions of their positions?

This volume was conceived as an attempt to clarify the diversity of perspectives that researchers adopt when approaching the study of emotional development. Theorists and researchers working in the field today were asked to define their positions with respect to three fundamental questions: To what do we refer when we speak of emotion? What develops in emotional development? What roles do developing emotions play in the lives of individuals? The responses they provided form the body of this volume. In posing these questions, we hoped to clarify points of agreement and disagreement about the nature of emotional development, provide examples of developmental trajectories in emotional processes, and raise further issues and questions for researchers addressing what it means to speak of emotions in the context of human development.

We are grateful to many individuals for the roles they have played in shaping this volume. We thank Carroll Izard and Jerome Singer for their helpful commentary in the early stages of the project, and for their contributions in bringing the project to fruition. Terry Brown, Robbie Case, Laura Craig-Bray, Kurt Fischer, Jerome Kagan, Bonnie Kanner, Jim Mancuso, and Theodore Sarbin provided helpful comments and encouragement at various stages of the project. Thomas Schoenfeld offered invaluable assistance in the review of Panksepp, Knutson, and Pruitt's thoroughgoing chapter on affective neuroscience and emotional development. We thank Pat Bowman-Skeffington, Mary O'Connell, and Bethany Parker for their able assistance in the coordination and preparation of manuscripts and correspondence with contributors. We would also like to thank Susan Haas for the splendid artwork that embellishes the cover of this volume. We would also like to express our thanks to Eliot Werner for his astute help and support throughout the development of this manuscript, and to Herman Makler for his able assistance in bringing the volume to print. Finally, we wish to thank our many graduate and undergraduate students and colleagues at Merrimack College and Clark University for their roles in learning with us about the development of emotions. Work on this project was supported by grants from Merrimack College to the first editor and from Clark University to the second editor.

Contents

12. The Narrative Construction of Emotional Life: Developmental Aspects 297

James C. Mancuso and Theodore R. Sarbin

VI. CONCLUSION AND INTEGRATION

13. Alternative Conceptions of Emotional Development: Controversy and Consensus 319

Michael F. Mascolo and Sharon Griffin

What Develops
in Emotional Development?

I

Introduction

On the Nature, Development, and Functions of Emotions

Sharon Griffin and Michael F. Mascolo

> What are emotions, anyway? Our culture sees this question as a deep
> and ancient mystery. Common-sense psychology has not even reached
> a consensus on which emotions exist. If there exists anger, what
> constitutes rage? How does fear relate to fright, terror, dread, dismay,
> and all such other awful things? Are these just various degrees of
> intensity and direction, or are they genuinely different entities that
> happen to be neighbors in an uncharted universe of the affections?
> Are hate and love quite separate things, or similarly, courage and
> cowardice—or are they merely pairs of extremes, each just the absence
> of its peer? What are emotions, anyway, and what are all the other
> things we label moods, feelings, passions, needs, or sensibilities?
>
> MARVIN MINSKY (1985, p. 172)

The study of emotions and emotional development has changed dramatically
in the past several decades. At the early and middle points of the century,
emotional processes were generally seen as secondary or even disruptive

Sharon Griffin • Frances L. Hiatt School of Education, Clark University, Worcester, Massachusetts 01610.   Michael F. Mascolo • Department of Psychology, Merrimack College,
North Andover, Massachusetts 01845.

What Develops in Emotional Development? edited by Michael F. Mascolo and Sharon Griffin.
Plenum Press, New York, 1998.

aspects of human functioning (e.g., Young, 1943). Today, emotional processes are no longer relegated to the periphery of psychological analysis. Instead, they are seen as central motivators and organizers of cognition, action, social interaction, and development itself (Campos, Campos, & Barrett, 1989; Lewis & Haviland, 1993; Thompson, 1993). However, despite widespread agreement about the importance of emotion in human functioning, the concept of emotion continues to be an elusive one, as Minsky (1985) indicates in the opening quotation. Theorists and researchers differ widely in their approaches to emotion and emotional development. As a result, there is a general lack of clarity with respect to a series of foundational issues: To what do we refer when we speak of emotions? What develops in emotional development? What is the role of developing emotions for individuals and those with whom they interact? Our purpose in organizing this volume was to provide a forum for a systematic examination of these issues from a variety of theoretical perspectives. In posing these questions, we hoped to clarify points of consensus and controversy concerning the nature of emotion and to explore the implications of different approaches for understanding the shapes of emotional development.

To illustrate existing diversity in the study of emotional development, we first describe the approaches to emotional development that provided the immediate context for the present volume. Thereafter, we examine points of controversy and unresolved issues in the current study of emotional development. We then provide an overview of the structure of the volume and a brief synopsis of the ways in which contributors address central issues about the nature, development, and functions of emotion.

A SELECTIVE REVIEW OF CURRENT APPROACHES TO EMOTIONAL DEVELOPMENT

Theorists and researchers have approached the study of emotional development from different perspectives. In this section, we examine several influential models of emotion that have contributed to the debate about the nature of emotional development and which have been foundational for much of the work described in this volume. We present five basic frameworks: (1) biological and differential emotions theory, (2) cognitive approaches, (3) structural–developmental approaches, (4) functionalist approaches, and (5) sociocultural approaches. In our analysis of each framework, we examine how the concept of emotion is defined, what it is that develops in emotional development, and the role that emotion plays in the psychological and social lives of developing individuals. To facilitate comparison among these different views, the answers provided by representative proponents of each framework are summarized in Table 1.

Table 1. Foundational Perspectives

Perspectives	What are emotions?	Function of emotions?	What develops?
Biological (e.g., Izard)	Discrete sets of neurochemical processes—expressive behaviors–feeling states • Each has its own neurophysiological substrate • Each independent of cognition	Send social signals; foster social interaction; motivate behavior and cognitive development	Connections with other systems are established • Emotions themselves are largely invariant over the life span
Cognitive (e.g., Kagan)	Superordinate categories representing varied relations among external incentives, thoughts, and detected changes in feeling states	Direct attention; motivate thought and action; support cultural values	Incentives that contribute to feeling states develop as a function of cognitive development • New emotions become possible
Structural-Developmental (e.g., Sroufe)	Subjective reactions to salient events characterized by physiological, experiential, and overt behavioral change	Communicate inner states; facilitate response to emergencies; promote environmental mastery; ensure reproductive success	Differentiated affective systems (e.g., joy, anger, fear), undergo developmental transformation from earlier to more advanced forms organized around an affective core
Functionalist (e.g., Campos & Barrett)	Patterns of interaction between organism and environment in service of a goal • Dependent on "appreciation" of relation of event to goal	Regulates flow of information, selection of response processes, and social and interpersonal behavior	Number and complexity of interaction patterns change as a function of socialization and cognitive development • Some "appreciations" exist at birth and are continuous over life span
Social–Cultural (e.g., Abu-Lughod & Lutz)	Socially or culturally constructed syndromes constituted by interaction of many components related to individuals in their social and physical context	Preserve social orders and prevailing sociomoral frameworks	Syndromes change as a function of socialization, discursive practices, and enculturation.

Biological Perspectives and Discrete Emotions Theory

Among the most influential classes of theories that have guided emotion research in recent years have been models that stress the biological founda- tions of emotional functioning or the functioning of discrete emotional sys- tems. In this class of models, emotions are conceptualized as innate, neuro- muscular processes, much of which remains stable throughout ontogenesis. Ekman (1984; Ekman, Friesen, & Ellsworth, 1972), Izard (1977; Izard, 1984; Izard & Malatesta, 1987), and Tomkins (1982, 1984) have been among the most persuasive proponents of this view. For example, in their elaboration of differential emotions theory, Izard and Malatesta (1987) define emotions as "a particular set of neural processes that lead to a specific expression and a corresponding specific feeling" (p. 496). As such, emotions are concep- tualized as discrete systems that are distinct from cognition and other psycho- logical processes, yet interact with cognition. Ten discrete emotions have been proposed—interest–excitement, enjoyment–joy, startle–surprise, distress– anguish, rage–anger, disgust–revulsion, contempt–scorn, fear–terror, shame– shyness–humiliation, and guilt–remorse—and each is seen to have its own neurophysiological substrate (Izard, 1977, 1984; Izard & Malatesta, 1987).

In this view, there are age-related changes in the neural and expressive (e.g., facial) components of emotion over the first few months of life. How- ever, this growth is largely determined by maturational constraints. The feeling component, described as a felt "sensation," or "quality of conscious- ness" consists of a "reflexive response to the other two components" and is invariant over the lifespan (Izard, 1984; Izard & Malatesta, 1987). Although the emotion system is seen as distinct from other systems (e.g., perceptual, behavioral, cognitive) from birth, with development, emotions interact and become increasingly connected with the cognitive and behavioral systems. The establishment of such connections enables the uncoupling of relations between emotion expression and feeling, permitting social control over emo- tions as well as emotion understanding. However, these and other changes that result are largely seen to reflect changes in more peripheral aspects of emotion, rather than changes in emotions per se.

From a differential emotions view, emotions function as primary motiva- tors of behavior and cognition. In addition, the expressive component of emotions serves critical adaptive functions in development. A large and growing body of research spawned by differential emotions theory demon- strates that emotion-related facial expressions regulate the quality and type of caregiver attention, the formation of social relationships, and other aspects of social communication from infancy onwards (Demos, 1986; Trevarthen, 1984). Thus, differential emotions theory and related models of emotional develop- ment provide a rich framework for explaining the functions of emotions in

children's development, especially with regard to facial expressivity in infancy (Camras, Malatesta, & Izard, 1991).

Cognitive Perspectives

Another class of models that emerged in the same time period as the
biological models are models that stress the cognitive foundations of emotional functioning. Although these models do not deny the role of biology in
human functioning, they conceptualize emotion quite differently from the
biological models and they have been equally influential in shaping much
subsequent work. In this class of models, emotions are conceptualized as a
function of cognition (Kagan, 1978, 1984), as a cognitive construction (Mandler, 1984, 1990), or as a social-cognitive construction (Mancuso, 1986; Weiner &
Graham, 1984).

Kagan (1978, 1984, 1994) has been a persuasive proponent of this view of
emotional development. For Kagan (1984), the term *emotion* refers to a superordinate category representing varied relations among (1) external incentives,
(2) thoughts, and (3) detected changes in internal feeling states, called "feeling
tone." Although Kagan recognizes a class of emotional phenomena in which
physiological changes (called "feeling tone") are undetected, he believes that
the detection of the feeling tone is of extreme importance for the subsequent
emotional state. Thus, detected and undetected changes in feeling tone de-
serve categorically different labels. In his view, relations among external
incentives, thoughts, and detected changes in feeling states form coherences
(i.e., a gestalt experience) to which we can assign labels. For example "seeing a
dangerous animal–expecting physical harm–perceiving an increase in heart
rate" forms one coherency. "Seeing a frown on the face of a loved one–
expecting rejection–noticing an increase in heart rate" forms another that
differs dramatically from the first in external incentive, in thoughts, and in
behavioral consequences. Because Kagan believes that even subtle changes in
any one component will render a different emotion experience, he advocates
abandoning the abstract emotion terms that are currently available in favor of
labeling feeling–event occurrences that show regularity and coherence. Thus,
rather than label joy and distress as emotion categories, Kagan prefers "joy of
understanding" and "distress to physical privation."

Emotional development occurs, in this view, as a function of cognitive
development and the acquisition of new knowledge. With the development of
new cognitive functions (e.g., the ability to evaluate self and to recognize
when social standards have been violated), the types of incentives that contribute to emotion states change, systematically, from external to internal.
These new acquisitions permit the individual to experience emotions that
would not be possible without them, and the resulting emotions are seen to be

qualitatively distinct from previous ones. In this view, emotions function to keep the mind focused on the desires and events of the moment, to direct the person to find ways to maintain the pleasant feelings and eliminate the unpleasant ones, and to support the enculturation of values.

Structural–Developmental Perspectives

A third class of emotion theories proceeds from an explicitly structural–developmental framework. These models are embodied in the works of Lewis (1990, 1995; Chapter 2, this volume; Lewis, Sullivan, Stanger, & Weiss, 1989), Sroufe (1979, 1984, 1996), Fischer (Fischer, Shaver, & Carnochan, 1990), Case (Case, Hayward, Lewis, & Hurst, 1988), and others (Cicchetti & Hesse, 1982; Piaget, 1981). For example, Sroufe's (1979, 1996) approach is based explicitly on a developmental orientation in which development is defined in terms of *directionality* and *structural transformation*. Any given psychological process is defined in terms of the organization of its elements, which undergo qualitative change in the direction of increased differentiation and integration (Werner & Kaplan, 1963/1984). As such, no psychological processes—even those that are postulated to be innate—emerge at a given point in development. Rather, all behavior undergoes a series of changes from simple and more global forms to increasingly complex and mature forms.

Sroufe's (1979, 1984, 1996) developmental model of emotion proceeds from the premise that emotional development is tied to changes in other domains, including neurophysiological, cognitive, and social development. Sroufe (1996) proposes a working definition of emotion as "a subjective reaction to a salient event, characterized by physiological, experiential and overt behavioral change" (p. 15, although he warns against any attempt to reduce emotion to a simple definition). Sroufe postulates a series of stage transitions in the development of three affect systems: joy, anger, and fear. Like differential emotions theory (Izard & Malatesta, 1987), Sroufe suggests that each system is differentiated from the other. However, unlike Izard's system, emotions within each system undergo developmental transformation from early to more advanced forms while preserving their basic affective core. In newborns, emotional reactions within each system are defined in terms of physiological states that are evoked by physical stimulation. Precursor emotions emerge subsequent to the newborn period, which are mediated by the meaning that an event has for the infant. Basic emotions of joy, anger, and fear emerge during the second half of the first year with the development of an infant's capacity for more immediate recognition of the meaning of a given event for the child. More mature forms of each emotion continue to evolve during the second year of life. Thus, any given level of emotional functioning is defined by different organizations among affect, cognition, physiological responsiveness, and behavior within a given social context. As such, emotions serve adaptive functions for individuals' attempts to adapt to their social communities. These include communicating inner states to others, facilitating responses to emergency situations, promoting environmental mastery, and ultimately ensuring reproductive success.

Other structural–developmental approaches proceed from slightly different assumptions. For example, in the Case et al. (1988) model, emotion is defined as "a distinctive internal experience that is rooted in the activation of a distinctive neurological system" (p. 10). Although this definition is similar to that offered by Izard (1977), Case et al. also suggest that the emotion system is linked directly to all of the other major systems at birth and can influence or be influenced by them in a direct fashion (see Lewis & Douglas, Chapter 7, this volume, for an elaboration of this position). As such, Case et al. (1988) claim that "from birth onwards, activation of any [cognitive] scheme is experienced as having a particular affective character, either positive, negative, or neutral" (p. 3). In this view, two pairs of emotions are present at birth: contentment–distress and sensory engagement–disengagement. All other emotions evolve out of these basic affective states as cognitive-affective systems undergo developmental transformation. First to emerge are rage, joy, fear and, considerably later, jealousy, shame, pride, and guilt. Cognitive development also results in changes in the types of situations in which an emotion can be experienced and in the control structures children develop to deal with the situation and the emotions they elicit. Thus, although emotion is independent of cognition, it is nevertheless intimately connected to it, and so emotion and cognition are seen as equal partners from birth onward. Within this partnership, emotion functions as an energizer and director of children's thought. Furthermore, it influences the course of cognitive growth by determining the amount of time children spend in epistemic activity (which will be less if children experience fewer emotional benefits) by channeling cognition and behavior in particular directions, and by increasing the efficiency of cognitive processes.

Functionalist Approaches

Functionalist models view emotions as organized ensembles of multiple component processes that serve adaptive functions in the context of personally significant events (Barrett & Campos, 1987; Campos, Barrett, Lamb, Goldsmith, & Stenberg, 1983; Frijda, 1986, 1988). For example, Barrett and Campos (1987) suggest that emotions involve physiological, experiential, appraisal, internal reaction, motive–action tendency, expressive, and social display components. Functionalist thinkers define emotions in terms of "modes of action readiness" (Frijda, 1986) or "processes that serve particular functions in connection with an organism's relationship to its environment (Barrett & Campos, 1987) rather than in terms of subjective feeling states. For example, Campos (1994) defines emotion as "the attempt by the person to establish, maintain, change, or terminate the relation between the person and the environment on matters of significance to the person" (p. 1). In this view, there are as many basic emotions as there are modes of adaptation to events. Elicitation of emotion is dependent on how the individual relates events to his or her goals or strivings. To accomplish this, a high level of cognition is not necessary. All that is needed is an "appreciation" of the relation of event to goal. Because some goals are prewired, some "appreciations" of the relation of events to goals may exist at birth and form "an invariant core of affective continuity throughout the lifespan" (Campos & Barrett, 1984, p. 249).

Several changes are seen to occur in the emotion system as a function of experience, cognitive development, and socialization. First, as appreciations become more sophisticated, new members of any given emotion family may be created. As a consequence, for example, adults are capable of experiencing kinds of fear (e.g., of personal failure) that are different from the primal fear of dark, looming objects experienced by infants. Second, the relationship between emotional expression and emotional experience changes as children learn display rules and become capable of controlling expression. Finally, coping responses to emotion and receptivity to the emotional expression of others change with development. Of course, from a functionalist perspective, emotions are inherently adaptive. Individual emotion families serve specific internal-, behavior-, interpersonal-regulatory functions.

Fischer, Shaver, and Carnochan (1990; Mascolo & Fischer, 1995) proposed a dynamic skills theory model of emotional development that integrates functionalist and neo-Piagetian approaches to development. Dynamic skills theory (Fischer, 1980) provides a set of conceptual and methodological tools for charting developmental transformations in an individual's capacity to coordinate behavioral elements into increasingly complex skills. Drawing from functionalist approaches (Barrett & Campos, 1987; Frijda, 1986) Fischer et al. (1990) hold that emotions consist of organized ensembles of appraisal, physiological reaction, and action-tendencies that function in the service of a person's motives and concerns. Drawing upon dynamic skills theory (Fischer, 1980), Fischer et al. (1990) suggest that elements that compose emotion-relevant appraisals and action-tendencies undergo structural transformation as individuals gain the capacity to organize their behavior into increasingly complex skills. For example, at sensorimotor levels, infant anger may involve vigorous vocal or motor protest following interference with goal-directed motor actions. Among adults, anger may involve action-tendencies to retaliate or seek revenge in the context of appraisals that events are illegitimate. Fischer et al. suggest that emotions not only function to organize action and thought within a given context, but they also help shape development itself. Because emotions organize an individual's activities within a given context, repeated evocation of a given emotion can channelize development along specific emotional pathways. For example, different types of parent–child attachment relationships can organize development around emotional experiences that differentially influence the quality of children's social competence, relationships, and style of self-regulation (Sroufe, 1984; Sroufe, Carlson, & Shulman, 1993). Alternatively, childhood abuse can organize development around negative emotions and promote various forms of dissociation and affective splitting (Fischer & Ayoub, 1994).

Sociocultural Perspectives

A fifth class of models consists of social process (Fogel et al., 1992), cultural (Lutz, 1988), and social constructionist (Averill, 1990; Harre, 1986; Lutz & Abu-Lughod, 1992) perspectives, all of which emphasize social or cultural contributions to the development and functions of emotions. From a social process view (Fogel et al., 1992), emotion consists of a "self-organizing system constituted by the interaction of many components related to individuals in their social and physical context" (p. 129). As such, emotion does not refer to any single component process, but instead to the dynamic relations among neural firing, experience, expression, and other components as they become organized over time within social interactions. From a social process view, because partners continuously influence each other's actions throughout the course of any given social interaction, social context exerts a direct influence on the formation of any given emotional reaction. As a result, any particular class of emotional reactions or components (e.g., facial actions) exhibits considerable variation with both social context and development. Furthermore, emotional reactions serve different functions in different interpersonal relationships and environments (see Dickson, Fogel, & Messinger, Chapter 10, this volume).

From sociocultural and social constructionist views, emotions refer to socially constructed syndromes (Averill, 1982), interpretive structures (Armon-Jones, 1986a; Shweder, 1994), or discursive practices (Abu-Lughod & Lutz, 1992) that reflect larger social, cultural, and political orders and meaning systems (Armon-Jones, 1986b; Harre, 1986; Sarbin, 1986, 1995; Shweder, 1994). Although sociocultural and social constructionist psychologists do not necessarily deny the role of biology in the formation of emotion, they stress cultural foundations of emotion that are largely ignored by more traditional models (Oatley, 1993). From a social constructionist view, different emotions are defined in terms of different socially and historically shaped attitudes, beliefs, and judgments rather than as innately given bodily states. For example, according to Harre and Finlay-Jones (1986), the medieval emotion of *accidie* can be defined as a sense of boredom, dejection, or disgust in fulfilling one's religious duty. Accidie was founded in social rules about the necessity of performing one's religious duties with joy rather than with indolence or sloth, and could not have been experienced in the absence of such social rules and meanings. As an extinct emotion, accidie provides an example of the ways in which emotions can be founded upon beliefs and judgments that are shaped by one's local sociomoral order. Although social constructionists do not focus directly on developmental changes in emotion, the assertion that emotions are founded in social judgments implies that they undergo development in ontogenesis. Furthermore, by focusing on cultural and historical differences and the social construction of emotion, these models imply that developmental changes in emotion would occur in the direction of culturally specified endpoints.

ISSUES IN THE ANALYSIS OF EMOTIONAL DEVELOPMENT

As illustrated in the foregoing discussion and in Table 1, there is considerable diversity in existing ways of approaching the study of emotion and its development. Some researchers define emotions in terms of discrete physiological states, others in terms of relations between cognition and feeling tone, others in terms of action-tendencies, others in terms of the patterned configurations of multiple subsystems, and still others in terms of discursive acts or social roles. Theorists vary in the extent to which they regard emotions as independent systems in their own right, or as derived experiences that are dependent on other psychological systems (e.g., cognition, action, social meanings, etc.). Some theorists view emotions as states existing within individuals, whereas others define emotion in terms of processes that occur between individuals. Some define emotion in terms of a relatively small number of central and tightly knit elements, and others suggest that no single attribute provides a necessary or sufficient condition for the attribution of emotion. As such, different theorists focus on different aspects of organismic functioning in defining the concept of emotion. Such lack of consensus is indicative of the elusive nature of the concept of emotion.

Beyond the confusion engendered by diverse ways of approaching the study of emotion, it is sometimes difficult to ascertain what is central and what is peripheral within particular accounts of emotion. For example, many theorists define emotion in terms of patterned configurations among many if not all organismic subsystems (e.g., social process, sociocultural, and to an extent, functionalist researchers). Given the diversity of elements deemed relevant to the characterization of emotion, one might ask how emotion differs from psychological functioning in general. If the concept of emotion is all encompassing, can it continue to serve a useful purpose? Or is it an anachronism, like fairies or elves, left over from previous centuries? Similarly, functionalist, social process, and other models maintain that feeling is but one part of a broader emotional reaction. If feeling is not a central component in the definition of emotion, then what is it that makes a reaction emotional? Furthermore, within cognitive approaches, emotion is understood in terms of relations between cognition, external incentives, and detected or undetected feeling tone. Does emotion refer to all of these processes together? Or are cognitive processes simply one of many types of process that have the capacity to evoke independent feeling states (Izard, 1993)? Also, there are cases in which people report rich emotional experiences in the absence of appraisal patterns that might normally be associated with such states (e.g., as in listening to music or great oratory). Is cognition or appraisal part of the definition of these experiences (Ellsworth, 1994)?

A different set of issues emerges with models that define emotion in terms of tightly knit sets of physiological, expressive, and subjective elements that are distinct from cognition and other processes (Izard, 1993; Tomkins, 1984). Whereas differential emotions theorists maintain that emotions form tightly knit and stable structures, others suggest that the elements that characterize any given category of emotions are at best only moderately correlated in any given context. Furthermore, there is disagreement between biologically and cognitively oriented theorists about the intentionality of emotions, and about the role of cognition in defining individual emotional states. For some theorists (e.g., Campos, 1994; Solomon, 1976), emotions are intentional states; that is, they are about something (i.e., I am not just angry, but angry *that* someone stole my wallet). Similarly, cognitive theorists suggest that certain appraisal-related "relational themes" provide part of the very meaning of various emotional experiences (e.g., blaming others in anger, loss in sadness, taking responsibility for a wrongdoing in guilt; see Lazarus, 1991; Smith & Lazarus, 1990). Whereas some cognitive theorists would claim that intentionality and appraisal-related themes constitute definitive properties of emotions themselves, differential emotions theorists would preserve the distinction between emotion and cognition by maintaining that such characteristics are best considered properties of affective–cognitive structures rather than properties of emotions per se (Izard, personal communication, April 25, 1997). Similarly, some theorists suggest that emotions are distinct from cognition yet, at the same time, so intimately connected to it that the very nature of emotion is transformed with changes in cognition (e.g., Case et al., 1988). These competing claims create the puzzling impression that emotions are both independent of and dependent on cognition.

Gaining clarity on questions of definition is important if one is to address questions about the nature of emotional development. Models that conceptualize emotion in terms of tightly knit sets of physiological, expressive, and subjective elements are likely to endorse the view that emotion feeling states remain largely invariant in ontogenesis (Izard & Malatesta, 1987; Tomkins,

1984). As researchers begin to conceive of emotion more broadly (e.g., Barrett & Campos, 1987; Sroufe, 1996), it becomes sensible to speak of developmental changes in emotional states and experiences. However, the study of developmental trajectories in emotional states and experiences is still in its infancy. Although theorists have proposed models consistent with the proposition that emotions undergo developmental change, with notable exceptions (Case et al., 1988; Lewis, 1995; Fischer et al., 1990; Sroufe, 1996), few have charted or proposed specific trajectories in the development of particular emotions or emotional components. Fewer researchers have addressed the issue of how developmental changes in one emotional component affects other emotional components. Thus, one might ask a series of important questions. Do emotions themselves undergo developmental change? Or does emotional development simply involve the attachment of basic feeling states to other developing psychological processes? Do only certain components of emotional reactions develop? If so, which ones? What types of trajectories occur in emotional states, processes, or components? Do changes in any given emotional component transform an emotional state? Is there evidence for broad stages of emotional development? Or do different components of emotion develop separately from one another? Do emotional processes change quantitatively, differing only in degree, or do they change qualitatively, differing in organization or type?

Given the absence of consensus on the prior two questions and the wide range of opinions that have been offered, it is surprising to discover that emotions are seen to serve similar functions by proponents of different perspectives. In short, emotions are generally seen to motivate and regulate thought and action and, in some perspectives, preserve cultural values as well. However, it is less clear how emotions, as construed in several perspectives, achieve these functions. For example, it remains unclear how emotional processes not only influence but are also influenced by cognition, behavior, and social interaction (see Lewis, Sullivan, & Michalson, 1984, for a discussion of this problem). An additional difficulty inherent in the task of understanding the nature, development, and functions of emotional processes is our inability to measure them directly. On this issue as well, none of the measurement tools that are presently available (e.g., measures of facial expression, physiological change, verbal reports) has been found adequate by the majority of researchers and each has been found wanting in serious ways (see Kagan, 1984, and Ortony, Clore, & Collins, 1988, for a discussion of this issue). However, until we know what it is that we are looking for, it will be difficult to construct useful tools to measure it. Thus, we seem to be trapped in a conundrum at present. Perhaps the only way out is to shed more light on the subject—to achieve greater clarity in definition—and this is a major purpose of the present volume.

AIMS AND ORGANIZATION OF THE VOLUME

It is difficult to make progress in any field of study if the meanings assigned to central constructs vary so widely across investigators. This volume was designed to systematize and help clarify the different ways in which emotion researchers approach fundamental questions about the nature of emotion and emotional development. Theorists and researchers adopting different theoretical orientations were asked to address three major questions about emotions and their development. These included the following:

1. According to your theoretical perspective, what is an emotion? Is there anything essential that makes an emotion an emotion; that is, what components, if removed from your definition, would render the state or experience nonemotional?
2. What about emotions, if anything, undergoes developmental change? Describe or propose types of transformations that may occur in an emotion, emotion family, or emotion component. If you believe that emotions generally remain invariant in ontogenesis, what, if anything, does change?
3. What are the functions of the changes that you describe for the psychological or social life of the child?

In posing these questions to contributors, we hoped to explore the implications of adopting different models of emotion for the issue of whether and how emotions change in development, and for understanding the role of developing emotions in psychological and social life. As such, the present effort seeks to (1) frame the debate about the nature of emotions, their development, and their roles in the psychological and social lives of persons; (2) organize existing theory and research; (3) chart developmental transformations in selected emotions and emotional components; and (4) provide theoretical grounding for new research where investigation is sparse. Furthermore, in analyzing trends in the study of emotional development, we can begin to determine whether it will be more profitable to sharpen distinctions among alternative models of emotional development or to begin to work toward synthesis.

The models that form the body of this volume vary along several dimensions. They run the gamut from biological perspectives to sociocultural perspectives, and they offer several unique perspectives along this continuum. In the remainder of this chapter, we provide an overview of each model included in this volume. In so doing, we examine the ways in which each set of contributors addressed the three questions that formed the basis of this volume. The responses provided by each set of contributors are also summarized in Table 2.

Table 2. Perspectives Represented in This Volume

Author	What are emotions?	Function of emotions?	What develops?
Michael Lewis	Assemblies of components including emotional *elicitors, receptors, states, expressions,* and *experience*	Communicates states and experience to others; socializes young	*Experience* undergoes structural change with socialization and the development of cognition and self, which then transforms elicitors, states, expressions
Panksepp, Knutson, & Pruitt	Separable neural circuits located in subcortical areas of the brain	Governs approach, withdrawal behavior; functions to prolong life and enable procreation	Neurochemical systems specific to emotional behaviors as a result of epigenetic interactions between genes and environment.
Ackerman, Abe, & Izard	Innate discrete states composed of neurochemical processes, expressive behaviors, and subjective experiences.	Motivates behavior, organizes cognition, sends social signals; functions as the fundamental building block of personality and cognitive organization	Core experience is invariant; affective–cognitive structures develop as a function of socialization and cognitive development
Barrett	Multicomponent processes defined in terms of *functions* they serve for the organism in the context of significant relations with the environment	Individual emotion families perform different functions in regulating behavior, social interaction, and internal processes.	All emotion components (e.g., appreciations, behaviors, displays, internal reactions) except for emotion-specific functions that emerge early
Kozak & Brown	Reactions to maladaption which consist of involuntary behavior, feelings, and reequilibration strategies	Initiate equilibration strategies to restore adaptive order; feelings act as evaluative heuristics that select perception and action	Decrease in the number and intensity of emotional reactions with the development of cognition and value structures; transformation of defensive strategies

Lewis & Douglas	Affective states involving specific feeling tone, physiology, and response tendencies that are evoked by specific classes of goal-related events	Facilitates coupling among cognitive elements; emotion–cognition interactions organize the development of personality and psychological defense	Links between emotions and cognitive systems (Emotional Interpretations), which self-organize into attractors and repellers with development
Mascolo & Harkins; Mascolo & Griffin	Patterned activity of multiple components (e.g., appraisal, physiological, action-tendency) that self-organize through mutual regulation in the context of notable changes in events	Serves adaptive functions defined by the organization of their components; emotional feelings select motive-relevant appraisals and action within a context	Changes in component systems (e.g., appraisal, action-tendencies) and their relations prompt changes in existing classes of emotion processes and the creation of new ones
Dickson, Fogel, & Messinger	Self-organizing, dynamic processes involving interacting constituents (e.g., bodily change, feelings, motives, appraisals, behavior) in social contexts	Has no function independent of its constituents; communicative and other functions emerge from interaction among all constituents in a social context	Change occurs in the self-organization of emotion constituents in real time, in development, and as a function of social context
Frijda & Mesquita	Event-elicited response set (e.g., concerns, appraisals, action readiness) involving one's relation to an object/person and a change in control precedence	Deal with significant events for the sake of one's concerns; motivate changes in action readiness; signal affect and intentions	All emotion components except arousal, as a function of socialization and cognitive development
Mancuso & Sarbin	Narrative constructions of mobilization reactions that occur in contexts involving social discrepancy	Facilitates action to reduce discrepancy between personal anticipatory constructions and event-related social input	Narrative structures a function of cognitive development and sociocultural processes; enactment of emotion in terms of social narratives

In Chapter 2, Lewis suggests that an emotion is comprised of five components (elicitors, receptors, states, expressions, and experiences) and their interconnections. He defines each component, reviews relevant research, and raises several intriguing developmental questions pertinent to each. In the ensuing discussion, it becomes clear that, in this framework, not all components are necessary for an emotion to occur and none of them, independently, appear to be sufficient. For example, emotion states (defined as changes in neurophysiological activity) are seen to accompany the activation of receptors. However, receptors are not necessarily activated by elicitors in a direct fashion, and it is possible that a generalized psychophysiological response may be common to many or all emotional states. Thus, elicitors may produce emotional responses through the mediation of general arousal and cognitions in context.

Lewis suggests that the most likely explanation of emotional development is that two basic emotion states that are present at birth (a negative/distress state and a positive/satiated state) become increasingly differentiated as a function of maturation, socialization, and cognitive development. In the process, positive and negative states are transformed into joy, sadness, anger, for example, in the first year of life; into embarrassment, pride and shame in the second year; and into guilt in the third year. Of particular interest is Lewis's analysis of the central role of self-awareness in the experience of emotion. Lewis maintains that the onset of self-awareness at around 15–20 months of age is a necessary condition for the experience of emotion. Finally, in this framework, emotions function to communicate states and experiences to others and to facilitate the socialization of infants into the culture in which they are raised.

Biological Approaches and Discrete Emotion Theory

In Chapter 3, Panksepp, Knutson, and Pruitt describe an approach to emotion research called *affective neuroscience*, which aims to elucidate emotion-relevant neurochemical processes that drive learning and specific classes of behavior. The approach taken in this chapter is to document the changing likelihood that mammals (e.g., rats, mice, guinea pigs) will display specific socioemotional behaviors (e.g., separation vocalizations, dominance displays, sexuality) across the lifespan, and to examine the neural and chemical changes that are present at onset and offset of these behaviors. It is assumed that these (and other) behaviors are emotional because, in humans, they are typically associated with states that are commonly called distress, assertiveness, and lust. From this perspective, emotions function to promote specific behaviors that enhance adaptation to the environment and procreation (e.g., approach, attack, flight, seeking, mating).

In this view, emotions are defined as integrative sensorimotor command systems, which are located in the subcortical area of the brain, and which organize a large variety of brain processes (including physiological arousal, feeling states, and species-specific behavioral displays). Emotional change is seen to arise from the neurochemical unfolding of genetically prescribed emotional systems, which are spontaneously active even *in utero*, and which are often present in fairly mature form at birth. Although Panksepp et al. primarily address biogenetic processes in the epigenesis of emotional behavior, they also describe the importance of interactions between biological and environmental factors. For example, an interesting finding of this research program is evidence that emotional change can also arise from environmental influences (e.g., handling of rats in the first week of life), which "mimic" neurochemical changes induced by early exposure to hormones, and which lead to similar outcomes in adulthood (e.g., improved learning).

In Chapter 4, Ackerman, Abe, and Izard provide a comprehensive elaboration of discrete emotion theory, which builds on previous versions of the theory (see earlier discussion), and which is more fully articulated. In their chapter, Ackerman et al. examine in detail the implications of viewing emotions as discrete, encapsulated systems that can function independently of cognition and other psychological systems. Ackerman et al. draw on evidence from a variety of sources to support their position that basic emotions operate as hardwired, fast-acting modular systems that emerge early in development and remain stable thereafter throughout ontogenesis. Although the emotion system is largely independent of cognition, emotion and cognition interact in ontogenesis to form affective–cognitive structures. However, in such interactions, cognition does not transform emotional states. Instead, invariant feelings become increasingly connected with changing thoughts and images. Furthermore, although basic emotions are seen as independent and modular systems, in this chapter, Ackerman et al. propose a new class of emotions called "dependent emotions" to account for emotions (i.e., shame, guilt, contempt) that were not easily handled in previous formulations. With this new construct, which appears to entail a shift in the way at least some emotions are defined, the theory gains still greater explanatory power.

Functionalist Approaches

For Barrett (Chapter 5), emotions are ensembles of multiple processes that occur in the context of significant person–environment interactions. Each emotion term (e.g., shame, fear) represents a family of related ensembles of emotional components that are defined by the three adaptive functions, namely, behavior regulation (e.g., avoidance), social regulation (e.g., shout to others), and internal regulation (e.g., attend to stimulus). In this view, there are very few psychological processes that do not involve emotion. A psychological process would be considered unemotional only if no ongoing relationship between person and environment is significant (e.g., driving to work "automatically"). In this view, three changes in emotion processes are seen to occur as a function of experience and socialization. First, more situations become capable of eliciting emotion. Second, the organism's repertoire for emotional responses, including coping behavior, increases. Third, certain emotion families that are highly dependent on socialization become evident for the first time. Barrett illustrates these changes with an analysis of the early emergence and development of shame and pride.

From this perspective, a high level of cognitive awareness is not necessary for the emergence of any given family of emotions, including pride and shame. In support of this view, Barrett reviews evidence to suggest that pride- and shame-relevant experiences may emerge quite early, even in the first year of life. She also suggests that after their emergence, pride and shame continue to change in ontogenesis as a result of changes in multiple processes (rather than just changes in cognition or any other single process). Such influences include changes in children's understanding of self and social standards, transitions in the significance of social rules to children, shifts in children's relationships with others, and the exposure of children to increasingly different social situations.

For Kozak and Brown (Chapter 6), emotions consist of reactions to adaptive malfunction. They are composed of intense feelings, involuntary behaviors (e.g., facial expression), and central and peripheral biological changes that are nonspecific but which aid the organism in carrying out its basic strategies of reequilibration. In this view, emotions occur only when primary and secondary regulators of conduct (i.e., cognitive and affective processes) fail, that is, when they are insufficient to the task at hand. In these situations, emotions—a third form of regulation—take over and produce a temporary disorganization (e.g., fight or flight) in order to reestablish adaptive equilibrium within a given context. With this formulation, Kozak and Brown place clear parameters around the construct of *emotion*, and specific conditions under which it can and cannot be said to exist.

A provocative contribution of Kozak and Brown's chapter is their differentiation of the concept of *emotion* from related concepts, such as *affect, feeling*, and *value*. Kozak and Brown maintain that although emotions involve feelings, emotion cannot be reduced to feeling. Feelings refer to the conscious aspects of a person's attempt to estimate the adaptive value of any given course of activity. As such, feelings play an important role in all decision-making (and thus cognitive) activity. Emotions, on the other hand, consist of more global processes that function to restore order, even if only to a lower level, in the context of maladaptation. With cognitive and affective development (i.e., changes in knowledge, feelings, and value structures), persons acquire more powerful modes of adapting to their environments. As a result, emotional reactions decrease in both frequency and intensity throughout ontogenesis. Emotional development also involves transformations in general strategies to restore individuals to adaptive equilibrium in the context of maladaptation.

Systems Approaches

In Chapter 7, Lewis and Douglas describe a dynamic systems approach to emotional development. In this view, as in Izard's discrete emotions theory, emotions are viewed as nonreducible affective states. However, Lewis and Douglas's dynamic systems approach takes cognitive-emotional interactions, rather than emotions themselves, as the units of analysis in the study of emotional development. In so doing, they hold that emotion-cognitive interactions self-organize into stable patterns (which they call emotional interpretations) in both in real time and in development. In this model, self-organization refers to the process whereby emotion and cognition influence each other continuously over time. For example, a cognitive appraisal (e.g., awareness of maternal absence) can evoke emotion (e.g., distress in an infant), which in turn directs and organizes further cognitive activity (e.g., looking for mother), which eventually crystallizes into a stable cognitive-emotion pattern for dealing with the class of events in question (e.g., looking away as a form of emotional defense). Thus, in their model, emotions function to organize cognitive activity. Lewis and Douglas illustrate their approach through an analysis of the self-organization of defensive reactions in infants in contexts involving maternal separation. The dynamic systems model that is presented in this chapter suggests the possibility of integrating aspects of differential emotions theory with cognitive and structural–developmental approaches to emotion.

In Chapter 8, Mascolo and Harkins propose a component systems approach to emotional development. Drawing upon systems metaphors, they propose that emotional reactions self-organize as appraisals, bodily reactions, action-tendencies, and feeling tone mutually influence each other within a given social context. Although emotional components can combine in a large number of different ways, because of the constraints they impose upon each other in a given context, they self-organize into a finite number of general patterns with a large number of local variations. From this view, social context is seen as a part of the emotion process, as it exerts an organizing influence on a child's emotion-relevant appraisals, physiological reactions, action-tendencies, and so on. The felt components of emotional reactions (i.e., feeling tone) function to select and organize appraisal and action; emotional action-tendencies serve communicative functions in the context of coregulated social interaction.

From a component systems viewpoint, the appraisal and action systems undergo systematic transformation as a function of biological, cognitive, and social development. With development, children become capable of making increasingly complex appraisals of their relations to their social environments and of displaying increasingly complex emotion-relevant action-tendencies. Mascolo and Harkins suggest that complex emotional reactions often have their origins in social interactions in which others provide "emotional scaffolding" that helps organize a child's appraisals and action-tendencies at a developmental level that is higher than what the child would be capable of producing alone. With development, children gain the capacity to reconstruct for themselves variations of emotion-relevant appraisals and action-tendencies that were initially coordinated in interactions with others. These changes are illustrated with an analysis of the development of pride-relevant appraisals and action-tendencies in 1- to 3-year-olds.

In Chapter 9, Mascolo and Griffin extend the component systems approach to an analysis of developmental changes in appraisal systems involved in anger states and experiences. Mascolo and Griffin argue that anger-relevant appraisals undergo nontrivial transformation in ontogenesis from simple want-violations in infancy to increasingly complex ought-violations in childhood and adulthood. In this chapter, Mascolo and Griffin describe three types of ought-violations that are relevant to an adult's experience of anger. These include personal violations (e.g., violations of personal boundaries), relational violations (e.g., failure to extend appropriate care or nurturance), and social–moral violations (i.e., violation of social or moral rules). Evidence is presented to show that these appraisal patterns differ across men and women in ways that are gender related but not gender specific. The authors also propose developmental sequences for each appraisal pattern from infancy to adulthood and suggest that each provides an alternative pathway to an adult anger episode. In this framework, different forms of anger function to remove different types of want- or ought-violations within different social contexts and interpersonal relationships.

Social and Cultural Approaches

In Chapter 10, Dickson, Fogel, and Messinger advance a social process theory of emotion. In so doing, they propose that emotions are not states but self-organizing dynamic processes created by an individual's activity in personally significant social contexts. As such, Dickson, Fogel and Messinger's model is at once a systems model and a social process viewpoint. In their view, emotions are composed of central nervous system (CNS) activation, autonomic nervous system (ANS) arousal, bodily change, feelings, motives, appraisals, and transactions between individual and environment. Because individuals are always meaningfully linked to an environment, and because constituents of emotion are continuously modified in social interaction, emotions are also seen as continuous and omnipresent. According to social process theory, although emotional processes serve adaptive and communicative functions in social contexts, those functions cannot be defined independently of their particular constituents. Thus, even the same class of emotional actions (e.g., different types of smiles) can serve different functions in different contexts.

In this view, development is conceptualized as a reorganization of constituent patterns when any control parameter reaches a critical level as a function of maturation, changes in neuromotor processes, or changes in the social context. Furthermore, any class of emotional reactions or actions may vary considerably with changes in social context. To illustrate these principles, Dickson, Fogel, and Messinger describe two studies on the social organization and development of smiling and laughing in infancy. In so doing, they report evidence that links different types of smiles to different types of social contexts in development, and which documents transitions in the relationship between smiling and laughing over the first year of life.

In Chapter 11, Frijda and Mesquita outline a componential model of emotion that is simultaneously functionalist and cultural. In so doing, they define emotion as an assembly of several components, including antecedent events, concerns, appraisals, action readiness, behavior, physiological response, belief changes, affect, and emotion experience. These components are seen to be only moderately correlated and hence, emotion names index concepts that are fuzzy and probabilistic. From this view, although all components are implicated in emotion, actin readiness appears to be the most important ("Emotions are, first of all, action dispositions"). Emotional experience "is no more than the experience of the other components coexisting in any given situation." Appraisals are seen to determine whether and what kind of emotional assembly is elicited. The resulting emotional ensembles function to deal with relevant events for the sake of one's goals, motives, and concerns.

In this chapter, the authors describe the ways various emotion components differ across cultures, as a function of cultural norms, values, and socialization practices. They indicate that cultural differences occur in each emotion component they analyzed, with the exception of physiological arousal, which they argue may be undifferentiated across emotional experiences. They suggest that each cultural difference described may have a counterpart in developmental differences. In addition, they suggest that, as appraisals, action-tendencies and concerns change, "particular kinds of emotions may radically change their nature over development." In articulating cultural differences in emotional components, Frijda and Mesquita demonstrate that there is both malleability and stability in emotional development.

Mancuso and Sarbin (Chapter 12) reject the idea that emotions exist as extant states or processes. Instead, they suggest that the concept of emotion is a socially constructed notion that people use to structure and give meaning to their bodily experiences within different social contexts. In elaborating upon this idea, Mancuso and Sarbin propose a model in which the registration of discrepancy between input and anticipatory constructions evokes mobilization reactions (i.e., alterations in the functioning of anatomical and physiological systems) that support an individual's effortful attempt to reduce discrepancy to a subjectively optimal level. Mobilization changes provide the bodily basis that underlies person's reports of "feelings." However, to be psychologically meaningful, persons must construe the input from mobilization reactions in terms of existing anticipatory constructions. As mobilization reactions evolve over time within socially structured contexts, persons build narrative structures to construe and thus experience their mobilization reactions as "emotion," "anger," "joy," or related concepts.

To Mancuso and Sarbin, emotional development consists of a process where children construct increasingly complex narratives that structure their emotional experiences in terms of socially available concepts of emotion. Because emotional life is construed as the "enactment of narrative," the manner in which narrative structures develop from infancy through early childhood is a central focus of this chapter. In this view, mobilization reactions that are evoked by the registration of discrepancy function to prepare individuals for effortful action aimed at reducing discrepancies to an optimal level. Socially constructed emotion narratives provide the primary means by which individuals experience their bodily reactions in terms of one or another category of emotion.

In their integrative chapter, Mascolo and Griffin (Chapter 13) compare the perspectives represented in this volume with respect to the answers provided for the three guiding questions. In so doing, they note points of similarity and difference, and they examine some common themes that run through the various contributions.

REFERENCES

Abu-Lughod, L., & Lutz, C. (1992). Introduction: Emotion, discourse, and the politics of everyday life. In C. Lutz & L. Abu-Lughod (Eds.), *Language and the politics of emotion* (pp. 1–23). Cambridge, UK: Cambridge University Press.
Armon-Jones, C. (1986a). The thesis of constructionism. In R. Harre (Ed.), *The social construction of emotions* (pp. 32–56). Oxford, UK: Basil Blackwell.
Armon-Jones, C. (1986b). The social functions of emotions. In R. Harre (Ed.), *The social construction of emotions* (pp. 57–82). Oxford, UK: Basil Blackwell.
Averill, J. R. (1982). *Anger and aggression: An essay on emotion.* New York: Springer-Verlag.
Averill, J. R. (1990). Emotions in relation to systems of behavior. In N. Stein, B. Leventhal, &

T. Trabasso (Eds.), *Psychological and biological approaches to emotion* (pp. 385–404). Hillsdale, NJ: Erlbaum.

Barrett, K. C., & Campos, J. J. (1987). Perspectives on emotional development: A functional approach to emotions. In J. D. Osofsky (Ed.), *Handbook of infant development* (2nd ed., pp. 555–578). New York: Wiley.

Campos, J. (1994, Spring). The new functionalism in emotion. *SRCD Newsletter*. Chicago: Society for Research in Child Development.

Campos, J., & Barrett, K. (1984). Towards a new understanding of emotions and their development. In C. Izard, J. Kagan, & R. Zajonc (Eds.), *Emotions, cognition and behavior* (pp. 229–263). New York: Cambridge University Press.

Campos, J. J., Barrett, K. C., Lamb, M. E., Goldsmith, H. H., & Stenberg, C. (1983). Socioemotional development. In P. H. Mussen (Ed.), *Handbook of child psychology* (Vol. 2, M. M. Haith, & J. J. Campos, Vol. Eds.), *Infancy and developmental psychobiology* (pp. 783–915). New York: Wiley.

Campos, J., Campos, R., & Barrett, K. C. (1989). Emergent themes in the study of emotional development and emotional regulation. *Developmental Psychology, 25*, 394–402.

Camras, L. A, Malatesta, C., & Izard, C. E. (1991). The development of facial expressions in infancy. In R. S. Feldman & B. Rime (Eds.), *Fundamentals of nonverbal behavior* (pp. 73–105). New York: Cambridge University Press.

Case, R., Hayward, S., Lewis, M., & Hurst, P. (1988). Toward a neo-Piagetian theory of affective and cognitive development. *Developmental Review, 8*, 1–51.

Cicchetti, D., & Hesse, P. (1982). Perspectives on an integrated theory of emotional development. In D. Cicchetti & P. Hesse (Eds.), *Emotional development* (pp. 3–48). San Francisco: Jossey-Bass.

Demos, V. (1986). Crying in early infancy: An illustration of the motivational function of affect. In T. B. Brazelton & M. W. Yogman (Eds.), *Affective development in infancy* (pp. 39–73). Norwood, NJ: Ablex.

Ekman, P. (1984). Expression and the nature of emotion. In K. R. Scherer & P. Ekman (Eds.), *Approaches to emotion* (pp. 319–343). Hillsdale, NJ: Erlbaum.

Ekman, P., Friesen, W. V., & Ellsworth, P. (1972). *Emotion in the human face: Guidelines for research and an integration of findings.* New York: Pergamon.

Ellsworth, P. C. (1994). Levels of thought and levels of emotion. In P. Ekman & R. J. Davidson (Eds.), *The nature of emotion: Fundamental questions* (pp. 192–196). New York: Oxford University Press.

Fischer, K. W. (1980). A theory of cognitive development: The control and construction of hierarchies of skills. *Psychological Review, 87*, 447–531.

Fischer, K. W., & Ayoub, C. (1994). Affective splitting and dissociation in normal and maltreated children: Developmental pathways for self in relationships. In D. Cicchetti & S. L. Toth (Eds.), *Rochester Symposium on Development and Psychopathology: Vol. 5. Disorders and dysfunctions of the self* (pp. 149–222). Rochester, NY: University of Rochester Press.

Fischer, K. W., Shaver, P. R., & Carnochan, P. (1990). How emotions develop and how they organize development. *Cognition and Emotion, 4*, 81–128.

Fogel, A., Nwokah, E., Dedo, J. Y., Messinger, D., Dickson, K. L., Matusov, E., & Holt, S. A. (1992). Social process theory of emotions: A dynamic systems approach. *Social Development, 1*, 122–142.

Frijda, N. H. (1988). The laws of emotion. *American Psychologist, 43*, 349–358.

Frijda, N. H. (1986). *The emotions.* New York: Cambridge University Press.

Harre, R. (1986). *The social construction of emotion.* New York: Basil Blackwell.

Harre, R., & Finlay-Jones, R. (1986). Emotion talk across times. In R. Harre (Ed.), *The social construction of emotion* (pp. 220–233). New York: Basil Blackwell.

Izard, C. (1984). Emotion–cognitive relationships and human development. In C. Izard, J. Kagan, & R. Zajonc (Eds.), *Emotions, cognition and behavior* (pp. 17–34). New York: Cambridge University Press.

Izard, C. E. (1977). *Human emotions.* New York: Plenum Press.

Izard, C. E. (1993). Four systems for emotion activation: Cognitive and noncognitive processes. *Psychological Review, 100*, 68–90.

Izard, C. E., & Malatesta, C. Z. (1987). Perspectives on emotional development: I. In J. D. Osofsky (Ed.), *Handbook of infant development* (2nd ed., pp. 494–554). New York: Wiley.

Kagan, J. (1978). On emotion and its development: A working paper. In M. Lewis & L. A. Rosenblum (Eds.), *The development of affect* (pp. 11–42). New York: Plenum Press.

Kagan, J. (1984). The idea of emotion in human development. In C. Izard, J. Kagan, & R. Zajonc (Eds.), *Emotions, cognition and behavior* (pp. 38–72). New York: Cambridge University Press.

Kagan, J. (1994). On the nature of emotion. In N. A. Fox (Ed.), The development of emotional regulation: Biological and behavioral considerations (pp. 7–24). *Monographs of the Society for Research in Child Development*, Serial No. 240, *59*.

Lazarus, R. (1991). Progress on a cognitive–motivational–relational theory of emotion. *American Psychologist, 46*, 819–834.

Lewis, M. (1990). The development of intentionality and the role of consciousness. *Psychological Inquiry, 1*, 231–248.

Lewis, M. (1995). Embarrassment: The emotion of self-exposure and evaluation. In J. P. Tangney & K. W. Fischer (Eds.), *Self-conscious emotions: The psychology of shame, guilt, embarrassment, and pride* (pp. 198–218). New York: Guilford.

Lewis, M., & Haviland, J. M. (Eds.). (1993). *Handbook of emotions*. New York: Guilford.

Lewis, M., Sullivan, M. W., & Michalson, L. (1984). The cognitive-emotional fugue. In C. Izard, J. Kagan, & R. Zajonc (Eds.), *Emotions, cognition and behavior* (pp. 264–288). New York: Cambridge University Press.

Lewis, M., Sullivan, M. W., Stanger, C., & Weiss, M. (1989). Self-development and self-conscious emotions. *Child Development, 60*, 146–156.

Lutz, C. A. (1988). *Unnatural emotions*. Chicago: University of Chicago Press.

Lutz, C. A., & Abu-Lughod, L. (Eds.). (1992). *Language and the politics of emotion*. Cambridge, UK: Cambridge University Press.

Mancuso, J. D. (1986). The acquisition and use of narrative grammar structure. In T. R. Sarbin (Ed.), *Narrative psychology: The storied nature of human conduct* (pp. 91–110). New York: Praeger.

Mandler, G. (1982). The construction of emotion in the child. In C. E. Izard (Ed.), *Measuring emotions in infants and children*. New York: Cambridge University Press.

Mandler, G. (1984). *Mind and body*. New York: Wiley.

Mandler, G. (1990). A constructivist theory of emotion. In N. L. Stein, B. Leventhal, & T. Trabasso (Eds.), *Psychological and biological approaches to emotion* (pp. 21–44). Hillsdale, NJ: Erlbaum.

Mascolo, M. F., & Fischer, K. W. (1985). Developmental transformations in appraisals for pride, shame and guilt. In J. Tangney & K. W. Fischer (Eds.), *Self-conscious emotions: The psychology of shame, guilt, embarrassment and pride* (pp. 64–113). New York: Guilford.

Minsky, M. (1985). *The society of mind*. New York: Simon & Schuster.

Oatley, K. (1993). Social construction of emotions. In M. Lewis & J. M. Haviland (Eds.), *Handbook of emotions* (pp. 341–352). New York: Guilford.

Ortony, A., Clore, G., & Collins, A. (1988). *The cognitive structure of emotions*. New York: Cambridge University Press.

Piaget, J. (1981). *Intelligence and affectivity*. Palo Alto, CA: Annual Reviews, Inc.

Sarbin, T. (1986). Emotion as situated action. In L. Cirillo & B. Kaplan (Eds.), *The role of emotions in ideal human development* (pp. 77–99). Hillsdale, NJ: Erlbaum.

Sarbin, T. (1995). Emotional life, rhetoric, and roles. *Journal of Narrative and Life History, 5*, 213–220.

Shweder, R. (1994). You're not sick, you're just in love: Emotion as an interpretive system. In P. Ekman & R. J. Davidson (Eds.), *The nature of emotion: Fundamental questions* (pp. 32–44). New York: Oxford University Press.

Smith, C. A., & Lazarus, R. S. (1990). Emotion and adaptation. In L. A. Pervin (Ed.), *Handbook of Personality: Theory and research* (pp. 609–637). New York: Guilford.

Solomon, R. (1976). *The passions*. New York: Anchor Press/Doubleday.

Sroufe, L. A. (1979). Socioemotional development. In J. Osofsky (Ed.), *The handbook of infant development* (pp. 462–516). New York: Wiley.

Sroufe, L. A. (1984). The organization of emotional development. In K. Scherer & P. Ekman (Eds.), *Approaches to emotion* (pp. 462–516). Hillsdale, NJ: Erlbaum.

Sroufe, L. A. (1996). *Emotional development: The organization of emotional life in the early years*. New York: Cambridge University Press.

Sroufe, L. A., Carlson, E., & Shulman, S. (1993). Individuals in relationships: Development from infancy through adolescence. In D. C. Funder, R. D. Parke, & Tomlinson-Keasy (Eds.), *Studying lives through time: Personality and development* (pp. 315–342). Washington, DC: American Psychological Association.

Tomkins, S. S. (1984). Affect theory. In K. R. Scherer & P. Ekman (Eds.), *Approaches to emotions* (pp. 163–196). Hillsdale, NJ: Erlbaum.

Tomkins, S. S. (1982). *Affect, imagery, consciousness* (Vol. 3). New York: Springer.

Trevarthen, C. (1984). Emotions in infancy: Regulators of contact and relationships with persons. In K. S. Scherer & P. Ekman (Eds.), *Approaches to emotion* (pp. 129–157). Hillsdale, NJ: Erlbaum.

Thompson, R. (1993). Emotional development: Enduring issues and new challenges. *Developmental Review, 13*, 472–504.

Weiner, B., & Graham, S. (1984). An attributional approach to emotional development. In C. Izard, J. Kagan, & R. Zajonc (Eds.), *Emotions, cognition, and behavior* (pp. 167–191). New York: Cambridge University Press.

Werner, H., & Kaplan, B. (1984). *Symbol formation*. Hillsdale, NJ: Erlbaum. (Original published 1963).

Young, P. T. (1943). *Emotion in man and animal: Its relation to attitude and motive*. New York: Wiley.

The Development and Structure of Emotions

Michael Lewis

In order to talk about what develops in emotional development, it is necessary
first to decompose the term *emotion* into its components, including (1) elicitors,
(2) receptors, (3) states, (4) expressions, and (5) experiences. In this chapter,
I address each of these components and pay most attention to states, experiences, and expressions. Having done so, I turn to the interconnections between components, and most specifically to how the development of consciousness gives rise to emotional states and expressions.

EMOTIONAL ELICITORS

In order for an emotion to occur, a stimulus needs to trigger a change in
the internal, physiological state of the organism. This event may be either an
external or an internal stimulus. External elicitors may be nonsocial (e.g., loud
noises) or social (e.g., separation from a loved one). Internal elicitors may
range from changes in specific physiological states (e.g., a drop in blood-sugar
level) to complex cognitive activities (e.g., problem solving). Since it is obviously much harder to identify and manipulate an internal elicitor than an
external one, most research deals with external stimuli, with attempts to

Michael Lewis • Institute for the Study of Child Development, Robert Wood Johnson Medical
School, New Brunswick, New Jersey 08903.

What Develops in Emotional Development? edited by Michael F. Mascolo and Sharon Griffin.
Plenum Press, New York, 1998.

determine precisely which features of the elicitor activate the emotion. A major problem in defining an emotional elicitor is that not all stimuli that produce a physiological change in the individual can be categorized as emotional elicitors. For instance, a blast of Arctic air may cause a drop in body temperature and elicit shivering, but one is reluctant to classify this occurrence as an emotional event. Consequently, the definition of an emotional elicitor tends to be circular, inasmuch as an elicitor is defined in terms of the consequences it produces.

What are the developmental issues associated with elicitors? First, there are classes of elicitors with little developmental history. A loud and sudden noise causes startling and possibly fear in organisms throughout their life. The sight of food, once associated with the relief of hunger, almost always serves as a positive elicitor if an organism is hungry. Thus, it is possible to imagine a class of events, either biologically determined or learned in the very beginning of life, that will consistently produce an emotional state.

Even for this class of automatic elicitors, however, the developmental experiences of organisms may be such as to inhibit or restrict the elicitor from operating; elicitors, if they could be measured, remain constant in their effect, but other aspects necessary for the organism to realize their effect may interfere. Alternatively, the effect of an elicitor may be modified by the deactivation of an emotional receptor and the resulting inhibition of the emotional state. For example, pain receptors can be deactivated by competing stimuli (e.g., loud music during dental surgery) or by drugs that inhibit receptor function at the central nervous system (CNS) level. In other words, the elicitor–response structure may remain constant but is overridden by other processes. This is the basic distinction between change and development. In the former, the structure remains but is subsumed by another process, whereas in the latter, the structure changes.

In the class of elicitors with a developmental course, the structure that supports the elicitor–response connection undergoes change. Within this class are elicitors that are biologically connected to a response, as well as elicitors that are connected to a response through learned associations. For example, infants' fear of strangers may be biologically programmed; over time, stranger fear may decline because the biological structure supporting the elicitor–response connection has broken down or has been altered through experience. Learned associations between elicitors and responses may also be subject to developmental change because new structures are formed or old ones are extinguished. For instance, the formation of new structures can be predicated on cognitive changes. The data from numerous sources suggest that important cognitive factors play a role in mediating the effects of classes of events in the elicitation of fear (Campos & Stenberg, 1981; Lewis, 1980; Schaffer, 1974).

EMOTIONAL RECEPTORS

Emotional receptors may be either (1) relatively specific loci or pathways in the CNS that mediate between elicitors and particular states or (2) non-specific general systems related to arousal and through arousal to particular states. Information about emotional receptors in scarce. Whether these receptors can even be located is open to question. The discussion of the developmental history of receptors, therefore, is speculative.

Specific receptors are select cells or neural structures located in the CNS. Their function is to detect and respond to certain classes of events. For example, an innate releasing mechanism (IRM) is thought to be an innate neural mechanism that operates as a specific receptor in response to highly specific environmental stimuli. When activated by a particular stimulus event (the "releaser"), the IRM responds through the release of instinctive behavioral patterns that presumably increase the organisms's chances of survival (Hess, 1970). It has been argued that the schema of the human face constitutes an innate releaser of the smiling response in babies (Spitz & Wolf, 1946; Wolff, 1963).

What these specific emotional receptors are like or where they may be located is still to be discovered, although research on anger and rage, as well as on pleasure (self-stimulation), implicates the hypothalamus. Studies have shown that the electrical stimulation of certain areas of the hypothalamus elicit a full-blown rage reaction, including attack (Akert, 1961; Hess, 1954, 1957). Whereas stimulation of the middle portion of the hypothalamus may produce rage, stimulation of the anterior hypothalamus produces fear ("flight behavior"), and stimulation of the posterior portion generates curiosity and alertness. The most critical region of the brain for self-pleasure stimulation seems to be the lateral hypothalamus (Olds, 1962). The effects of hypothalamic lesions on emotional behavior have confirmed, for the most part, the results of these stimulation experiments (Bard, 1928; Wheatley, 1944).

More recent findings, based on electrical recordings (EEG) suggest the existence of specific brain centers for different emotions (Davidson, 1992, 1993). The findings remain controversial. Only more work will show whether there are specific sites for specific emotions.

One neurological model that supports the notion of specific emotional receptors derives from research on the responses of specific visual cortex cells to specific stimuli. Theories of specific cells in perception suggest that there are specific neurons devoted to detecting highly specific events. Hubel and Wiesel (1962, 1968) have identified cells in the visual cortex of the cat that are activated only when a bar of light is presented at a certain angle. Different cells respond to different angles. Other cells respond only to movement through the visual field and movement only in a single direction. Some cells are so highly specialized that they are activated only by a line in a particular orientation and of a specific length and width. Other cells in the visual cortex respond to patterns such as curves and angles. In monkeys, some cells may be so finely tuned that they respond only to specific shapes and objects (Gross, Rocha-Miranda, & Bender, 1972).

Tomkins (1981) promoted the idea of affect receptors and has speculated on the role they might play; "organized sets of responses are triggered at subcortical centers where specific 'programs' for each distinct affect are stored" (Tomkins, 1980, p. 142). The activation of these centers is thought to be innate; that is, there are certain classes of events that automatically trigger these centers. Since the role of learning is not emphasized, it is uncertain whether new receptors develop.

Little attention has been paid to developmental issues pertaining to specific receptors. In general, these receptors are thought to be in place at birth and to be biologically determined and genetic in origin. Speaking about the programs of these receptors and the consequences of their elicitation, Tomkins (1980) stated that these programs are "innately endowed and have been genetically inherited" (p. 142). Thus, there may be little reason to postulate a developmental course in the maturation of specific receptors.

Yet the developmental course of an IRM is such that it may become increasingly selective toward releasers during the course of the organism's life (Hess, 1970). This increased selectivity may be due either to a narrowing of the range of effective eliciting stimuli through the elimination of individual stimuli (e.g., in the cases of the habituation to specific releasers or the strong negative conditioning of aversive stimuli) or to the selection and strengthening of a few releasers from a large range of potential releasers (e.g., the social imprinting of presocial bird species; Lorenz, 1965). The human face becomes more effective as an elicitor of the smiling response in babies, and, at the same time, smiling becomes increasingly selective as a function of age (Ahrens, cited in Hess, 1970). The notion of increasing selectivity as a consequence of the experience of the individual would appear to apply generally across IRMs.

Although there is little information on this topic, it is possible to imagine the development of specific neurological centers. There is no reason to assume that all centers exist at or soon after birth and develop at the same time or rate. In this case, two distinct courses of development can be hypothesized, one biological and the other culturally interactive. In the first, neurological development might proceed independent of experience. Thus, although all centers are not present at the same time, the unfolding of each may take place almost exclusively within a biological time frame. In the second, the neurophysiological development of these centers might interact with either social or subsequent biological experiences.

Much of the early research on emotion was predicated on the notion of specific brain receptors that produce specific responses. However, until recently, the data failed to confirm the notion of specificity. When a particular elicitor was presented to subjects, psychophysiological measures failed to show any distinct patterns corresponding to discrete emotions. Although Ax (1953) reported some evidence of physiological differentiation between anger and fear, other research has failed to uncover any autonomic response patterns that correlate with particular emotional response (e.g., Lacey & Lacey, 1958). Recently, Davidson and others have shown differential EEG patterns to several different emotions (Davidson, 1992, 1993). Davidson (1992) has argued that approach-related behavior and positive emotions, such as joy, appear to be a left-hemispheric response, whereas withdrawal-related behavior and negative emotions, such as fear, appear to be a right-hemispheric response. The research, while promising, still has a long way to go to demonstrate different brain sites. Much of the work in this area suggests that a generalized psychophysiological response may be common to all emotion-producing stimuli (Strongman, 1978). Thus, emotional elicitors may produce emotional responses through the mediation of a general arousal and cognitions in context (Ortony, Clore, & Collins, 1988; Schachter & Singer, 1962).

EMOTIONAL STATES

I will define an emotional state as a particular constellation of changes in somatic and/or neurophysiological activity. Emotional states can occur without the organism's perception of these changes. Thus, an individual can be angry as a consequence of a particular elicitor and yet not perceive its angry state. A specific emotional state may involve changes in neurophysiological and hormonal responses as well as changes in facial, bodily, and vocal behavior. However, facial, bodily, and vocal behaviors are treated as emotional expressions in a separate section.

Two views exist concerning emotional states. According to the first, these states are associated with specific receptors; indeed, they are the activation of these receptors (Izard, 1977; Tomkins, 1962, 1963). In the second, emotional states are not associated with specific receptors and do not exist as specific changes. Instead, a general receptor system (arousal) is thought to underlie all emotional states (Mandler, 1975, 1980; Ortony et al., 1988; Schachter & Singer, 1962). Other processes, such as cognitive evaluation, may produce the specific emotion.

Cognitive processes may play several roles in emotional states. Certain elicitors may evoke cognitive processes, which in turn elicit specific emotional states. In such cases, cognition is necessary for the elicitation of a specific state. Shame is a good example. One must have certain cognitions for shame to occur, since it is the perceived transgression of particular rules that produces the shame state (Lewis, 1992). Transgression and responsibility imply an elaborate cognitive process in which an individual compares an action with some standard and finds the two discrepant. The cognition (i.e., the perceived transgression) acts as the elicitor of or the mediator between specific behaviors and the specific state. The behaviors themselves that proceed the state do not lead directly to the state itself. Rather, they must be interpreted for the specific state to occur.

When receptors are activated, an emotional state, either a specific or general state, is produced. Critical to this definition is a focus on changes from previous levels of activation rather than on the absolute level. Change can occur as either an increase or a decrease in activity level. For example, heart rate increases have been associated with anxiety and fear (Campos, Emde, Gaensbauer, & Henderson, 1975; Weathers, Matas, & Sroufe, 1975), whereas heart rate decreases have been associated with attention or interest (Graham & Clifton, 1966; Lacey, Kagan, Lacey, & Moss, 1963; Lewis, Kagan, Kalafat, & Campbell, 1966).

Emotional states, then, are for the most part transient, patterned alterations in ongoing levels of neurophysiological and/or somatic activity. Is it possible that organisms are always in an emotional state? Although it is difficult to imagine, if one considers the variety of different states possible (e.g., interest, anxiety, happiness, passion, boredom), the notion of perpetual emotional states becomes more viable. Thus, it becomes difficult to imagine being awake and not being in some emotional state or at some level of arousal. It is important to remember that an emotional state is not the same as an emotional experience. Thus, an individual need not be aware of the state for it to occur.

It is not likely that all neurophysiological and/or somatic changes constitute emotional states. Which changes are critical, however, is unknown. If specific affect receptors exist, then any change in these would be sufficient to produce an emotional state. If there are no specific receptors and only a general receptor system, it is less clear whether every change in the general system constitutes an emotional state.

In discussing the developmental issues pertaining to emotional states, two issues need to be addressed. The first concerns the nature of different states and how they are derived. The second pertains to the developmental course of states once they emerge. Some of the issues raised in the discussion of receptor development appear again in discussions of emotional states. For example, if emotional states are viewed as specific, the question of how specific states are derived must be addressed. Two general models are possible. According to one, specific emotional states are derived from developmental processes, purely maturational processes, or they may be interactive, involving the organism with its environment. The second model does not depict a role for development in the emergence of specific states. Rather, discrete emotional states are assumed to be innate.

In the first model, the infant has two basic states (or one bipolar state) at birth, a negative or distress state and a positive or satiated state. Subsequent states emerge through the differentiation of this basic bipolar state. Such differentiation theories focus on both the modulation of the bipolar state and the general arousal system (Bridges, 1932). See also Spitz (1965), Sroufe (1979), and Emde, Gaensbauer, and Harmon (1976), who have added a contextual dimension to the basic scheme developed by Bridges (1932).

How general states develop into specific emotional states remains speculative. It has been argued that both mother–child interaction and maturation underlie the process of differentiation (Als, 1975; Brazelton, Koslowski, & Main, 1974; Sander, 1977). The regulation of the child's state (i.e., arousal and hedonic tone) may be the mechanism leading to differentiation. Although some theorists stress that emotional differentiation is determined more by biological than by interactive factors (Emde et al., 1976), the combination of the two forces seems most likely. Although the regulation of hedonic tone and arousal through caregiver–child interactions certainly modifies or alters the intensity and quality of each dimension, the derivation of specific emotional states remains without empirical support.

A much simpler developmental model concerning differentiation could be considered from a purely biological perspective. For instance, a simple biological model can be imagined in which undifferentiated emotion becomes differentiated as a function of maturation. According to such a view, the rate of differentiation and the unfolding of differentiated emotional states is programmed according to some physiological timetable. There are no examples of such a process, although one might examine the "pleasure" areas within the brain to see whether they have a developmental course. The differentiation from general to specific structures is common in morphology; there is no reason not to consider such a possibility in emotional development. The most likely explanation of emotional development is that the differentiation of emotional states occurs as a function of maturation, socialization, and cognitive development. Whatever processes underlie this differentiation, the model is developmental in nature.

An alternative model is that emotional states are discrete states that are preprogrammed in some sense and need no further differentiation (Izard, 1978; Izard & Buechler, 1979). They exist at birth, even though they may not emerge until a later point in development. This view is unlike the differentiation model in that discrete emotional states do not develop from an original undifferentiated state but are innate at birth in an already differentiated form. In the "discrete systems model" (Izard, 1978), specific emotional states emerge either in some predetermined order or as needed in the life of the infant. They may co-occur with the emergence of other structures, although they are independent of them. The emotion system essentially operates according to biological directives.

Some investigators claim that infants exhibit highly differentiated emotional expressions at birth or shortly thereafter and that these differentiated expressions reflect differentiated states. Oster (1978), for example, believes that eyebrow knitting is an expression of puzzlement related to problem solving. The connection between this facial expression and such a complex emotion exemplifies the discrete-emotions theory. Parents certainly think that their children are capable of highly differentiated emotions quite early. Pannabecker, Emde, Johnson, Stenberg, and Davis (1980) reported that parents believed that infants as young as 12 weeks have 10 of the 11 emotions asked about in their questionnaire. Clearly, parents expect to see a variety of emotions in infants earlier than Bridges's (1932) differentiation hypothesis would predict.

Izard has examined in much detail the facial musculature patterns of young infants through an elaborate measurement system (Izard, 1979; Izard & Dougherty, 1982; MAX). Using this coding system, he has demonstrated the existence of several discrete emotional expressions in infants as young as 1 month. There is little evidence, however, that these discrete emotional expressions correspond to internal emotional states this early in life.

A modification of this strong biological-determinism model is one in which distinct emotional states exist early in life but unfold in interaction with other processes. Emotional states are not produced in a developmental sense, but they cannot emerge until other structures have matured. For example, guilt and shame occur as a consequence of some violation of a standard. When the prerequisite cognitive capacities have developed, they may activate an already existing guilt or shame state. It is as if there exists a button called "shame/guilt" and the pushing of this button awaits the development of a set of cognitions. In contrast, one might posit that the developing cognitive capacities themselves produce the emotion; that is, the shame or guilt button does not exist as a prewired structure but emerges as a consequence of cognitive development. These models of cognitive growth that activate emotional states already programmed can be contrasted with developmental models in which discrete emotional states are the product of biological determinism.

These different models address the conceptual difference between experience and structure found in the arguments of Hume and Kant. In one case, experience produces a structure (Hume, 1739/1888). In the other case, experience is assimilated into innate structures (Kant, 1781/1958). In the study of emotional development, the question that one must address is whether emotional states are preformed and depend only on the development of cognitions or cognitions themselves produce the emotional states (structures).

The theoretical importance of the distinction can be illustrated in the study of fear. Is each fear state the same as other fear states, regardless of the circumstances, or do fear states differ as a function of the elicitor? For example, is the fear state produced by a loud noise the same as the fear state produced by the association of a white laboratory coat with the pain of a needle? Are emotional states independent of or dependent on particular elicitors? If emotional states are independent, they need not be created by the elicitor.

This distinction appears repeatedly in discussions of development as the fundamental issue concerning the role of experience in the production or change of a structure. Beilin (1971) suggested that Piaget's theory is a preformational one: Although experience is necessary for the production of a structure, the structure exists independent of the experience. In the same way, cognition may be necessary for the emergence of emotional states, but emotional states may not be produced by the cognitions.

The first major issue related to the topic of emotional states concerned the origin of discrete emotional states. The second major issue focuses on the developmental changes in emotional states once they have emerged. For example, 8-month-old children may show behaviors reflecting fear at the appearance and approach of a stranger, and 2-year-old children may exhibit fear behaviors when they have broken their parents' favorite lamp. Do similar fear states underlie the fear expressions in both cases? Although the elicitors of states and the children's cognitive capacities are different in these two cases, the emotional states may be similar.

Major developmental changes may occur in (1) the events that produce emotional states, (2) the behavioral responses used to reference states, and (3) the cognitive structures of children. Whether the emotional state itself changes as a function of development is difficult to determine. However, there may well be important physiological and neural changes that differentiate young and old organisms. Age changes in heart rate variability (Lewis, Wilson, Ban, & Baumel, 1970) and changes in cortisol levels (Lewis & Ramsay, 1995) are two physiological processes associated with emotional states that change over time. These and other changes may be such that once an emotional state emerges, it does not remain constant over time. Rather, the constancy of an emotion may be a function of the experience of it.

The issues related to the development of emotional states are complicated by the fact that emotional states are internal processes for which there are no good measures. Moreover, emotional states are often confused with emotional expressions. Although it is possible to measure emotional expressions, the correspondence between the two is not necessarily perfect (Lewis & Michalson, 1983). Thus, the development of emotional states remains to be explored.

EMOTIONAL EXPRESSIONS

Emotional expressions are those potentially observable surface changes in face, voice, body, and activity level that accompany emotional states.

Emotional states are considered constellations of changes in somatic and/or physiological activity that accompany the activation of receptors. Emotional expressions are the manifestation of these state changes. Elaborate coding systems have been developed for measuring facial muscular action (Ekman & Friesen, 1978, FACS; Izard & Dougherty, 1982; MAX).

Other manifestations of emotional states, such as bodily postures, have been described in terms of emotional states (Argyle, 1975). Sitting upright and forward when someone is speaking is associated with interest and attention, whereas slouching and turning away may indicate boredom. Some bodily postures convey sexual interest (Birdwhistell, 1970). More work on bodily manifestations of internal states (particularly fear, aggression, and sexuality) has been conducted with animals than with humans. This may be the case because the facial expressions of animals are less differentiated than those of humans. As a consequence, the emotional states of animals may be better reflected in bodily expressions than in facial movements. However, it is likely that for humans, too, there are elaborate bodily displays of emotion in need of greater clarification.

Vocalizations are one of the least understood aspects of emotional expression, although they seem to be important conveyors of emotional states. Indeed, vocal expressions are extremely powerful and may have as a property the ability to elicit similar emotional states in others. They may be much more contagious than facial or bodily expressions of emotion. For example, movies are much funnier when seen with others who laugh out loud than when seen in a silent theater. Because of their contagious nature, vocal expression may be the target of early socialization efforts to eliminate them from children's behavioral repertoire. Although not well understood, it seems to be the case that vocal displays of emotion are considered inappropriate in many cultures, certainly in the middle-class American culture. People are not supposed to laugh too loudly when happy, to cry too intensely when sad or frustrated, to growl when angry or revengeful, or to groan in pain. Adults report that the vocal manifestations of emotions are particularly embarrassing. Scherer (1979, 1982) developed some techniques for analyzing the frequency patterns in infants' vocal expressions, and these patterns have been related to different emotional states. For example, average pitch frequencies can be used to determine the anxiety or tension level of the vocal expression.

Locomotion and spatial location may be other modes of expressing emotions; running away from and running toward an object are locomotive responses associated with negative and positive emotions (Ricciuti & Poresky, 1972). Indeed, it is infants' movement away from an unfamiliar toy or person, independent of facial expression, that is often used to reference fear (Schaffer, Greenwood, & Parry, 1972).

Although there are some data on emotional expressions in each of these four different modalities (facial, postural, vocal, and locomotor), the relations among them have received almost no attention. It seems reasonable to assume that sobering, crying, and running away form a cohesive pattern of responses that reflect the emotional state of fear. On the other hand, the particular modality used to express an emotion might be a function of specific rules of socialization or a response hierarchy in which one modality has precedence over another. It may be the case that the least intense emotional states are expressed first in facial, then bodily, then vocal behaviors. Such a hierarchy might be determined either by a set of biological imperatives or by a set of socialization rules. In the absence of empirical data on this problem, the relationship among these different expressive modalities remains speculative. It is reasonable to suppose that the more intense the emotional state, the greater the number of different modalities that would be used to express that state.

The use of one or more channels to express a particular emotion may be determined by a complex set of interactions. One issue of particular interest is the effect on some expressions when one modality is inhibited. Inhibition in a particular modality can be experimentally produced by, for example, preventing children from moving about. Such conditions of inhibition may modify or alter the use of uninhibited modalities. For instance, if children are prevented from running away from an approaching stranger because they are restrained in a high chair, they may express their internal state more intensely through alternative means, such as facial musculature changes. Thus, facial expressions may be affected by whether an individual can express emotion through other channels.

Parenthetically, the total inhibition of the expression of emotion may force individuals to manifest their internal states in other ways, such as in the somaticizing of these states and the development of psychosomatic disorders. There is some evidence that people who are not very expressive in external modes (e.g., facial musculature) have more intense manifestations of emotional response in other channels of expression, such as the ANS. Buck, Miller, and Caul (1974) reported that facially unexpressive persons tend to have larger skin conductance and heart rate responses to emotional stimuli than do expressive persons. Lewis, Ramsay, and Kawakami (1993) have shown that although Japanese infants show few emotional expressions of pain, they have higher adrenocortical responses reflecting internal stress.

The communicative function of emotional expression is still poorly understood. How people respond to particular expressions varies as a function of their values, culture, and age. The communicative function has at least two parts. One is an elicitor of empathic behavior and the other is an information exchange. The empathic function serves to elicit in another the particular emotion that one is feeling and may elicit that feeling in them (contagion). For example, an angry expression may elicit anger in another, or a distress reaction may elicit distress in others. The information function serves to tell others what the person is feeling and allows him or her to adjust, to facilitate, to inhibit the emotion and alter his or her as well as the other's behavior. Emotional expressions can be intentionally produced in the absence of emotional states in order to influence those to whom the expressions are directed. Feigning disappointment or anger, for example, can be used to manipulate other people. Such deceptions serve a wide set of social needs (see Lewis & Saarni, 1993).

The communicative value of expressions involves what people know about other people's knowledge of expression and the meaning of that expression. It also involves the ability to control and manipulate one's own behavior intentionally. Thus, any discussion of the communicative function must consider the cultural rules involving deception. Such a discussion underscores the fact that emotional expressions are separate from emotional states and experiences. Furthermore, it suggests that one of the primary socialization tasks is learning the rules of emotional expression in particular situations (Saarni, 1979).

Theories of the development of emotional expressions depend on whether emotional expressions are believed to be directly connected to emotional states. Even more central to the issue of the development of emotional expression is the particular system used to measure expressions. Because the measurement systems for coding expressions other than facial ones are scarce, little is known about the development of other expressions. Historically, more attention has been paid to facial expression; most of the information about emotional development derives from their study.

The development of emotional expressions can be considered in terms of both the ability to produce various expressions and the ability to recognize or discriminate among expressions. The study of facial expression indicates that, for the most part, the facial expressions of joy, anger, fear, sadness, interest, and disgust are present quite early, at least by 6 months of age (Lewis, 1993). One problem with the studies that support these findings is the fact that "true" facial expressions, those that capture the definition proposed by the coding schemes, are relatively rare. Blends of expressions or partial expressions appear more to be the rule. Thus, scoring system disagreements suggest that even the expression of these emotions early in life may be questioned.

Besides these early emotions, more complex ones, those involving self-reference and cognitive rules and standards, appear toward the end of the second year. Darwin called them self-conscious emotions and they have recently come under study (Lewis, 1992; Lewis, Alessandri, & Sullivan, 1992; Lewis, Sullivan, Stranger, & Weiss, 1989; Stipek, Recchia, & McClinton, 1990). Using a facial, bodily, and language/communication scoring system, it appears that embarrassment emerges earlier than the rest, with pride, shame, and guilt emerging by 3 years of age.

Although there is a considerable literature on children's ability to discriminate facial expressions as well as their differential preference for certain facial expressions, little systematic work has been done on the nature of the discriminable aspects of those features. There is little conclusive evidence about when infants are able to discriminate gross facial configurations (Oster, 1981). Many studies do not find clear evidence of infant discrimination of positive or negative expressions before 5 or 6 months (Charlesworth & Kreutzer, 1973), although LaBarbera, Izard, Vietze, and Parisi (1976) reported that 4-month-olds preferred looking at joyous faces to looking at angry or neutral faces. YoungBrowne, Rosenfeld, and Horowitz (1977) also found that infants as young as 3 months could distinguish happy faces from surprised faces, although they could not discriminate happy faces from sad faces. Caron, Caron, and Myers (1982) introduced a series of controls in the investigation of facial discrimination in order to separate what they considered the irrelevant aspects of facial expressions from the more critical features. Their work suggests that not until 7 or 8 months of age can infants discriminate facial expressions independently of such irrelevant details at "toothy smiles." The careful demonstration of the role of superfluous stimuli in facial discrimination studies underscores the problems in studying facial discrimination. Infants do not discriminate expressions much before the beginning of the second half of the first year of life.

The development of facial expression is one of the areas of research receiving the most attention. With the more elaborate measurement systems currently being developed, along with the exploration of contextual variables that influence expressions, a more complete description of emotional expressions is likely. The major developmental issue related to emotional expressions appears to concern the time of their first emergence. Once produced, their expression and developmental course may be primarily a function of the contextual and socialization factors.

EMOTIONAL EXPERIENCES

Emotional experience involves turning attention on the self in order to interpret and evaluate perceived emotional states and expressions. Emotional experience requires that individuals attend to emotional states and expressions. The attending refers to the turning of one's consciousness toward the self as a referent. It is not automatic. Emotional experience may not occur because of competing stimuli to which the organism's attention is drawn. For example, the car a woman is driving suddenly has a blowout in the front tire. The car skids across the road, but the woman succeeds in bringing it under control and stopping the car on the shoulder of the road. Measurement of her physiological state as well as of her facial expression might show that while bringing the car under control, her predominant emotional state was fear. Because her attention was directed toward controlling the car, however, she is not aware of her internal state or expression. She only experiences fear after she gets out of the car to examine the tire.

Emotional experience is the consequence of attending to one's condition. Without attention, emotional experiences may not occur, even though an emotional state may exist. Thus, patients may not experience pain at the dentist if they are distracted through the use of earphones and loud music. This is not to say that at some level a painful state does not exist. Rather, it is simply not experienced as pain.

Emotional experience is very much like consciousness. When I say "I am sad," it means that I am in a state of sadness and I am experiencing the sadness. I may be in a sad state and not experience it (Lewis, 1990). Emotional experiences occur at different levels of consciousness. Such an analysis forms the basis of much psychoanalytic thought. For example, an individual may be in an emotional state of anger; that is, with the proper measurement techniques, one would find a pattern of internal physiological responses indicative of anger. Moreover, this person may act toward those objects or persons who have made her angry in a way that suggests she is intentionally behaving in response to an internal state of anger. Nonetheless, the person may deny that she feels angry or is acting in an angry fashion. Within the therapeutic situation, such people might be shown that (1) they are angry, and (2) they are responding intentionally as a consequence of that anger. The therapeutic process may further reveal that unconscious processes are operating in a fashion parallel to conscious ones. Defense mechanisms function to separate levels of consciousness. However, the power of repression is such that unconscious awareness still exerts powerful effects. Slips of the tongue, accidents, and classes of unintentional (conscious) behavior may be all manifest unconscious awareness (Freud, 1960). Thus, people may experience their internal states and expressions and therefore be conscious of this experience, they may not be conscious of the state, or they may be conscious of them but stop attending to them later. The problem of unconscious experience remains a significant problem in Western thought.

Emotional experience occurs through the interpretation and evaluation of states and expressions. Thus, emotional experience is dependent on cognitive processes. It is impossible to talk about interpretation and evaluation without discussing both the ability to interpret and evaluate (i.e., the cognitive processes involved) and the rules governing the interpretation and evaluation that are the product of socialization. Cognitive processes involving interpretation and evaluation include various perceptual, memory, and elaboration processes. Events need to be perceived and compared with previous experience. Thus, for example, changes in autonomic activity must be perceived and evaluated against prior state conditions. Interpretation involves comparisons with other events. Evaluation and interpretation not only involve cognitive processes that enable organisms to act on information (i.e., changes in emotional states), but also are very much dependent on socialization to provide the content of the emotional experience. The particular socialization rules are little studied (Lewis & Saarni, 1985).

For some, the emotional experience is a necessary part of feeling. James (1890) defined emotions as "the bodily changes [that] follow directly the perception of the exciting fact and our feeling of the same changes as they occur" (p. 449). In order to experience an emotion, a precipitating event ("exciting fact") must occur and cause a bodily change. The conscious feeling of that change is the emotional feeling. Thus, emotion is neither the precipitating event, nor the bodily change associated with that event, but the conscious feeling of that bodily change. Although the nature of the bodily change has been questioned, proponents of James's theory have maintained that the conscious feeling of bodily changes is as central to the concept of emotion as are the bodily changes themselves (Lewis, 1992; Lewis & Michalson, 1983).

The conscious feeling of James has become, at least for some (e.g., Ortony et al., 1988; Schachter & Singer, 1962), a cognitive-evaluative process that determines what to call the physiological change. Schachter and Singer follow a long tradition of investigators who have maintained that the somatic change is not specific to any particular emotional experience but is a general arousal state. This conclusion, in part, is based on the fact that sets of physiological responses that covary with any given emotional experience have not been found. The nature of any specific emotion is thought to be determined by the organism's evaluation of its aroused condition. This evaluation may involve contextual cues, past experience, and individual differences.

The theories of James and of Schachter and Singer are similar in that the elicitor produces a bodily change, which is experienced by the organism. The experience of the organism, defined as a conscious feeling by James or a cognitive-evaluative feeling by Schachter and Singer, is the feeling or emotion. For Schachter and Singer, the evaluation and interpretation are dependent on the context in which the change takes place. Thus, for experiences of either joy or fear, there may be a general, undifferentiated state change. What differentiates these experiences is the context in which the state change takes place. The sight of a mother who has been away may be interpreted as joy, whereas the sight of a stranger constitutes fear.

Not all theories of emotional experience need be as tied to the context, nor do all suggest that the underlying emotional state is the same. However, all emotional experience does involve an evaluation and interpretation of an internal state, the context, and the immediate eliciting stimulus. The context might constitute the social environment, a particular location, the type and number of others available, and the internal states and eliciting stimuli. Emotional experience is therefore not an automatic response connected in a one-to-one relationship to emotional state (Lewis & Michalson, 1983). Rather, emotional experience, more than any other component of emotional activity, is the most cognitive and learned aspect of the emotional process. Cultural and individual differences are apt to be most apparent in this aspect of emotion.

The development of emotional experiences is one of the least understood aspects of emotion. The development of experience or consciousness has received some attention (Lewis, 1995). Emotional experiences do not necessarily have a one-to-one relationship with emotional states. The development of experiences may occur long after the emergence of emotional states. Therefore, although newborns may show an emotional state of pain when pricked with a pin, it would not necessarily follow that they have an emotional experience of pain.

Emotional experiences require that the organism possess some fundamental cognitive abilities, including the ability to perceive and discriminate, recall, associate, and compare. Emotional experiences also require a particular cognitive ability, which is associated with the development of the concept of consciousness or what I have called self or "me" (Lewis, 1995). As I have already discussed, emotional experiences take the linguistic form, "I am frightened" or "I am happy." In all cases, the subject and the object are the same—oneself. Until an organism is capable of self-referential behavior or consciousness, such subjective experiences may not be possible (Lewis & Brooks-Gunn, 1979a). Finally, emotional experiences are learned through the behavior of others toward oneself. They are a consequence of how others interpret one's emotional states and expressions.

Emotional experiences require a set of stimulus changes that are located in the body and that are evaluated by the person. Both location and evaluation assume that a notion of self exists. Somatic changes are internal stimulus changes located only within one's own body, a location synonymous with "me." Evaluation of these changes assumes consciousness as well as cognitive ability. In addition, the evaluation process itself requires an agent of evaluation. It is most difficult to construct a sentence about the evaluation of internal stimuli that does not use a self-referent. The phrase "I am experiencing some internal changes, X," means "I am feeling X." The source of the stimuli and the agent evaluating the stimuli are the same; this interface is the self. To understand the development of emotional experiences, it is necessary to understand the development of self.

Before we go on to a discussion of self, it is important to consider, at least for a bit, the role of the social environment or experience. Emotional experience is also derived through the social world; emotional experiences are the social consequence of how other people interpret one's states and expressions (Lewis & Michalson, 1983; Lewis & Saarni, 1985).

The development of emotional experience may depend on how the social world responds to children's emotional states and expressions, and to the context in which they occur. For example, a caregiver seeing an infant cry in response to a pinprick may interpret the emotional state of the infant as pain. The caregiver's interpretation may be both verbal and behavioral. Different responses will be elicited by different sets of expressions in different contexts. These expressions and the contexts in which they occur are what adults use to interpret their own internal states and those of others. In this way, infants become, in part, what others think them to be (Lewis & Brooks-Gunn, 1979b; Mead, 1934). Thus, the very act of interpretation and evaluation by the social environment provides the rules by which children learn to evaluate and interpret (i.e., to experience) their own behaviors and states.

This model can be used to understand the development of emotional experience. Contextual cues are determined by infants' interactions with and knowledge about their social world. The caregiver provides the bulk of both the early knowledge and the interactions. Infants' evaluations are determined initially by (1) the elicitor, which produces (2) bodily changes, and (3) the responses (both verbal and nonverbal) of the caregiver in response to these bodily changes. The correlation between infants' overt expressions, the emotional feelings, and the caregiver's verbal labeling (e.g., "Don't be afraid") and behavioral responses (e.g., holding and comforting) may provide the information necessary for children to form an emotional experience, one that is consistent with what others expect. There are also indications that the social world, through misinterpretations and other difficulties, causes the pathological development of emotional experiences (see Lewis & Michalson, 1984).

The evaluative aspects of emotion (e.g., Schachter & Singer, 1962), the conscious feeling (James, 1890; Lewis, 1995), need further study in terms of the development of particular emotional experiences. Emotional experiences can occur only after certain cognitive and social underpinnings are present. Over the first 2 years of life, children acquire these faculties and, with them, the ability to experience emotions. Whereas emotional elicitors may produce specific emotional states and expressions, it is not until consciousness exists that one can speak of infants as having certain emotional experiences.

EXPERIENCES AND THE DEVELOPMENT OF THE SELF

Emotional experience has been defined as individuals' interpretation and evaluation of their perceived emotional state and expression. To have an emotional experience requires that the person be able to attend to and differentiate a set of internal events, processes that require specific cognitive capacities, to make reference to the fact that it is "I" to whom these events are happening. Finally, people must interpret these events in the context of the meaning systems that they have acquired through interactions with others. These capacities involve the development of a referencing self, a metacognition such as the memory of a memory.

The development of the self over the first 3 years has received attention

(Kagan, 1981; Lewis, 1992; Lewis & Brooks-Gunn, 1979a; Lewis & Michalson, 1983). Lewis and Brooks-Gunn (1979a) have tried to trace the developmental course of the self-concept, and Lewis and Michalson (1983) and Lewis (1992) have related its development to emotional experiences and to cognitive development in general. Studies of the development of the self have as their focus self-referential behavior, particularly the ability to recognize oneself. Featural descriptions of the self require only rudimentary forms of social knowledge. The use of self-recognition provides an opportunity to explore empirically what otherwise is a metaphysical issue, especially in organisms too young to speak about complex topics.

The self is conceived of as having two features. Lewis (1995) has labeled one the "machinery of the self," which includes regulation functions and even high order learning. The other he has labeled "consciousness" or the "idea of me." This idea has an existential (subjective) aspect, the idea that "I am." It also has an objective or categorical self, a self of characteristics, such as gender, competence, worth, and so on. These characteristics may be universal, but they may also be particular to a culture and to a historical time. The categorical self has a developmental sequence: Some characteristics emerge early and remain invariant (e.g., gender); some emerge early and are variant (e.g., age); and some emerge later and are variant (e.g., strength).

Although an objective self can be studied, it implies the existential self; however, study of an object self requires language. This makes the study of the onset of an existential self difficult to do. Lewis and Brooks-Gunn (1979a) argued that the study of the existential or conscious self is possible if we assume that recognition of "that's me" is an appropriate measure. In a series of studies involving mirrors, still photographs, and video feedback, Lewis and Brooks-Gunn demonstrated that infants recognize themselves between 15 and 24 months (see also Amsterdam, 1972; Bertenthal & Fischer, 1978).

Emotional experiences can be independent of emotional states (Lewis, 1992; Lewis & Michalson, 1983). The model in regard to development suggests that before 15 months, children have emotional states but do not have experiences of them. After this developmental milestone, the early emotional states, such as those of anger, sadness, fear, disgust, and happiness, also have associated with them emotional experiences.

This new cognitive capacity not only changes the nature of the earlier emotional states but, more importantly, acts to create new emotional states and experiences. Thus begins the emergence of what has been called secondary emotions (Plutchik, 1980) or self-conscious emotions (Darwin, 1872; Lewis, 1992; Lewis & Michalson, 1983). These new emotional states and experiences have particular expressions, although not only on the face. They are elicited by complex cognitive processes that themselves are dependent on the "idea of me," since they involve the knowledge about my actions and the evaluation of my actions against my standards. These standards, now internalized, are socialized through the child's commerce with its social environment, including parents, siblings, peers, and other adults such as teachers. These evaluation processes involve the "idea of me" as well as other cognitive processes such as memory and comparison. These self-conscious emotions emerge between 18 and 36 months and include embarrassment (Lewis et al., 1989) as well as pride, shame, and guilt (Lewis, 1992; Lewis et al., 1992).

As we can see, emotional life is dependent on emotional experiences, that is, the development of the idea of me, which, whether through maturation or some combination of maturation and socialization, comes into existence in the second year of life. It is the development of experience that is likely to exert the most powerful force in the development of emotional life.

REFERENCES

Akert, K. (1961). Diencephalon. In D. E. Sheer (Ed.), *Electrical stimulation of the brain.* Austin: University of Texas Press.

Als, H. (1975). *The human newborn and his mother: An ethological study of their interaction.* Ph.D. dissertation, University of Pennsylvania.

Amsterdam, B K. (1972). Mirror self-image reactions before age two. *Developmental Psychology, 5,* 297–305.

Argyle, M. (1975). *Bodily communication.* New York: International Universities Press.

Ax, A. F. (1953). The physiological differentiation of fear and anger in humans. *Psychosomatic Medicine, 15,* 433–442.

Bard, P. (1928). A diencephalic mechanism for the expression of rage with special reference to the sympathetic nervous system. *American Journal of Physiology, 84,* 490–515.

Beilin, H. (1971). Developmental stages and developmental processes. In D. R. Green, M. P. Ford, & G. B. Flamer (Eds.), *Measurement and Piaget* (pp. 24–56). New York: McGraw-Hill.

Bertenthal, B. I., & Fischer, K. W. (1978). Development of self-recognition in the infant. *Development Psychology, 14,* 44–50.

Birdwhistell, R. L. (1970). *Kinesics and context.* Philadelphia: University of Pennsylvania Press.

Brazelton, T. B., Koslowski, B., & Main, N. (1974). The origins of reciprocity: The early mother–infant interaction. In M. Lewis & L. Rosenblum (Eds.), *The effect of the infant on its caregiver* (pp. 49–76). New York: Wiley.

Bridges, K. M. B. (1932). Emotional development in early infancy. *Child Development, 3,* 324–334.

Buck, R. W., Miller, R. E., & Caul, W. F. (1974). Sex, personality, and physiological variables in the communication of affect via facial expression. *Journal of Personality and Social Psychology, 30,* 587–596.

Campos, J. J., Emde, R., Gaensbauer, R., & Henderson, C. (1975). Cardiac and behavioral interrelationships in the reactions of infants to strangers. *Developmental Psychology, 11,* 589–601.

Campos, J., & Stenberg, C. (1981). Perception, appraisal, and emotion: The onset of social referencing. In M. E. Lamb & L. R. Sherrod (Eds.), *Infant social cognition: Empirical and theoretical considerations* (pp. 273–314). Hillsdale, NJ: Erlbaum.

Caron, R. F., Caron, A. J., & Myers, R. S. (1982). Abstraction of invariant face expressions in infancy. *Child Development, 53,* 1008–1015.

Charlesworth, W. R., & Kreutzer, M. A. (1973). Facial expressions of infants and children. In P. Ekman (Ed.), *Darwin and facial expression: A century of research in review* (pp. 91–168). New York: Academic Press.

Darwin, C. R. (1872). *The expression of the emotions in man and animals*. London: John Murray.

Davidson, R. J. (1992). Anterior cerebral asymmetry and the nature of emotion. *Brain and Cognition, 20*, 125–151.

Davidson, R. J. (1993). Cerebral asymmetry and emotion: Conceptual and methodological conundrums. *Cognition and Emotion, 7*(1), 115–138.

Ekman, P., & Friesen, W. V. (1978). *The Facial Action Coding System (FACS)*. Palo Alto, CA: Consulting Psychologists Press.

Emde, R. N., Gaensbauer, T., & Harmon, R. (1976). Emotional expression in infancy: A biobehavioral study. *Psychological Issues. 10*(1, Whole No. 37).

Freud, S. (1960). *The psychopathology of everyday life* (A Tyson, trans.). New York: Norton.

Graham, F. K., & Clifton, R. K. (1966). Heart-rate change as a component of the orienting response. *Psychological Bulletin, 65*, 305–320.

Gross, C. J., Rocha-Miranda, C. E., & Bender, D. B. (1972). Visual properties of neurons in inferotemporal cortex of the macaque. *Journal of Neurophysiology, 35*, 96–111.

Hess, W. R. (1954). *Diencephalon: Autonomic and extrapyramidal functions*. New York: Grune & Stratton.

Hess, W. R. (1957). *The functional organization of the diencephalon*. New York: Grune & Stratton.

Hess, E. H. (1970). Ethology and developmental psychology. In P. H. Mussen (Ed.), *Carmichael's manual of child psychology* (pp. 1–38). New York: Wiley.

Hubel, D. H., & Weisel, T. N. (1962). Receptive fields, binocular interaction, and functional architecture in the cat's visual cortex. *Journal of Physiology, 160*, 106–154.

Hubel, D. H., & Weisel, T. N. (1968). Receptive fields and functional architecture of money striate cortex. *Journal of Physiology, 195*, 215–243.

Hume, D. (1888). *A treatise of human nature* (L. A. Selby-Bigge, Ed.). Oxford: Clarendon. (Originally published 1739)

Izard, C. E. (1977). *Human emotions*. New York: Plenum Press.

Izard, C. E. (1978). Emotions and emotion–cognition relationships. In M. Lewis & L. A. Rosenblum (Eds.), *The development of affect* (pp. 389–413). New York: Plenum Press.

Izard, C. E. (1979). *The Maximally Discriminative Facial Movement Coding System (MAX)*. Newark, DE: Instructional Resources Center, University of Delaware.

Izard, C. E., & Buechler, S. (1979). Emotion expressions and personality integration in infancy. In C. E. Izard (Ed.), *Emotions in personality and psychopathology*. New York: Plenum Press.

Izard, C. E., & Dougherty, L. M. (1982). Two complementary systems for measuring facial expressions in infants and children. In C. E. Izard (Ed.), *Measuring emotions in infants and children* (pp. 97–126). New York: Cambridge University Press.

James, W. (1890). *The principles of psychology*. New York: Holt.

Kagan, J. (1981). *The second year: The emergence of self-awareness*. Cambridge, MA: Harvard University Press.

Kant, I. (1781/1958). *Critique of pure reason* (Kemp Smith, trans.). New York: Macmillan.

LaBarbera, J. D., Izard, C. E., Vietze, P., & Parisi, S. A. (1976). Four- and six-month-old infants' visual responses to joy, anger, and neutral expressions. *Child Development, 47*, 535–538.

Lacey, J. I., & Lacey, B. C. (1958). Verification and extension of the principle of autonomic response stereotype. *American Journal of Psychology, 71*, 50–73.

Lacey, J. I., Kagan, J., Lacey, B. C., & Moss, H. A. (1963). The visceral level: Situational determinants and behavioural correlates of autonomic response patterns. In P. H. Knapp (Ed.), *Expressions of the emotions in man* (pp. 72–94). New York: International Universities Press.

Lewis, M. (1980). Developmental theories: Issues in the development of fear. In I. L. Kutash & L. B. Schlesinger et al. (Eds.), *Handbook on stress and anxiety* (pp. 48–62). San Francisco: Jossey-Bass.

Lewis, M. (1990). Thinking and feeling—the elephant's tail. In C. A. Maher, M. Schwebel, & N. S. Fagley (Eds.), *Thinking and problem solving in the developmental process: International perspectives (the WORK)* (pp. 89–110). Hillsdale, NJ: Erlbaum.

Lewis, M. (1992). *Shame, the exposed self*. New York: Free Press.

Lewis, M. (1993). The emergence of human emotions. In M. Lewis & J. Haviland (Eds.), *Handbook of emotions* (pp. 223–235). New York: Guilford.

Lewis, M. (1995). Aspects of self: From systems to ideas. In P. Rochat (Ed.), *The self in early infancy: Theory and research* (pp. 95–115). Advances in Psychology Series. North Holland: Elsevier Science Publishers.

Lewis, M., Alessandri, S., & Sullivan, M. W. (1992). Differences in shame and pride as a function of children's gender and task difficulty. *Child Development, 63,* 630–638.

Lewis, M., & Brooks-Gunn, J. (1979a). *Social cognition and the acquisition of self.* New York: Plenum Press.

Lewis, M., & Brooks-Gunn, J. (1979b). Toward a theory of social cognition: The development of self. In I. Uzgiris (Ed.), *New directions in child development: Social interaction and communication during infancy* (pp. 1–20). San Francisco: Jossey-Bass.

Lewis, M., Kagan, J., Kalafat, J., & Campbell, H. (1966). The cardiac response as a correlate of attention in infants. *Child Development, 37,* 63–71.

Lewis, M., & Michalson, L. (1983). *Children's emotions and moods: Developmental theory and measurement.* New York: Plenum Press.

Lewis, M., & Michalson, L. (1984). The socialization of emotional pathology in infancy. *Infant Mental Health Journal, 5*(3), 121–134.

Lewis, M., & Ramsay, D. S. (1995). Developmental change in infants' responses to stress. *Child Development, 66,* 657–670.

Lewis, M., Ramsay, D. S., & Kawakami, K. (1993). Differences between Japanese infants and Caucasian American infants in behavioral and cortisol response to inoculation. *Child Development, 64,* 1722–1731.

Lewis, M., & Saarni, C. (Eds.). (1985). *The socialization of emotion.* New York: Plenum Press.

Lewis, M., & Saarni, C. (Eds.). (1993). *Lying and deception in everyday life.* New York: Guilford.

Lewis, M., Sullivan, M. W., Stanger, C., & Weiss, M. (1989). Self-development and self-conscious emotions. *Child Development, 60,* 146–156.

Lewis, M., Wilson, C. D., Ban, P., & Baumel, M. H. (1970). An exploratory study of resting cardiac rates and variability from the last trimester of prenatal life through the first year of postnatal life. *Child Development, 41*(3), 800–811.

Lorenz, K. A. (1965). *Evolution and modification of behavior.* Chicago: University of Chicago Press.

Mandler, G. (1975). *Mind and emotion.* New York: Wiley.

Mandler, G. (1980). The generation of emotion: A psychological theory. In R. Plutchik & H. Kellerman (Eds.), *Emotion: Theory, research, and experience,* Vol. 1 (pp. 219–244). New York: Academic Press.

Mead, G. H. (1934). *Mind, self, and society: From the standpoint of a social behaviorist.* Chicago: University of Chicago Press.

Olds, J. (1962). Hypothalamic substrates of reward. *Physiological Review, 42,* 554–604.

Ortony, A., Clore, G. L., & Collins, A. (1988). *The cognitive structure of emotions.* New York: Cambridge University Press.

Oster, H. (1978). Facial expression and affect development. In M. Lewis & L. A. Rosenblum (Eds.), *The development of affect* (pp. 43–76). New York: Plenum Press.

Oster, H. (1981). "Recognition" of emotional expression in infancy? In M. E. Lamb & L. R. Sherrod (Eds.), *Infant social cognition: Empirical and theoretical considerations* (pp. 85–126). Hillsdale, NJ: Erlbaum.

Pannabecker, B. J., Emde, R. N., Johnson, W., Stenberg, C., & Davis, M. (1980, April). *Maternal perceptions of infant emotions from birth to 18 months. A preliminary report.* Paper presented at the International Conference of Infant Studies, New Haven, CT.

Plutchik, R. (1980). *Emotion: A psychoevolutionary synthesis.* New York: Harper & Row.

Ricciuti, H. N., & Poresky, R. H. (1972). Emotional behavior and development in the first year of life: An analysis of arousal, approach–withdrawal, and affective responses. In A. D. Pick (Ed.), *Minnesota Symposium on Child Psychology* (Vol. 6) (pp. 116–139). Minneapolis: University of Minnesota Press.

Saarni, C. (1979). Children's understanding of display rules for expressive behavior. *Developmental Psychology, 15,* 424–429.

Sander, L. W. (1977). Infant and caretaking environment: Investigation and conceptualization of adaptive behavior in a system of increasing complexity. In E. J. Anthony (Ed.), *The child psychiatrist as investigator.* New York: Plenum Press.

Schachter, S., & Singer, J. E. (1962). Cognitive, social, and physiological determinants of emotional state. *Psychological Review, 69,* 379–399.

Schaffer, H. R. (1974). Cognitive components of the infant's response to stranger. In M. Lewis & L. A. Rosenblum (Eds.), *The origins of fear* (pp. 11–24). New York: Wiley.

Schaffer, H. R., Greenwood, A., & Parry, M. H. (1972). The onset of wariness. *Child Development, 43,* 165–175.

Scherer, K. R. (1979). Nonlinguistic vocal indicators of emotion and psychopathology. In C. E. Izard (Ed.), *Emotions in personality and psychopathology* (pp. 85–102). New York: Plenum Press.

Scherer, K. R. (1982). The assessment of vocal expression in infants and children. In C. E. Izard (Ed.), *Measuring emotions in infants and children.* New York: Cambridge University Press.

Spitz, R. A. (1965). *The first year of life.* New York: International Universities Press.

Spitz, R. A., & Wolf, K. M. (1946). The smiling response: A contribution to the ontogenesis of social relations. *Genetic Psychology Monographs, 34,* 57–125.

Sroufe, L. A. (1979). Socioemotional development. In J. Osofsky (Ed.), *The handbook of infant development* (pp. 462–516). New York: Wiley.

Stipek, D. J., Recchia, S., & McClinton, S. (1990). *Achievement-related self-evaluation in young children.* Unpublished manuscript.

Strongman, K. T. (1978). *The psychology of emotion* (2nd ed.). New York: Wiley.

Tomkins, S. S. (1962). *Affect, imagery, consciousness: Vol. 1. The positive affects.* New York: Springer.

Tomkins, S. S. (1963). *Affect, imagery, consciousness: Vol. 2. The negative affects.* New York: Springer.

Tomkins, S. S. (1980). Affect as amplification: Some modifications in theory. In R. Plutchik & H. Kellerman (Eds.), *Emotion: Theory, research, and experience,* Vol. 1 (pp. 141–164). New York: Academic Press.

Tomkins, S. S. (1981). The quest for primary motives: Biography and autobiography of an idea. *Journal of Personality and Social Psychology, 41,* 306–329.

Waters, E., Matas, L., & Sroufe, L. A. (1975). Infants' reactions to an approaching stranger: Description, validation and functional significance of wariness. *Child Development, 46,* 348–356.

Wheatley, M. E. (1944). The hypothalamus and effective behavior in cats: A study of the effects of experimental lesions, with anatomic correlations. *Archives of Neurological Psychiatry, 52,* 296–316.

Wolff, P. H. (1963). Observations on the early development of smiling. In B. M. Foss (Ed.), *Determinants of infant behavior* (Vol. 2) (pp. 214–239). New York: Wiley.

YoungBrowne, G., Rosenfeld, H. M., & Horowitz, F. (1977). Infant discrimination of facial expressions. *Child Development, 48,* 555–562.

II

Biological and Differential Emotions Perspectives

3

Toward a Neuroscience of Emotion
The Epigenetic Foundations of Emotional Development

Jaak Panksepp, Brian Knutson, and Douglas L. Pruitt

NATURAL FOUNDATIONS OF EMOTION

Affective neuroscience is an emerging field that promises to illuminate the neural bases of emotional change over the life span in all mammals (Panksepp, 1998). It offers a complementary alternative to behavioral neuroscience (which, like behaviorism, denies emotional experience as a valid area of study) and cognitive neuroscience (which concerns itself more with cortical mechanisms involved in symbolic processing). Rather than simply focusing on behavioral indices of learning, affective neuroscience aims to elucidate the emotional processes that *drive* learning—the ancient programs laid down by our mammalian genetic heritage, which channel the unfolding of emotional experience and behavior over the course of the life span (see also Panksepp, 1991, 1995). In order to understand emotional development, we must consider not only changes associated with pervasive environmental influences, but

Jaak Panksepp, Brian Knutson, and Douglas L. Pruitt • Department of Psychology, Bowling Green State University, Bowling Green, Ohio 43402.

What Develops in Emotional Development? edited by Michael F. Mascolo and Sharon Griffin. Plenum Press, New York, 1998.

also changes associated with the natural emergence of the various emotional programs of the brain. Affective neuroscience focuses more on the half of the brain–behavior equation that is due to nature, while always accepting and acknowledging that nurture inevitably molds and modulates specific expressions of these organismic potentials. Although it is evident that all higher brain functions are epigenetically controlled, it will be impossible to disentangle those processes unless we appreciate the genetically provided hardware that allows animals to perceive, feel, and behave in characteristic ways.

The present thesis, amplified in detail elsewhere (Panksepp, 1998), is that distinct emotional operating systems in the brain orchestrate a variety of changes in behavior, various automatic bodily functions, as well as subjectively experienced affective states. These systems are generally subcortically localized in the brain, descending from amygdala, basal forebrain, and septal regions mostly to the hypothalamus (which communicates with the body via the pituitary portal to the bloodstream) and the periventricular gray (which communicates with the body via the spinal nerves). The upper regions of these systems also interact with various paleocortical areas (cingulate, frontal, and periamygdaloid) to interact with cognitive processes. However, these emotional systems do not appear to be either strictly cognitive or behavioral, but rather integrative sensorimotor command systems that organize a large variety of brain processes. These executive systems arouse coherent psychobehavioral syndromes (including autonomic arousal, feeling states, and species-typical behavioral displays), which have served the adaptive functions of prolonging life and enabling procreation over the history of a given mammalian species. Artificial arousal of these systems, as can be achieved with localized electrical stimulation of the brain, induces strong positive and negative affective consequences for both animals (Panksepp, 1981) and humans (Panksepp, 1985), which clearly indicates that we are dealing with emotional as opposed to mere behavioral control systems. In summary, these emotional systems have (1) strong evolutionary/genetic antecedents; (2) anatomically separable subcortical circuit components, (3) the ability to generate subjective feeling states, and (4) the ability to coordinate multiple behavioral outputs.

Modern biological psychiatry's success in developing mood-altering drugs through the study of the brain substrates of animal behaviors also strongly affirms that all mammals share similar affectively valenced brain functions. The striking anatomical resemblances of the human brain to that of other mammals, especially in ancient subcortical areas where the basic emotions are elaborated, further supports this thesis. The existence of a variety of neuropeptide systems provides credible neural substrates around which discrete emotional and motivational processes are organized (Panksepp, 1993a). Thus, it has now become clear that we can learn a great deal about the deep evolutionary sources of human emotional experience by studying the brains of other mammalian species. Also, because it is now well accepted that neural systems exhibit spontaneous firing before birth and throughout all stages of life, we have to accept a new perspective on the epigenetic origins of emotions. Not only are there strong genetic components to basic emotional responses, but also the intrinsic activities of many systems within the brain create a dynamic internal environment that is not typically considered when people use epigenetic concepts. Not only are these circuits molded by external environments in which organisms must subsist, but they may also be modified by the spontaneously active internal environments of brain and body.

Emerging neuroscientific methods are finally enabling us to disentangle emotional brain mechanisms in mammalian models. For instance, we can now ask whether early experiences modify the ramification of the underlying emotional circuits using various long-lasting cell-tracing procedures that can highlight neuronal morphology for a sufficiently long time to capture the long-term impact of environmental influences. We can ask whether experiences change the presynaptic neurotransmitter and postsynaptic receptor characteristics of neural circuits, as well as their electrical activity. We can even ask whether early experiences change the dynamic expression of genetic information within neurons, as monitored with *in situ* hybridization and other specialized tools of molecular biology (see Panksepp, 1991, 1998). Because of such breakthroughs, the existence of environmentally linked internal representation in animals, as well as evolutionarily dictated affective representation, is a less controversial topic today than it was just a few years ago. However, obvious ethical concerns preclude neural studies of many of the mechanistic issues underlying emotion in humans. We can only monitor some traces of emotional experience with electroencephalographic (EEG) techniques and other modern imaging procedures that can access the functional terrain within the living human brain (Dawson & Fisher, 1994; Kertesz, 1994; Posner & Raichle, 1994).

In our discussion of neural correlates of emotional development, we first describe a strategy for functional analysis and briefly summarize present knowledge about the neural substrates of some representative socioemotional processes. Later, we outline findings regarding the development of transmitter chemistries, receptors, and brain morphologies. Specific examples accompany some of the more extensively studied systems. Finally, we close by way of example, with an empirically based template for an emotional system. In this short chapter, our coverage cannot be comprehensive, but by integrating many critical lines of evidence related to emotional development, we seek to highlight promising paths for future investigations.

DEVELOPMENTAL PATTERNS OF SOCIOEMOTIONAL BEHAVIORS

Most mammalian emotional behaviors occur in the context of social interactions. This makes adaptive sense, because young mammals depend on their parents for survival and older mammals must garner the interest of mates and compete for resources to ensure the survival of their young. The changing likelihood that a mammal will display specific socioemotional behaviors can be approximately traced across the life span. Although the presence of conspecifics triggers the expression of these behaviors and hones their coordination, certain laboratory animals that have had no directly relevant social experience will readily display them when given their first opportunity (e.g., rough-and-tumble play: Ikemoto & Panksepp, 1991; separation distress: Panksepp et al., 1980), which suggests that these repertoires possess highly sophisticated, innate components for integration of emotional tendencies. Thus, a systematic ethological description of their occurrence across the life span should provide some basis for eventually linking neural systems to specific forms of socioemotional development. To help visualize such issues, we have plotted idealized ethological trajectories of several mammalian socioemotional behaviors (see Figure 1) and provide a brief description of developmental changes in expression and neural correlates of each. Because of the abundance of data, our examples will primarily highlight development in the laboratory rat. However, we include other species as needed for clarity.

Distress Vocalizations

When young mammals are separated from their primary caregiver, they typically vocalize. These protest vocalizations are thought to signal a state of distress. For instance, rats show distress vocalizations (DVs) during the first 2 weeks of life in the absence of their mother, despite the presence of adequate heating and comfort (Archer & Hansen, 1991). As summarized in Figure 1, the propensity of different types of mammals to exhibit DVs depends on the species. As a general rule, precocial species such as the guinea pig, which are born ambulatory, tend to vocalize much more and for longer periods than altricial species such as the rat, which remain put in their nests for some time after birth (Pettijohn, 1979). This serves an adaptive purpose, because precocial infants are more likely to wander into potentially dangerous situations and thus require ia strong "monitoring system" for parental protection.

---→

Figure 1. An idealized schematic summary of the approximate trajectories of emotional development in laboratory rats as a function of their life span. Y axis is on an arbitrary scale. The SEEKING, FEAR, and RAGE systems are projections that are not based on a solid database, and dotted lines in the other systems also indicate phases of life where there are little data. Since the intensity of separation–distress appears to exhibit great species diversity (as measured by separation–distress vocalization), another species, guinea pigs, are indicated to demonstrate a more typical response pattern. The early peak in NURTURANCE reflects a period of time when young rats exhibit strong maternal urges, as indicated by high levels of interactions with neonates.

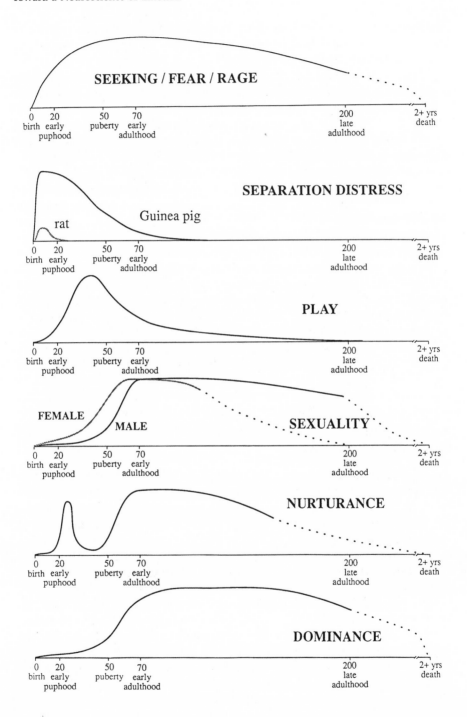

Unfortunately, because of their limited display of this behavior, rats make less-than-optimal models for the study of separation distress (see Panksepp, Newman, & Insel, 1992, for a discussion of this controversy).

The main trajectory of the distress vocalization system ascends from evolutionarily ancient mesencephalic brain areas that mediate pain to the dorsomedial thalamic and preoptic hypothalamic areas, which transmit information to various forebrain areas, especially the cingulate cortex. Electrical stimulation of these brain areas produces DVs even in adult animals (Herman & Panksepp, 1981). Several pharmacological manipulations exert profound effects on the expression of DVs in mammals without affecting other behaviors such as motor activity. For instance, low doses of opiates can selectively inhibit DVs, whereas opiate antagonists increase them (Panksepp, Normansell, Herman, Bishop, & Crepeau, 1988). The peptides oxytocin and prolactin also powerfully reduce DVs when injected directly into the brain (Winslow & Insel, 1992; Panksepp, 1988; Panksepp, Nelson, & Siviy, 1994). This is not surprising, because rat oxytocin receptors are abundant on cingulate and thalamic neurons that comprise the putative separation-distress/social-bonding circuit during the first few weeks of life when mother–infant bonding occurs. Only later, during sexual maturity, do these receptors dynamically shift in distribution to the ventromedial hypothalamus and the ventral hippocampal areas (Björklund, Hökfelt, & Tohyama, 1992; Insel, 1992), presumably to subserve other sociosexual and social-memory functions. On the other hand, agonists of the simple amino acid neurotransmitter glutamate or corticotrophin releasing factor dramatically enhance DVs when injected into avian (Panksepp et al., 1988) and mammalian brains (Archer & Hansen, 1991).

Rough-and-Tumble Play

Until the last two decades, play behavior has been relatively neglected by both human and animal ethologists, but rough-and-tumble play appears in most mammals between late infancy and puberty, when it can serve as a powerful reinforcer. For instance, young rats who have been socially isolated prefer areas where they have played before (Schechter & Calcagnetti, 1993) and will work for an opportunity to play with a conspecific (Ikemoto & Panksepp, 1992; Normansell & Panksepp, 1990). Furthermore, in humans, such play is typically associated with feelings of excitement and joy. Play behavior is especially prominent in altricial, predatory mammals, which show an extended period of childhood (or neoteny) compared to precocial, herbivorous mammals (Fagen, 1992). No one has yet empirically demonstrated the adaptive function of rough-and-tumble-play, but it surely provides an early exercise of social interaction skills, which may prepare animals for later friendly and agonistic encounters with conspecifics (Panksepp, Siviy, & Normansell, 1984; Panksepp, 1993b; Thor & Holloway, 1984).

Neuroanatomically, an intact cortex is not essential for the expression of rough-and-tumble play, because neonatally decorticated rats exhibit play at levels comparable to sham-operated controls (Panksepp et al., 1994; Pellis, Pellis, & Whishaw, 1992). A pathway through the parafascicular area of the thalamus seems especially important in the elaboration of play—if this area is damaged, play behavior is specifically reduced (Siviy & Panksepp, 1987). Play relies on a delicate balance of brain chemistry, because most pharmacological manipulations can reduce play (Panksepp, 1993b). However, low doses of morphine can increase play, whereas opiate antagonists such as naltrexone decrease it, suggesting a specific modulating role by opioid systems (Panksepp, Jalowiec, DeEskinazi, & Bishop, 1985). In summary, rough-and-tumble play represents a developmentally bounded socioemotional behavior that is ripe for rigorous neural and functional analysis.

Sexuality

At puberty, which usually occurs earlier in females than males, young animals begin to exhibit sexual behaviors. In humans, these behaviors are typically accompanied by feelings of lust and attraction for the opposite sex. As mammals age, their sexual vigor gradually declines. Sex is the evolutionary paragon of all social behaviors, though different species often exhibit distinct sexual repertoires. On one end of the spectrum are "tournament" species, where males and females tend to differ greatly in size, "alpha" males commonly mate with many females, and infant care is generally the exclusive province of females. At the other end of the spectrum are "pair-bonded" species, where males and females resemble each other in size, sometimes bond for life, and share infant-rearing more equally (Sapolsky, 1993). But despite such differences, to the best of our knowledge, the basic neural ground plan for sexual urges is remarkably similar for all mammals (Carter, 1992; Carmichael et al., 1987; LeVay, 1993). Only the details differ.

The neural substrates of sexual behavior have been more clearly detailed than any other socioemotional behavior discussed here. Sexual maturation depends on a two-stage sequence of neural events. In the rat, the "organizational" stage occurs during the third trimester of pregnancy, when the developing infant's testes secrete testosterone that is aromatized to estrogen and subsequently promotes the growth of male-specific circuits in the brain such as the medial preoptic area of the hypothalamus (MPOA), while the 5-α-reductase product of testosterone metabolism, dihydrotestosterone, guides the molding of the male body (LeVay, 1993). The ensuing "activational" stage of sexual development that accompanies puberty is characterized by a series of well-mapped brain and hormonal processes, which differ for females and males. For instance, when the female rat's vagina opens at puberty under the influence of hypothalamic releasing factors, the endogenous brain receptivity cycle of estrus begins, which is marked hormonally by the cyclic 4–5 day surges of estrogen release, followed by progesterone spikes from the maturing ovarian follicles. At that point, females simultaneously become fertile and sexually receptive. At sexual maturity, male rats' testes begin to release testosterone, which activates male sexual behavior. Testosterone targets both the MPOA, which is necessary for the proper execution of copulation, and also amygdaloid and lateral hypothalamic circuits, which stimulate seeking behaviors for sexual partners in both males and females (Everitt & Bancroft, 1991). Human sexuality differs from other mammals, largely because of more complex learning factors as well as a chronically receptive state in females that is controlled more by adrenal androgens than by the cyclic ovarian hormones (Burger, Hailes, Nelson, & Menelaus, 1987; Morris, Udry, Khan-Dawood, & Dawood, 1987; Sherwin & Gelfand, 1987).

Sexual behavior can also be modulated by several neurochemical systems. For instance, increased dopaminergic tone via amphetamine sensitization enhances seeking of sexual contact with male rats (Nocjar, Panksepp, & Conner, 1995). On the other hand, increases in serotonergic tone via serotonin-specific reuptake inhibitors decreases sexual behaviors, whereas pharmacological lesions of the serotonin system increase sexual behavior in both males and females (Tsutsui, Shinoda, & Kondo, 1994). Furthermore, many peptides play key roles in the expression of both male and female sexual behaviors. For instance, estrogen promotes the brain production of oxytocin, which increases female sexual receptivity as well as penile erection (Björklund et al., 1992), whereas testosterone promotes the brain production of vasopressin, which enhances both male–female sexual assertiveness and intramale sexual possessiveness (Björklund et al., 1992; Winslow, Hastings, Carter, Harbaugh, & Insel, 1993).

Nurturance

All mammalian mothers care for their young by providing milk. However, both male and female mammals also care for their young in less obvious ways, such as keeping them warm, protecting them, playing with them, and teaching them by example—in a word, by nurturing their offspring. Human parents readily attest to the deep bonds of affection that they feel for their own children, and other mammals also show behavioral signs of positive feelings of attachment at discrete periods during the life cycle. Some species, such as sheep, have narrow windows of bonding opportunity, whereas others, such as rats, seem to be willing to care for any pup that appears in their nest (Kendrick, Levy, & Kaverne, 1992). Presumably, these behaviors reflect an age- and hormone-delimited nurturance "drive." For instance, as depicted in Figure 1, juvenile rats show a transient but intense interest in infant rats, at a time that may correspond to the period when young human children show an interest in dolls (Björklund et al., 1992). This interest rapidly disappears and does not typically resurface until rats have given birth to their own young, but it can be induced by sufficiently long exposure to rat pups. An emerging neuroscientific literature suggests that distinct neural changes underlie, modulate, and direct these expressions of affection (Bridges & Mann, 1994; Krasnegor & Bridges, 1990; Numan, 1988; Winberg & Kjellmer, 1994).

A few days prior to birth, female rats exhibit intense cleaning and nest-building behaviors, which can be triggered by a specific milieu of hormonal changes marked by low levels of progesterone and high levels of estrogen, prolactin, and oxytocin. Immediately after birth, a number of hormones and peptides act in concert to help prepare new mothers for the care of their young. In the estrogen-primed female, oxytocin plays a major role in the initiation of maternal care. Peripherally, oxytocin enables the birthing process and release of milk from the mammary glands, whereas in the brain, it establishes a central psychobehavioral state that makes maternal activities more probable. It is also noteworthy that vaginal stimulation and the baby's suckiing on the mother's breast releases oxytocin in the mother's brain in a time-locked fashion (Pederson, Caldwell, Jirikowski, & Insel, 1992). This may well facilitate maternal feelings of affection toward the pup, because in pups, oxytocin specifically mediates mother–infant bonding (Nelson & Panksepp, 1995), and in adults, brain oxytocin arousal facilitates partner preferences (Gavish, Carter, & Getz, 1985).

Although oxytocin promotes the initiation of maternal behavior, prolactin and endogenous opioids appear to play a permissive role in allowing it to continue (Bridges & Mann, 1994; Panksepp et al., 1994). In fact, brain opioids have been implicated in social bonding for some time (Panksepp, 1981), and there is some evidence that opiate antagonists can reduce imprinting in young birds (Panksepp, Siviy, Normansell, White, & Bishop, 1982) and infant–mother bonding in young rats (Panksepp et al., 1994). In one rodent model of infant–mother bonding, rat pups are reunited with a mother whose ventrum has been sprayed with a distinctive odor after a short period of separation. Several days later, the pups' attraction to that odor is measured in a runway. As summarized in Figure 2, when pups' opioid receptors had been blocked with naloxone, approach to the conditioned smell was significantly reduced.

Interestingly, these hormone and peptide target areas of the hypothalamus are implicated in female sexual receptivity, which suggests that the substrate of maternal nurturance and social bonding may have arisen from brain circuits that originally subserved female-typical sexual function. However, oxytocin may also have affiliative effects on male rats, because it can facilitate the nurturant responsivity of male rats to unfamiliar infants (a phenomenon known as "sensitization" or "concaveation"), which is especially strong in young rats (e.g., 3–4 weeks of age; Brown, 1986; Brunelli, Shindledecker, & Hofer, 1987). This latter developmental phase may be reflected in the very high tendency of young children between 9 and 24 months of age to exhibit high levels of helping behavior (Hoffman, 1981), and this may

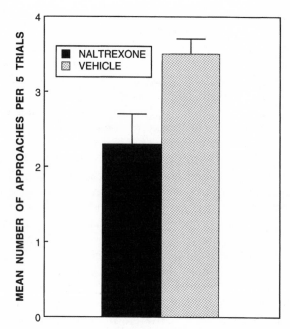

Figure 2. Eleven-day-old rat pups ($n = 44$) were removed from their mothers, and reunited for half-hour periods three times at 3-hour intervals. Prior to each reunion period, the mothers were sprayed on the ventrum with orange extract. Before each reunion, half the animals were injected with 0.5 to 1.0 mg/kg of naltrexone, while the control animals received equivolumetric injections of the vehicle. Twenty-four hours later, animals were given five odor-approach trials in a straight runway. Animals that had experience maternal reunion when their opioid system was blocked with naltrexone exhibited weaker approach than control animals ($t(42) = 2.42$, $p < .05$). Data adapted from Panksepp, Nelson, and Siviy (1994).

be due to changes in brain affiliative systems such as those organized around oxytocin. A surge of oxytocin release in the brain accompanies ejaculation in the male rat, and periods of free access to sexual gratification can increase brain oxytocin levels by a factor of three (Pedersen et al., 1992). Accordingly, sexual activity reduces male rats' tendency to kill unfamiliar rat pups, and this suppression is most potent 3 weeks after copulation, which nicely corresponds with the gestational term of female rats (Kennedy & Elwood, 1988; Mennella & Moltz, 1988).

Dominance

Agonistic behavior, colloquially known as "intermale fighting," emerges first in pubertal male rats and somewhat later in lactating females. This disputatious behavior commonly occurs in the context of competition for resources or status and thus serves the adaptive function of facilitating access to valuable commodities (Adams & Boice, 1989). For male rats, the prototypical valued resources are mates and territory, whereas for females they are pups and nest sites. Chimpanzees fight for similar reasons (Goodall, 1992) and so, probably, do humans. During a fight, mammals undoubtedly experience the "fight or flight" emotions of anger and fear, depending on who is winning. These emotions will be discussed in the next section. However, in humans, the decision to engage in an offensive attack presumes an initial feeling of assertiveness or agency on the part of the initiator. Emerging empirical evidence indicates that this assertive state may have a neural basis (Albert, Walsh, & Jonik, 1993; Compaan, Wozniak, DeRuiter, Koolhaas, & Hutchinson, 1994).

As with sexual behavior, the onset of dominance behavior in male rats is controlled to some extent by the neural organizational effects of a pubertal testosterone surge. Moreover, at sexual maturity, testosterone activates brain vasopressinergic circuits that synapse on areas of the hypothalamus associated with male sexual behavior. In the hamster, vasopressin placed into the brain enhances territorial marking and can even determine the winner of a territorial dispute (Ferris & Delville, 1994). Additionally, vasopressin can enhance male sexual possessiveness in rats, because males will attack competitors for females with whom they have copulated or even those in whose presence they have merely received brain infusions of vasopressin (Winslow et al., 1993). Indeed, measurement of these neurohormones in the brain suggests that maternal aggression may also be caused by a shift of brain oxytocin/vasopressin distributions from a female-typical pattern to a male-typical one (Pederson et al., 1992). Thus, just as nurturant behavior appears to rise out of a substrate of female-typical sexuality, dominant behavior may rise out of a substrate of male-typical sexuality. Interestingly, there is some evidence that social outcomes reciprocally affect the long-term functioning of these dominance systems. For instance, defeat during intermale fighting leads to a reduction in plasma testosterone (Olweus, Mattsson, Schalling, & Low, 1988), which may lead to altered levels of vasopressin (Sachser, Lick, & Stanzel, 1994). Clearly, more work needs to be done to link natural dominance outcomes to steroid receptor-mediated shifts in neurochemistry.

DEVELOPMENTAL PROGRESSION OF "BASIC" EMOTIONAL BEHAVIORS

We have discussed some prominent socioemotional behaviors that change in characteristic ways across the mammalian life span. However, when most human emotion researchers talk about emotion, they refer not to feelings associated with the specific social behaviors listed earlier, but rather to a less socially delimited group of "basic" emotions such as anger, happiness, fear, and sadness (e.g., Ekman, 1992). Psychologists often use facial and vocal expressions as markers for the onset of these "basic" emotions in children (though physiological measures have also been used; see Fox & Calkins, 1993). For instance, Ahadi and Rothbart (1994) outline a developmental sequence of human emotional development based on some of these expressive markers: The newborn infant immediately shows signs of distress; smiling can occur 2 to 12 hours after birth; anger/frustration reactions have been observed at 2 months of age, whereas anxious inhibition in response to fearful or novel stimuli does not occur until 8 to 9 months of age.

In contrast to human infants, rats and other "lower" mammals exhibit comparatively few facial or complex vocal signs of their emotional experience (with the exception of DVs). However, one can infer a rat's emotional state without facial or vocal cues by observing certain fundamental behavioral trajectories related to some "basic" emotions. Take, for instance, the three emotions that even John Watson, the archbehaviorist, admitted that humans feel: love, anger and fear. Specifically, the desirous component of love involves "approach" or moving toward an object with the apparent intent to incorporate it into one's environment. Anger involves "attack" or moving toward an object with the apparent intent to remove it from one's environment. Slight fear involves "freezing" or a rigid, static stance with the intent to locate a potentially harmful object, and extreme fear involves "flight" or moving away from the vicinity of that object with the intent to avoid it. All of these behavior patterns can be elicited toward initially neutral stimuli via electrodes implanted in the brain in specific and distinct circuits (Panksepp, 1982, 1991). This argues that some "basic" emotional behaviors are triggered not only by the external features of an object, but also require the activation of distinct emotional circuits.

In order to link brain activity to "basic" emotional behaviors, one must address the same questions as posed earlier: (1) When does the behavior appear? (2) When does it disappear? (3) What are neural correlates of the behavior's onset and offset? As depicted in Figure 1, "basic" emotional behaviors show a broader and less well-defined course than some of the more time-delimited socioemotional behaviors. However, these are idealized curves for two reasons. First, no one has established an indisputable link between the behavioral tendencies described and the basic emotions as experienced in animals. For instance, to what extent does the appearance of these behaviors mark the development of motoric ability versus an emotional state? We assume that animals experience these emotions because electrical and pharmacological stimulation of these same circuits have powerful emotional effects in humans (Panksepp, 1985; Penfield, 1992). As a second caveat, much less research exists that has ethologically mapped the developmental trajectories of these "basic" emotional behaviors. For instance, we know of no integrated emotional test battery that assesses desire, anger, and fear behaviors in male and female rats, though promising neuroethological progress is being made on this front (see Olivier et al., 1994). Nonetheless, we hope that this theoretical sketch of the idealized trajectories of these "basic" emotional behaviors will facilitate thought and research on the topic.

Desire/Seeking

Rats as young as 11 days have been shown to traverse a runway for nipple attachment (McDougall, Nonneman, & Crawford, 1991). Clearly, at age 15, by eye opening, young rats begin to explore beyond the confines of their nest, and they will wean themselves naturally starting at about 21 days of age. Approach behaviors solidify with age, probably peaking at puberty. Data on approach behavior in old age are scarce, but the decline is undoubtedly significant with age.

More than any other system, the mesolimbic dopaminergic projections that course from the ventral tegmental area through the lateral hypothalamus to the limbic system and forebrain have been implicated in desirous seeking behaviors. These projections are an integral part of the major lateral-hypothalamic self-stimulation system of the brain that has previously been proposed to mediate "expectancy" processes (Panksepp, 1981, 1982). Under specific circumstances, animals will forego all other pleasures (e.g., food, sex, drink) to stimulate this system. Thus, it is no surprise that the activation of this system is intimately associated with the addictive potential of cocaine and amphetamines (Robinson & Berridge, 1993; Wise & Bozarth, 1987). However, this system seems to motivate appetitive "seeking" or "desire" rather than consummatory reward or "satisfaction." Electrical stimulation of this system elicits active foraging and search behaviors. For instance, this circuit becomes quite active when the male rats approach an estrus female, but does not increase in activity during copulation (Pfaus & Phillips, 1991). Also, although the seeking behavior evoked by stimulation of this system generally remains constant, a stimulated animal will switch from one specific goal to another, depending on stimulus availability (e.g., from eating to drinking to gnawing; see Berridge & Valenstein, 1991; Panksepp, 1982).

The details of this system are presently being revealed. Dopaminergic transmission activates several receptor subtypes of which D1 receptors have been predominantly implicated in anticipation of reward, whereas D2 receptors have been primarily implicated in the motoric onset of seeking behavior. Interestingly, both young (11 days) and older (60 days) rats require activation of both dopamine receptor subtypes to demonstrate fully expressed seeking behavior, but rats at 17–21 days of age require only stimulation of the D1 receptors (Pruitt, Bolanos, & McDougall, 1995). This augmented responsiveness of the seeking system may spur young rats to leave the nest and seek out new, though less dependable, sources of sustenance.

Anger/Attack

Although little is known regarding anger-mediated behaviors prior to puberty, full-fledged attack behavior associated with intense anger in humans usually peaks with the onset of puberty in male rats and at the time of lactation in females, as noted earlier. Similarly, little is known about the ethological prevalence of affective attack in older animals. Males typically show more aggression than females throughout the life span, with the exception of lactation, when female brain chemistry coincidentally shifts to a more male-like pattern (see Pedersen et al., 1992). Nonetheless, the neural substrate underlying affective attack is similar for both males and females (Siegel & Pott, 1988).

One can elicit affective attack (as opposed to instrumental/predatory attack) via stimulation of neural pathways that descend from the central and medial amygdaloid nuclei through the stria terminalis to the medial hypothalamus and terminate in the periventricular gray (Bandler, 1988). In addition to stimulating seeking behavior, dopaminergic activation can also increase affective attack. This is not surprising, because both behaviors involve a prominent behavioral approach component. However, a lack of serotonergic activation may distinguish desirous approach from angry approach. Low brain serotonin has consistently been linked to elevated aggressiveness in the mammalian brain research literature (Valzelli, 1984). Moreover, several environmental contingencies that lower brain serotonin, such as social isolation and low dietary availability of serotonin precursors, also increase affective attack behavior (Olivier, Mos, & Miczek, 1991). In areas of the brain implicated in motor commands, serotonin interacts with dopamine and has been shown to turn behaviors "off" once initiated (Barber, Teicher, & Baldessarini, 1989). Thus, affective attack may present a natural example of the emotional consequences of frustrating intense approach behavior.

Fear/Freezing and Flight

As mentioned earlier, fearful behavior consists of both freezing and flight. The two coexist under one emotional heading because one can elicit freezing with slight stimulation of the same circuitry that elicits flight at higher amplitudes, suggesting that both behaviors are expressions of the same qualitative emotional state (Panksepp, 1990; Panksepp, Sacks, Crepeau, & Abbott, 1991). Accordingly, young rats (16 days old) respond to a conditioned fear stimulus with slowed heartbeat and freezing, whereas adolescent rats (30 days old) respond to the same conditioned fear stimulus with heart-beat acceleration and flight (Kurtz & Campbell, 1994).

The neural wiring of fear circuitry runs parallel but somewhat lateral to that of anger (Siegel & Pott, 1988). Benzodiazepine receptors are well represented in this circuitry, and benzodiazepine receptor agonists such as diazepam quell both freezing and flight behavior in rats as well as feelings of anxiety in humans. Conversely, several centrally administered agents precipitate extreme fearful behavior in mammals. For example, direct administration of glutamate agonists can induce both freezing and flight in rats, as does corticotrophin-releasing factor (CRF; Kalin & Takahashi, 1990). Interestingly, when two rats fight, both show a rise in blood levels of corticosterone (which is triggered by central CRF), but only the loser continues to show enhanced corticosterone long after the fight has ended (Schuurman, 1980). There are many nonspecific brain factors that control all of the aforementioned emotional behaviors. For instance, pharmacological manipulations that increase noradrenergic activity in rats can potentiate fearful behaviors, but this probably results from a general modulatory effect, because norepinephrine modulates many other emotional behaviors as well (e.g., separation distress: Panksepp, Yates, Ikemoto, & Nelson, 1991).

Overview

These brief sketches of brain emotional systems raise some important questions for understanding the natural biological progression of emotional development. For instance, do the anatomical growth and myelinization of these basic emotional brain circuits or changes in neurochemical activities and sensitivities mark important developmental changes in emotional behavior? Conversely, how do specific, unconditional emotional stimuli and the consequences of learning affect the functioning of these systems, both in the short-term and over the life span? Answers to such questions will require more extensive ethological analysis of basic emotional behaviors and further characterization of the underlying neural substrates.

EXAMPLES OF NEUROCHEMICAL CHANGES AND THEIR IMPACT ON EMOTIONAL BEHAVIOR

In the past 20 years, developmental psychology has preferentially focused on issues of nurture, such as the interaction of environmental vectors and the learning potentials of the individual child (however, there is also a rich developmental tradition that focuses on nativism; cf. Blurton-Jones, 1972; Broman & Grafman, 1994). At the same time, there has been a growing database on the massive neuronal changes that naturally occur as the brain develops throughout childhood. The young of most species are born with essentially a full complement of neuronal elements. Those elements continue to mature via the extension of nerve processes (axons and dendrites); progressive increases in myelinization, the selective death of neurons, synaptic proliferation and pruning, the development of a large number of synaptic chemistries, neuronal metabolic abilities, and the functional maturation and coordination of the electrical activities of the brain (Dawson & Fisher, 1994). Indeed, some of these changes progress for periods of time that just a decade ago would have been considered unbelievable. For instance, the myelinization of inputs to the hippocampus progresses well into adulthood (Benes, 1989), which may influence the expression of psychiatric disorders such as schizophrenia (Benes, 1991).

Because the strongest linkages between human developmental issues and animal brain research are likely to be found at the neurochemical level (especially with regard to pharmacological treatment of childhood psychiatric problems), we will briefly highlight some of the many developmental changes that have been characterized in animal models. Although we can presently only make a few linkages to human data, it is likely that these patterns will eventually elucidate the types of changes that are also occurring in the human brain. Because much of this literature has been covered in detail elsewhere (see Benes, 1994; Björklund et al., 1992), we only provide a brief outline of the development of several neurochemical systems, including the major amino acids of the brain (gamma-aminobutyric acid [GABA], glutamate, and glycine), the biogenic amine systems (dopamine, norepinephrine, and serotonin), and, finally, some additional neuropeptides that are especially important for regulating emotional processes (Panksepp, 1993a). Eventually, we would like to link the developmental patterns described in Figure 1 to specific changes in brain anatomy, electrophysiology, and chemistry. But for now, we can only present a few specific examples of linkages and promising directions for future research.

Amino Acids

Glutamate and GABA are the most important excitatory and inhibitory neurotransmitters in the brain. They are expressed in widespread circuits that participate in every emotional and cognitive function that has been studied. Just like the other transmitters already covered, they are present at birth but continue to mature for up to several months following birth, often in an inverted U-type manner. For instance, glutamate receptors increase for the first 2 or 3 weeks of life and then decline to adult levels (Baudry, Arst, Olivier, & Lynch, 1981; Schliebs, Kullman, & Bigl, 1986). GABA shows a slightly different pattern, with a gradual increase in synthetic enzymes for the first 3 weeks of life, leading to approximately adult levels at 2 weeks of life (Coyle & Enna, 1976; Rozenburg, Robain, Jardin, & Ben-Ari, 1989; Seress & Ribak, 1988). Receptors also proliferate dramatically during the first few weeks of life, and then continue to increase gradually thereafter until puberty (Candy & Enna, 1976). Also, one should note the existence of functional plasticity in these systems, because animals reared in the dark exhibit decrements in synthetic enzyme activities for GABA within the visual cortex (Fosse, Heggelund, & Fonnum, 1989).

Glycine, the simplest of the natural amino acids, serves two distinct major functions in the brain. It both inhibits motor processes in the lower reaches of the brain and facilitates glutamate transmission in the higher reaches, where glutamate is a major cortical transmitter. Without adequate glycine transmission, as occurs when a glycine receptor antagonist is administered, organisms tend to be prone to seizures and excessive reflex responses. For instance, inhibition of glycine markedly facilitates startle responses, a reflex that has been used very effectively to study fear processes in the brain. Mutations of the glycine receptor produce neurological disorders such as hyperekplexia (startle disease) as well as various forms of motor abnormalities characterized by hypertonia and hyperexcitability, yielding strains of mice with colorful names such as *spastic*, *spasmodic*, and *oscillator* mice (Becker, 1995). Remarkably, the glycine receptor comes in two distinct forms, one being the "neonatal" form, which is highest at birth and gradually disappears by 2 weeks of age, and an "adult" form, which is low at birth and increases to adult levels at about the time the neonatal form has died out (Becker, Schmieden, Tarroni, Strasser, & Betz, 1992). Presumably, these two receptors have distinct developmental functions, but it is not yet clear what they are. However, in the aforementioned mutants, the symptoms of their disease do not start until about 2 weeks after birth, when the "neonatal" form of the glycine receptor has died out and the aberrant adult form of the receptor prevails in controlling glycinergic transmission in the brain (Becker, 1995). Although the implications for treatment of human startle disorders remains obscure, one might imagine that genetic manipulations that would sustain the neonatal form of the receptor might ameliorate the progression of those neurological abnormalities, but this speculation remains empirically untested at present.

Acetylcholine

Acetylcholine neurons are already in place at birth (Bayer, 1985), but rat pups do not begin to synthesize substantial amounts of the transmitter until the second week of life. Further increases in acetylcholine activity are seen until 30 days or a bit later (Björklund et al., 1992). Receptor densities continue to increase until puberty (Coyle & Yamamura, 1976). The fact that acetylcholine appears to be especially important in attentional processes that are necessary for responding well to emotional stimuli, and the fact that anterior hypothalamic cholinergic systems have been implicated in vocal and other behaviors such as fear and or aversive responses (Golebiewski & Ramaniuk, 1985), suggest that it mediates emotional responses during the earliest periods of life. This is in general agreement with the early development of various fear responses in humans as well (see Marks, 1987). Interestingly, when the developmental trajectory of this system is envisioned, one can readily see that it mirrors the ontogeny of play in rats. Robust play behavior is first noted at about 20–21 days of age, peaks at 30–35 days, and gradually declines quite slowly until at approximately 58 days it has returned to a more or less baseline level (Panksepp, 1981). The notion that the cholinergic system may underlie the expression of play is supported by the fact that anticholinergic agents antagonize play with unparalleled efficacy (Beatty, 1983). In humans, acetylcholine synthesis increases until about 10 years of age (Diebler, Farkas-Bargeton, & Wehrle, 1979), whereas receptor densities are highest at birth and gradually decline until old age (Ravikumar & Sastry, 1985). Although clearly untested, such parallelism invites the supposition that perhaps the same neurochemistries affecting play in the rat may mediate such behavior in humans.

Biogenic Amines

Serotonin, norepinephrine, and dopamine cell groups are fairly mature at birth, even though the axons continue to grow and mature in their respective target areas. Serotonergic innervation of the cortex continues to mature for several months after birth in rats (Deguchi & Barchas, 1972; Johnston, 1988) as well as in primates (Goldman-Rakic & Brown, 1982). Norepinephrine circuits are more extensive at birth than at maturity (Coyle & Molliver, 1977) even though norepinephrine-producing enzymes continue to develop until puberty (Johnston & Coyle, 1980). Although the full complement of dopamine cells exist at birth, dopamine innervation of cortex requires up to 3 weeks to mature (Berger & Verney, 1984). Dopamine receptors, although plentiful at birth, also continue to proliferate until adolescence, whereas transmitter levels do not reach full expression until adulthood (Bruinink, Lishtensteinger, & Schlumpf, 1983; Deskin, Seidler, Whitmore, & Slotkin, 1981). There is evidence that several of the biogenic amines, especially serotonin and norepinephrine, are trophic factors for the maturation of other systems (D'Amato et al., 1987; Kasamatsu & Pettigrew, 1976). Also, we might mention that the hormone melatonin, which is synthesized from serotonin, is abundantly available in early development where it serves a variety of poorly understood developmental functions, including the proper myelinization of the brain (Björklund et al., 1992).

Some effects of dopaminergic manipulations on emotional development have been mentioned earlier, but genetic alterations of the serotonin system can also have profound emotional consequences later in life. In 1993, Brunner, Nelen, Breakefield, Ropers, and van Oost identified a cohort of related Dutch males characterized by mild mental retardation and a tendency toward aggressive outbursts, particularly during times of emotional stress. Genetic analysis indicated that these men lacked a gene that codes for the production of monoamine oxidase A (MAO-A). This enzyme selectively breaks down serotonin and norepinephrine in the brain. Additionally, the Dutch cohort had reduced urine metabolites of serotonin (5-HIAA) and other monoamine metabolites. Low cerebrospinal levels of 5-HIAA have been specifically linked to impulsive aggressive behavior in other studies of humans (Coccaro, 1989). Accordingly, Cases et al. (1995) created a mouse strain with the same genetic alteration as the Dutch cohort by using a genetic knockout procedure. The MAO-A–deficient mice also showed impulsive aggressive behavior. For instance, adult mutants had more bite wounds from cagemates and attacked nest intruders more readily. Although they also had low brain levels of 5-HIAA, the report did not specify exactly how this long-term metabolic imbalance had functionally affected the serotonin system. However, the emotional consequences of a genetic mutation that focally compromises serotonin function can now be simulated and examined quite effectively in a murine model.

Peptides

The developmental patterns of many neuropeptides have recently been documented (Björklund et al., 1992), and there is no general principle that covers them all. Some, like neurotensin, are very elaborate prior to birth and then diminish throughout early development. Although most are abundant at birth, some, like cholecystokinin, are quite limited at birth and exhibit progressive elaboration as animals age. Many exhibit transient expressions during certain phases of development, presumably serving some temporary developmental function and then disappearing from the face of the brain. Certain components of endogenous opioid and somatostatin systems exhibit such patterns. Only a few items have been linked credibly to the maturation of functions, such as the sudden appearance of vasopressin in the suprachiasmatic nucleus at about the time rat pups begin to exhibit a strong circadian cycle (Reghunandanan, Reghunandanan, & Marya, 1991). In general, a cornucopia of developmental neuropeptide expression patterns have been described at the basic neuroscientific level, but not at the functional level, which creates a major challenge for affective neuroscientists and developmental psychologists alike.

One of the more striking developmental effects of neuropeptides has been the recent demonstration that endogenous opioids are a major developmental control factor in maturing mammals. Chronic opioid exposure tends to dramatically reduce physical and psychological development (Zagon, Zagon, & McLaughlin, 1989), whereas opiate antagonists can promote both neural and physical development. These types of changes have been connected to pervasive developmental disorders such as autism (Zagon, Gibo, & McLaughlin, 1991), and recent work demonstrates that opiate antagonists can provide some benefit in the treatment of such disorders (Kolmen, Feldman, Handen, & Janosky, 1995; Leboyer et al., 1992; Panksepp, Lensing, Leboyer, & Bouvard, 1991).

EXAMPLES OF EARLY EMOTIONAL INTERVENTIONS

In addition to emotional changes that arise from the neurochemical unfolding of genetically prescribed emotional systems, environmental factors undoubtedly have a profound impact on the emotional development of the young mammal. However, investigators who do not ascribe to dualism must acknowledge that all environmental influences ultimately modify behavior by leaving imprints on the brain. In fact, the ability to emotionally respond to environmental contingencies is surely one of the most primary and powerful learning tools within the mammalian brain. Next, we discuss some examples of early environmental influences on emotional behavior and some common brain vectors that may mediate them.

Effects of Early Handling and Stress

Among the earliest and most comprehensive lines of comparative research was work that chronicled the effects of early handling and how early hormone treatment increased exploration and reduced responsivity to fearful stimuli, whereas in the long term, early handling conferred stress-resiliency (Meany et al., 1991). Apparently, the early handling mimicked stress, because early injections of the adrenal steroid corticosterone could simulate the latter stress-inoculating effect of early contact. Interestingly, the effects of handling could only be obtained if animals received extra stimulation during a "sensitive period" lasting the first week of life. During the second week, the same manipulations were much less effective, and lack of a response is now known to be due to a normal period of adrenal insensitivity that typically occurs during the second week of life in the normal development of young rats (O'Grady, Hall, & Menzies, 1993). We do not know the adaptive value of this insensitive period, but perhaps it reduces steroid output during a time when such stressors might prove neurotoxic to newly developing cognitive functions. For instance, excessive levels of adrenal steroids are neurotoxic to cells, especially in sensitive brain areas such as the hippocampus (Sapolsky, 1993). We do not know whether human infants undergo a similar period of development; however, extra tactile stimulation has beneficial effects on premature babies.

Effects of Early Peptide Administration

Considering the probability that many specific emotional systems of the brain are organized around specific neuropeptide circuits (Panksepp, 1993a), it is of some interest in the present context to summarize what we know of neonatal peptide treatments on subsequent development. As already mentioned, there is a great deal of data regarding the developmental effects of early exposure to endogenous opioids on rats, and other provocative findings suggest that early exposure to other neuropeptides can also produce lifelong changes in learning abilities, emotional, and sensory responsivities. For instance, early exposure to the endogenous opioid β-endorphin can increase pain-sensitivity and open-field activity in adulthood (Zadina & Kastin, 1986). Treatment of infants with alpha melanocyte–stimulating hormone (α-MSH) yields animals that exhibit a broad spectrum of changes, including improved learning abilities (McBride et al., 1994). Treatment with melanocyte-stimulating-hormone inhibiting factor (MIF-1) and tyrosine-MIF-1 can modify the effects of opioids and accelerate various indices of brain and behavioral development (Galina & Kastin, 1986). Similar effects can be obtained with thyroxine, and it is well known that thyroid deficits lead to developmental disorders (Hulse, 1983). Early exposure to the stress hormone CRF can apparently have broad developmental effects, so that treated rat infants exhibit accelerated eye opening and decreased body weight. In adulthood, they show changes in open-field activity and responsivity to opiates (Zadina & Kastin, 1986). Although the meaning of these developmental effects for emotional maturation is not known, it is clear that the environmental events that induce similar neurochemical changes could easily lead to lifelong modifications of the temperamental style of individuals.

Effects of Repeated Electrical Stimulation

A general principle that seems to be emerging from several avenues of neuroscientific research is that even modest, direct arousal of emotional systems, as with localized electrical stimulation of specific brain areas, can have lifelong consequences for an animal. Perhaps the most compelling data have come from two procedures that have come to be known as *kindling* and *limbic permeability*. Essentially, kindling is the tendency of artificially stimulated brain systems to develop the ability to gradually initiate seizure activity in specific circuits of the brain (Adamec, 1990). One of the brain areas that kindles most readily is the amygdala, yielding a seizure pattern that resembles natural limbic epilepsy (i.e., psychomotor fits). Once these circuits have been kindled, cats and rats tend to exhibit chronic emotional changes, such as persistent fearfulness and increases in aggressiveness (Adamec, 1990). Animals that were previously fairly nonchalant in response to environmental challenges develop emotionally reactive response tendencies that are hard to extinguish. To obtain these effects, one does not even have to induce full-blown seizure activity.

The ability of a few brief stimulations of the amygdala to open an "arousal doorway" to lower emotional circuits has been called *limbic permeability*. This phenomenon can be seen using electrical evoked-potential procedures as well as behavioral measures. For instance, there is a strong input from the basolateral amygdala to the ventromedial area of the hypothalamus, and after a few brief stimulations of those amygdaloid sites, one obtains expanded field potentials in medial hypothalamic recording sites. When this happens, cats also tend to become hyperdefensive, showing more fear behavior toward other cats, experimenters, and even rats. Simply exposing these animals to the sounds of conspecifics fighting is enough to make them timid and hypervigilant. A very similar effect can be obtained with anxiogenic "inverse agonists" of the benzodiazepine receptor, such as FG-7142. This pattern of brain and behavioral changes resembles that seen in posttraumatic stress disorder (PTSD). In other words, neural inputs from higher processes (presumably cognitive representations of possible harm) tend to gain much easier access to the basic diencephalic circuits for fear and anger (Adamec, 1990).

These emotional personality changes can last a lifetime in animals, and an especially important avenue of future inquiry will be to determine how such changes might be reversed. Through a willingness to appreciate the relevance of such animal models, great progress can be made in understanding how various emotional stressors early in life may change the trajectories of emotional development in humans.

CONCLUSION

In summary, certain emotional tendencies are innate in mammals although they change developmentally, as a function of environmental as well as internal brain experiences, across the life span. Such changes can now be characterized and detailed in a variety of animal models. Although we have long appreciated the role of experience in psychological maturation, we can finally begin to incorporate the natural unfolding of neurobiological processes that underlie emotional development into such epigenetic perspectives. A marriage of ethology and neuroscientific methods will allow us to link changes in emotional behaviors to environmental and brain changes over the life span.

As an example of this type of integration, we present a model of the social affect system, which incorporates the multiple levels of analysis that must be addressed in any emotional system (Figure 3). Specifically, the basic social motivation system has complex evolutionary sources and various sensory controls that are responsive to many subtle environmental cues (some unconditionally, but all potentially conditionally). Evolutionarily, these cues signal social connectedness at one end of the spectrum and separation at the other. Our working hypothesis is that this emotional system is to a substantial degree confluent with the distress vocalization circuit that courses between higher areas such as cingulate, septal, and preoptic brain areas and lower representations in the periventricular gray. This brain system controls various subfunctions, including feeling states, which have important behavioral consequences and, ultimately, implications for life-span development. We assume that the biological nature of the "secure base" and "insecure attachment" are embedded within such circuits. Because the social motivation system is attuned to both social connection and separation, associated feelings are probably bidimensional and operate according to opponent-process principles. For instance, humans report both distress at perceived social abandonment and comfort in the presence of familiar others, which may represent a basic form of love. Finally, the social affect system generates coherent behavioral (e.g., DVs, searching followed by depressive stasis) and physiological (e.g., autonomic arousal) responses to separation from caretakers (Hofer, 1984, 1994; Panksepp et al., 1988). Relevant details of this system are more fully discussed elsewhere (Panksepp, 1981, 1991; Nelson & Panksepp, 1996).

Because of the diversity of sensory controls for the social affect system, species can vary widely in response to the various available inputs. This variance can help explain some of the species differences that have been documented in the literature, such as the neurochemical paradoxes that appear to exist between infant rats and most other mammals (Nelson & Panksepp, 1996; Panksepp et al., 1992). Also, different species may vary in terms of the strength with which the social affect system is coupled with more ancient precursor systems. For instance, even though the evolutionary substrates for this emotional system can only be a matter of theoretical speculation at the present time, it may well be that nest-dwelling animals such as rats have stronger linkages between ancient place–attachment mechanisms and the social affect system, whereas more ambulatory and herbivorous mammals such as guinea pigs may show stronger connections between antecedent pain mechanisms and the social affect system. This may help explain why infant rats exhibit less distress upon separation from their caretaker than do guinea pigs.

Although there are few data on place-attachment substrates, our brain

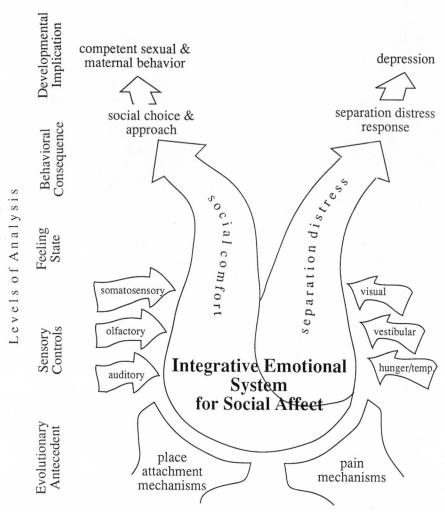

Figure 3. A schematic summary of the organization of the integrative emotional system that is envisioned to mediate social affect. The system mediates a two-pronged affective response, and there are multiple sensory controls that interact with the emotional system. The roots of the system go back evolutionarily to ancient pain and place-attachment mechanisms. Because the system can be analyzed at various levels of analysis, it is important to recognize the diversity of controls that contribute to the overall intergrative response.

mapping of separation calls does suggest that some of the roots of the social attachment system are anatomically related to primitive pain mechanisms deep in the brain stem (Panksepp et al., 1988). The phenomenological similarity between pain and social loss has allowed knowledge concerning the neurochemistry of pain to guide research on the neural basis of separation distress (Panksepp, 1981). Thus, the social affect system meets the criteria for emotional systems listed in the introduction. Specifically, it has (1) evolutionary antecedents, (2) a subcortical neural basis, (3) a concomitant feeling state, and (4) a syndrome of coordinated behavioral outputs. Multilevel characterization of the other emotional systems will doubtless add richness and depth to our understanding of how emotional capacities naturally unfold in various environments over the course of mammalian development.

Furthermore, such knowledge will eventually enable us to address important mental health issues. For example, one could frame the perennial quest for the fountain of youth in neuroscientific terms: What are the brain substrates implicated in a youthful state of emotional vigor? Some intriguing possibilities lie on the horizon. For instance, facilitation of dopaminergic tone within the brain can promote youthfulness: Old animals whose dopaminergic tone has been heightened pharmacologically exhibit revitalized interest in sex and live longer (Ivy, Rick, Murphy, Head, & Reid, 1994; Knoll, 1988). One can also promote physiological indices of youth in aging animals with hormones such as melatonin and dihydroepiandrosterone (Hermida, Halberg, & Halberg, 1986; Regelson, Loria, & Kalimi, 1988). We are currently investigating the possibility that receptor stimulants of endogenous cannabinoid activity (i.e., anandamide; Childers, Sexton, & Roy, 1993) may promote youthful, playful states of mind, and so far we have observed that cannabinoid stimulants can increase playfulness in aging rats. Findings like these may have important implications not only for enhancing the quality of life during normal aging, but also for remediating disorders caused by pervasive delays in neural development (Broman & Grafman, 1994; Schopler & Mesibov, 1987).

Although our coverage of the basic emotional systems of the mammalian brain in this chapter has not focused sufficiently on the many environmental factors that help guide the maturation of the underlying brain systems, the present view adds a new dimension to the widely accepted idea that an epigenetic perspective is essential for an adequate understanding of all developmental processes. Contrary to earlier perspectives, most neuroscientists now recognize that the brain is a spontaneously active organ, even *in utero*. As is being increasingly emphasized (e.g., van Pelt, Corner, Uylings, & da Silva, 1994), this active internal environment must also be considered in modern conceptualizations of epigenesis. An understanding of the spontaneous neurodynamics of the brain is as essential for our understanding of psychological matters as the ever-present external environmental events that entice our senses and hence unfairly capture most of the ongoing research effort to achieve a scientific appreciation of the developing mind.

ACKNOWLEDGMENTS. Preparation of this review and the research summarized herein were supported by the Memorial Foundation for Lost Children, Bowling Green, OH, 43402, as well as NIH Grant HD-30387 and Navy Wright-Patterson Contract #F336019 MU146 & MT702 to J.P. and NIMH postdoctoral fellowship #T32MH18931 to B.K.

REFERENCES

Adamec, R. E. (1990). Kindling, anxiety and limbic epilepsy: Human and animal perspectives. In J. A. Wada (Ed.), *Kindling 4. Advances in behavioral biology* (pp. 329–341). New York: Plenum Press.

Adams, N., & Boice, R. (1989). Development of dominance in domestic rats in laboratory and seminatural environments. *Behavioral Processes, 19,* 127–142.

Ahadi, S. A., & Rothbart, M. K. (1994). Temperament, development, and the Big Five. In C. F. Halverson & G. A. Kohnstamm (Eds.), *The developing structure of temperament and personality from infancy to adulthood* (pp. 189–207). Hillsdale, NJ: Erlbaum.

Albert, D. J., Walsh, M. H., & Jonik, R. H. (1993). Aggression in humans: What is its biological foundation? *Neuroscience and Biobehavioral Reviews, 17,* 405–425.

Archer, T., & Hansen, S. (Eds.). (1991). *Behavioral biology: Neuroendocrine axis.* Hillsdale, NJ: Erlbaum.

Bandler, R. (1988). Brain mechanisms of aggression as revealed by electrical and chemical stimulation: Suggestion of a central role for the midbrain periaqueductal grey region. In A. N. Epstein & A. R. Morrison (Eds.), *Progress in psychobiology and physiological psychology* (Vol. 13, pp. 67–154). New York: Academic Press.

Barber, N. I., Teicher, M. H., & Baldessarini, R. J. (1989). Effects of selective monoaminergic reuptake blockade on activity rhythms in developing rats. *Psychopharmacology, 97,* 343–348.

Baudry, M., Arst, D., Olivier, M., & Lynch, G. (1981). Development of glutamate binding sites and their regulation by calcium in rat hippocampus. *Developmental Brain Research, 1,* 37–48.

Bayer, S. A. (1985). Neurogenesis of the magnocellular basal telecephalic nuclei in the rat. *International Journal of Developmental Neuroscience, 3,* 229–243.

Beatty, W. W. (1983). Scopolamine depresses play fighting: A replication. *Bulletin of the Psychonomic Society, 21,* 315–316.

Becker, C.-M. (1995). Glycine receptors: Molecular heterogeneity and implications for disease. *Neuroscientist, 1,* 130–141.

Becker, C.-M., Schmieden, V., Tarroni, P., Strasser, U., & Betz, H. (1992). Isoform-selective deficit of glycine receptors in the mouse mutant spastic. *Neuron, 8,* 283–289.

Benes, F. M. (1989). Myelinization of cortical-hippocampal relays during late adolescence: Anatomical correlates to the onset of schizophrenia. *Schizophrenia Bulletin, 15,* 585–594.

Benes, F. M. (1991). Toward a neurodevelopmental understanding of schizophrenia and other psychiatric disorders. In D. Cicchetti (Ed.), *Developmental psychopathology* (pp. 161–184). Hillsdale, NJ: Erlbaum.

Benes, F. M. (1994). Development of the corticolimbic system. In G. Dawson & K. W. Fisher (Eds.), *Human behavior and the developing brain* (pp. 176–206). New York: Guilford.

Berger, B., & Verney, C. (1984). Development of the catecholamine innervation in rat neocortex:

Morphological features. In L. Descarries, T. R. Reader, & H. H. Jasper (Eds.), *Monoamine innervation of cerebral cortex* (pp. 95–121). New York: Alan R. Liss.

Berridge, K. C., & Valenstein, E. S. (1991). What psychological process mediates feeding evoked by electrical stimulation of the lateral hypothalamus. *Behavioral Neuroscience, 105,* 3–14.

Björklund, A., Hökfelt, T., & Tohyama, M. (Eds.). (1992). *Handbook of chemical neuroanatomy: Vol. 10. Ontogeny of transmitters and peptides in the CNS.* New York: Elsevier.

Blurton-Jones, N. (Ed.). (1972). *Ethological studies of child behavior.* London: Cambridge University Press.

Bridges, R. S., & Mann, P. E. (1994). Prolactin-brain interactions in the induction of maternal behavior in rats. *Psychoneuroendocrinology, 19,* 611–622.

Broman, S. H., & Grafman, J. (Eds.). (1994). *Atypical cognitive deficits in developmental disorders.* Hillsdale, NJ: Erlbaum.

Brown, R. E. (1986). Paternal behavior in the male Long–Evans rats (*Rattus norvegicus*). *Journal of Comparative Psychology, 43,* 36–42.

Bruinink, A., Lichtensteinger, W., & Schlumpf, M. (1983). Pre- and postnatal ontogeny and characterization of dopaminergic D2, serotonergic S2 and spirodecan on binding sites in rat forebrain. *Journal of Neurochemistry, 40,* 1227–1237.

Brunelli, S. A., Shindledecker, R. D., & Hofer, M. A. (1987). Behavioral responses of juvenile rats (*Rattus norvegicus*) to neonates after infusion of maternal blood plasma. *Journal of Comparative Psychology, 101,* 47–59.

Brunner, H. G., Nelen, M., Breakefield, X. O., Ropers, H. H., & van Oost, B. A. (1993). Abnormal behavior associated with a point mutation in the structural gene for monoamine oxidase A. *Science, 262,* 578–580.

Burger, H., Hailes, J., Nelson, J., & Menelaus, M. (1987). Effect of combined implants of estradiol and testosterone on libido in postmenopausal women. *British Medical Journal, 294,* 936–939.

Candy, J. M., & Enna, S. (1976). Neurochemical aspects of the ontogenesis of GABAergic neurons in the rat brain. *Brain Research, 111,* 119–133.

Carmichael, M. S., Humbert, R., Dixen, J., Palmisano, G., Greenleaf, W., & Davidson, J. M. (1987). Plasma oxytocin increases in the human sexual response. *Journal of Clinical Endocrinology and Metabolism, 64,* 27–31.

Carter, C. S. (1992). Oxytocin and sexual behavior. *Neuroscience and Biobehavioral Reviews, 16,* 131–144.

Cases, O., Seif, I., Grimsby, J., Gaspar, P., Chen, K., Pournin, S., Muller, U., Aguet, M., Babinet, C., Shih, J. C., & de Meyer, E. (1995). Aggressive behavior and altered amounts of brain serotonin and norepinephrine in mice lacking MAOA. *Science, 268,* 1763–1766.

Childers, S. R., Sexton, T., & Roy, M. B. (1993). Effects of anandamide on cannabinoid receptors in rat brain membranes. *Biochemical Pharmacology, 47,* 711–715.

Coccaro, E. F. (1989). Central serotonin and impulsive aggression. *British Journal of Psychiatry, 155,* 52–62.

Compaan, J. C., Wozniak, A., DeRuiter, A. J., Koolhaas, J. M., & Hutchison, J. B. (1994). Aromatase activity in the preoptic area differs between aggressive and nonaggressive male house mice. *Brain Research Bulletin, 35,* 1–7.

Coyle, J. T., & Enna, S. J. (1976). Neurochemical aspects of the ontogenesis of gabanergic neurons in the rat brain. *Brain Research, 111,* 119–133.

Coyle, J. T., & Molliver, M. (1977). Major innervation of newborn rat cortex by monoaminergic neurons. *Science, 196,* 444–447.

Coyle, J. T., & Yamamura, H. I. (1976). Neurochemical aspects of the ontogenesis of cholinergic neurons in the rat brain. *Brain Research, 118,* 429–440.

D'Amato, R. J., Blue, M., Largent, B., Lych, D., Leobetter, D., Molliver, M., & Snyder, S. (1987). Ontogency of the serotonergic projection of rat neocortex: Transient expression of a dense innervation of primary sensory areas. *Proceedings of the National Academy of Sciences USA, 84,* 4322–4326.

Dawson, G., & Fisher, K. W. (Eds.). (1994). *Human behavior and the developing brain.* New York: Guilford.

Deguchi, T., & Barchas, J. (1972). Regional distribution and developmental change in tryptophan hydroxylase in rat brain. *Journal of Neurochemistry, 19,* 927–929.

Deskin, R., Seidler, F. J., Whitmore, W. L., & Slotkin, T. A. (1981). Development of noradrenergic and dopaminergic receptor systems depends on maturation of their presynaptic nerve terminals in the rat brain. *Journal of Neurochemistry, 36,* 1683–1690.

Diebler, M. F., Farkas-Bargeton, E., & Wehrle, R. (1979). Developmental changes of enzymes associated with energy metabolism and synthesis of some neurotransmitters in discrete areas of human neocortex. *Journal of Neurochemistry, 32,* 429–435.

Ekman, P. (1992). An argument for basic emotions. *Cognition and Emotions, 6,* 169–200.

Everitt, B. J., & Bancroft, J. (1991). Of rats and men: The comparative approach to male sexuality. *Annual Review of Sex Research, 2,* 77–117.

Fagen, R. (1992). Play, fun, and communication of well-being. *Play and Culture, 5,* 40–58.

Ferris, C. F., & Delville, Y. (1994). Vasopressin and serotonin interactions in the control of agonistic behavior. *Psychoneuroendocrinology, 19,* 593–601.

Fosse, V. M., Heggelund, P., & Fonnum, F. (1989). Postnatal development of glutamatergic, GABAergic and cholinergic neurotransmitter phenotypes in the visual cortex, lateral geniculate nucleus, pulvinar and superior colliculus in cats. *Journal of Neurochemistry, 9,* 426–435.

Fox, N. A., & Calkins, S. D. (1993). *Multiple measure approaches to the study of infant emotion.* In M. Lewis & J. M. Haviland (Eds.), *Handbook of emotions* (pp. 167–184). New York: Guilford.

Galina, Z. H., & Kastin, A. J. (1986). Existence of antiopiate systems as illustrated by MIF-1/Tyr-MIF-1. *Life Sciences, 39,* 2153–2159.

Gavish, L., Carter, C. S., & Getz, L. L. (1983). Male–female interactions in prairie voles. *Animal Behavior, 31,* 511–517.

Goldman-Rakic, P. S., & Brown, R. M. (1982). Postnatal development of monoamine content and synthesis in the cerebral cortex of rhesus monkey. *Developmental Brain Research, 4,* 339–349.

Golebiewski, H., & Romaniuk, A. (1985). The participation of serotonergic system in the regulation of emotional–defensive behavior evoked by intrahypothalamic carbachol injections in the cat. *Acta Neurobiologiae Experimentalis, 45,* 25–36.

Goodall, J. (1992). *Through a window: My thirty years with the chimpanzees of Gombe.* Boston: Houghton Mifflin.

Herman, B. H., & Panksepp, J. (1981). Ascending endorphinergic inhibition of distress vocalization. *Science, 211,* 1060–1062.

Hermida, R. C., Halberg, F., & Halberg, E. (1986). Chronoendocrine relations to personality validated by circannual and circadian bootstrapping. *New Trends in Experimental and Clinical Psychiatry, 2,* 113–130.

Hofer, M. A. (1984). Relationships as regulators: A psycholobiologic perspective on bereavement. *Psychosomatic Medicine, 46,* 183–197.

Hofer, M. A. (1994). Early relationships as regulators of infant physiology and behavior. *Acta Paediatrica* (Suppl. 379), 9–18.

Hoffman, R. (1981). Is altruism part of human nature? *Journal of Personality and Social Psychology, 40,* 121–137.

Hulse, A. (1983). Congenital hypothyroidism and neurological development. *Journal of Child Psychology and Psychiatry and Allied Disciplines, 24,* 629–635.

Ikemoto, S., & Panksepp, J. (1992). The effects of early social isolation on the motivation for social play in juvenile rats. *Developmental Psychobiology, 25,* 261–274.

Insel, T. R. (1992). Oxytocin: A neuropeptide for affiliation-evidence from behavioral, autoradiographic and comparative studies. *Psychoneuroendocrinology, 17,* 3–35.

Ivy, G. O., Rick, J. T., Murphy, M. P., Head, E., & Reid, C. (1994). Aging. In I. Nagy, H. Denham, & K. Kenichi (Eds.), *Pharmacology of aging processes: Methods of assessment and potential interventions* (pp. 45–59). New York: New York Academy of Sciences.

Johnston, M. V. (1988). Biochemistry of neurotransmitters in cortical development. In A. Peters & E. G. Jones (Eds.), *Cerebral cortex: Vol. 7. Development and maturation of cerebral cortex* (pp. 211–236). New York: Plenum Press.

Johnston, M. V., & Coyle, J. T. (1980). Ontogeny of neurochemical markers for noradrenergic, GABAergic and cholinergic neurons in neocortex lesioned with methylozoxy methanol acetate. *Journal of Neurochemistry, 34,* 1429–1441.

Kalin, N. H., & Takahashi, L. K. (1990). Fear-motivated behavior induced by prior shock experience is mediated by corticotropin-releasing hormone systems. *Brain Research, 509,* 80–81.

Kasamatsu, T., & Pettigrew, J. W. (1976). Depletion of brain catecholamines: Failure of monocular dominance shift after monocular occlusion in kittens. *Science, 194,* 206–209.

Kendrick, K. M., Levy, F., & Kaverne, E. B. (1992). Changes in the sensory processing of olfactory signals induced by birth in sheep. *Science, 256,* 833–836.

Kennedy, H. F., & Elwood, R. W. (1988). Strain differences in the inhibition of infanticide in male mice. *Behavioral and Neural Biology, 50,* 349–353.

Kertesz, A. (1994). *Localization and neuroimaging in neuropsychology.* San Diego: Academic Press.

Knoll, J. (1988). Extension of lifespan of rats by long-term (–)deprenyl treatment. *Mount Sinai Journal of Medicine, 55,* 67–74.

Kolmen, B. K., Feldman, H. M., Handen, B. L., & Janosky, J. E. (1995). Naltrexone in young autistic children: A double-blind, placebo-controlled crossover study. *Journal of American Academy of Child and Adolescent Psychiatry, 34,* 223–231.

Krasnegor, N. A., & Bridges, R. S. (Eds.). (1990). *Mammalian parenting: Biochemical, neurobiological and behavioral determinants.* New York: Oxford University Press.

Kurtz, M. M., & Campbell, B. A. (1994). Paradoxical autonomic responses to aversive stimuli in the developing rat. *Behavioral Neuroscience, 108,* 962–971.

Leboyer, M., Bouvard, M., Launay, J., Tabuteau, F., Waller, D., Dugas, M., Kerdelhue, B., Lensing, D., & Panksepp, J. (1992). Brief report: A double-blind study of naltrexone in infantile autism. *Journal of Autism and Developmental Disorders, 22,* 309–319.

LeVay, S. (1993). *The sexual brain.* Cambridge, MA: MIT Press.

Marks, I. M. (1987). The development of normal fear: A review. *Journal of Child Psychology and Psychiatry and Allied Disciplines, 28,* 667–697.

McBride, R. B., Beckwith, B. E., Swenson, R. R., Sawyer, T. K., Hadley, M. E., Matsurage, T. O., & Hruby, V. J. (1994). The actions of melanin-concentrating hormone (MCH) on passive avoidance in rats: A preliminary study. *Peptides, 15,* 757–759.

McDougall, S. A., Nonneman, A. J., & Crawford, C. A. (1991). Effects of SCH 23390 and sulpiride on the reinforced responding of the young rat. *Behavioral Neuroscience, 105,* 744–754.

Meany, M. J., Mitchell, J. B., Aitken, D. H., Bhatnagar, S., Bodnoff, S. R., Iny, L. J., Sairieau, A. (1991). The effects of neonatal handling on the development of the adrenocortical response to stress. Implications for neuropathology and cognitive deficits in later life. *Psychoneuroendocrinology, 16,* 85–103.

Mennella, J. A., & Moltz, H. (1988). Infanticide in rats: Male strategy and female counterstrategy. *Physiology and Behavior, 42,* 19–28.

Morris, N., Udry, J., Khan-Dawood, F., & Dawood, M. (1987). Marital sex frequency and midcycle female testosterone. *Archives of Sexual Behavior, 16,* 27–37.

Nelson, E., & Panksepp, J. (1995). Central oxytocin antagonism blocks preweanling rat pups' acquisition of preference for maternally associated odor. *Abstracts, Society for Neuroscience, 21,* 756.

Nelson, E., & Panksepp, J. (1997). Brain substrates of infant–mother attachment in mammals. *Neuroscience and Biobehavioral Reviews.* In press.

Nocjar, C., Panksepp, J., & Conner, R. L. (1995). Effect of chronic psychostimulant and opiate treatment on subsequent long-term appetitive behaviors for drug, sexual and food reward: Interaction with environmental variables. *Abstracts, Society for Neuroscience, 21,* 1466.

Normansell, L., & Panksepp, J. (1990). Effects of morphine and naloxone on play-rewarded spatial discrimination in juvenile rats. *Developmental Psychobiology, 23,* 75–83.

Numan, M. (1994). Maternal behavior. In E. Knobil & J. D. Neill (Eds.), *The physiology of reproduction* (Vol. 2, pp. 221–302). New York: Raven Press.

O'Grady, M. P., Hall, N. R., & Menzies, R. A. (1993). Interleukin-1 beta stimulates adrenocorticotropin and corticosterone release in 10-day-old rat pups. *Psychoneuroendocrinology, 18,* 241–247.

Olivier, B., Molewijk, E., Van Oorschot, R., Van der Poel, R., Guus, P., Zethof, T., van der Heyden, J., & Mos, J. (1994). New animal models of anxiety. *European Neuropsychopharmacology, 4,* 93–102.

Olivier, B., Mos, J., & Miczek, K. A. (1991). Ethopharmacological studies of anxiolytics and aggression. *European Neuropsychopharmacology, 1,* 97–100.

Olweus, D., Mattsson, A., Schalling, D., & Low, H. (1988). Circulating testosterone levels and aggression in adolescent males: A causal analysis. *Psychosomatic Medicine, 50,* 261–272.

Panksepp, J. (1981). The ontogeny of play in rats. *Developmental Psychobiology, 14,* 327–332.

Panksepp, J. (1982). Toward a general psychobiological theory of emotions. *Behavioral and Brain Sciences, 5,* 407–467.

Panksepp, J. (1985). Mood changes. In P. J. Vionken, G. W. Bruyn, & H. L. Klawans (Eds.), *Handbook of clinical neurology. Vol. 1. (45): Clinical Neuropsychology* (pp. 271–285). Amsterdam: Elsevier Science Publishers.

Panksepp, J. (1988). Posterior pituitary hormones and separation distress in chicks. *Abstracts, Society for Neuroscience, 14,* 287.

Panksepp, J. (1990). The psychoneurology of fear: Evolutionary perspectives and the role of animal models in understanding human anxiety. In R. Burrow (Ed.), *Handbook of anxiety* (pp. 3–58). Amsterdam: Elsevier/North-Holland Biomedical Press.

Panksepp, J. (1991). Affective neuroscience: A conceptual framework of the neurobiological study of emotions. In K. T. Strongman (Ed.), *International review of studies on emotion* (Vol. 1, pp. 59–99). Chichester, UK: Wiley.

Panksepp, J. (1993a). Neurochemical control of moods and emotions: Amino acids to neuropeptides. In M. Lewis & J. M. Haviland (Eds.), *Handbook of emotions* (pp. 87–107). New York: Guilford.

Panksepp, J. (1993b). Rough and tumble play: A fundamental brain process. In K. MacDonald (Ed.), *Parent–child play: Descriptions and implications* (pp. 147–184). New York: State University of New York Press.

Panksepp, J. (1994). Prolactin reduces separation-distress in young domestic chicks. *Abstracts, Society for Neuroscience, 20,* 811.

Panksepp, J. (1995). Affective neuroscience: A paradigm to study the animate circuits for human emotions. In R. D. Kavanaugh, B. Zimmerberg, & S. Fein (Eds.), *Emotions: An interdisciplinary approach* (pp. 29–60). Hillsdale, NJ: Erlbaum.

Panksepp, J. (1998). *Affective neuroscience: The foundations of human and animal emotions.* New York: Oxford University Press.

Panksepp, J., Herman, B. H., Vilberg, T., Bishop, P., & DeEskinazi, F. G. (1980). Endogenous opioids and social behavior. *Neuroscience and Biobehavioral Reviews, 4,* 473–487.

Panksepp, J., Jalowiec, J., DeEskinazi, F. G., & Bishop, P. (1985). Opiates and play dominance in juvenile rats. *Behavioral Neuroscience, 99,* 441–453.

Panksepp, J., Lensing, P., Leboyer, M., & Bouvard, M. P. (1991). Naltrexone and other potential new pharmacological treatments of autism. *Brain Dysfunction, 4,* 281–300.

Panksepp, J., Nelson, E., & Siviy, S. (1994). Brain opioids and mother–infant social motivation. *Acta Paediatrica, 83* (Suppl. 397), 40–46.

Panksepp, J., Newman, J. D., & Insel, T. R. (1992). In K. T. Strongman (Ed.), *International review of studies on emotion* (Vol. 2, pp. 51–72). Chichester, UK: Wiley.

Panksepp, J., & Normansell, L. (1990). Effects of ACTH (1–24) and ACTH/MSH (4-10) on isolation-induced distress vocalization in domestic chicks. *Peptides, 11,* 915–919.

Panksepp, J., Normansell, L., Cox, J. F., & Siviy, S. M. (1994). Effects of neonatal decortication on the social play of juvenile rats. *Physiology and Behavior, 56,* 429–443.

Panksepp, J., Normansell, L., Herman, B., Bishop, P., & Crepeau, L. (1988). Neural and neurochemical control of the separation distress call. In J. D. Newman (Ed.), *The physiological control
of mammalian vocalization* (pp. 263–299). New York: Plenum Press.

Panksepp, J., Sacks, D. S., Crepeau, L. J., & Abbott, B. B. (1991). The psycho- and neurobiology of
fear systems in the brain. In M. R. Denny (Ed.), *Fear, avoidance, and phobias* (pp. 7–59).
Hillsdale, NJ: Erlbaum.

Panksepp, J., Siviy, S., & Normansell, L. (1984). The psychobiology of play: Theoretical and
methodological perspectives. *Neuroscience and Biobehavioral Reviews, 8,* 465–492.

Panksepp, J., Siviy, S., Normansell, L., White, K., & Bishop, P. (1982). Effects of β-chlornaltexamine
on separation distress in chicks. *Life Sciences, 31,* 2387–2390.

Panksepp, J., Yates, G., Ikemoto, S., & Nelson, E. (1991). Simple ethological models of depression:
Social-isolation induced "despair" in chicks and mice. In B. Olivier, J. Mos, & J. L. Slanger
(Eds.), *Animal models in psychopharmacology* (pp. 161–181). Basel, Switzerland: Birkhauser Verlag.

Pedersen, C. A., Caldwell, J. D., Jirikowski, G., & Insel, T. R. (Eds.). (1992). *Annals of the New York
Academy of Sciences: Vol. 652. Oxytocin in maternal, sexual and social behaviors.* New York: New
York Academy of Sciences.

Pellis, S. M., Pellis, V. C., & Whishaw, I. Q. (1992). The role of the cortex in play fighting in rats.
Brain Behavior and Evolution, 39, 270–284.

Penfield, W. (1992). The mind and the brain. In F. G. Worken, J. P. Swazxey, & G. Adelman (Eds.),
The neurosciences: Paths of discovery (pp. 437–454). Boston: Birkhauser.

Pettijohn, T. F. (1979). Attachment and separation distress in the infant guinea pig. *Developmental
Psychobiology, 12,* 73–81.

Pfaus, J., & Phillips, A. (1991). Role of dopamine anticipatory and consummatory aspects of sexual
behavior in the male rat. *Behavioral Neuroscience, 105,* 727–743.

Posner, M. I., & Raichle, M. E. (1994). *Images of mind.* San Francisco: Scientific American Library
(Freeman).

Pruitt, D. L., Bolanaos, C. A., & McDougall, S. A. (1995). The effects of dopamine D1 and D2
antagonists on cocaine-induced place preference conditioning in preweanling rats. *European
Journal of Pharmacology, 283,* 125–131.

Ravikumar, B. V., & Sastry, P. S. (1985). Muscarinic cholinergic receptors in human foetal brain:
Characterization and ontogeny of [3H]quinuclidinyl benzilate binding sites in frontal cortex.
Journal of Neurochemistry, 44, 240–246.

Regelson, W., Loria, R., & Kalimi, M. (1988). Hormonal intervention: "Buffer hormone" or "state
dependency." *Annals of New York Academy of Sciences, 521,* 260–273.

Reghunandanan, V., Reghunandanan, R., & Marya, R. K. (1991). Vasopressin: Its possible role in
circadian time keeping. *Chronobiologia, 18,* 39–47.

Robinson, T., & Berridge, K. (1993). The neural basis of drug craving: An incentive–sensitization
theory of addiction. *Brain Research Reviews, 18,* 247–291.

Rozenberg, F., Roabain, O., Jardin, L., & Ben-Ari, Y. (1989). Distribution of GABAergic neurons in
late fetal and early postnatal rat hippocampus. *Developmental Brain Research, 50,* 177–187.

Sachser, N., Lick, C., & Stanzel, K. (1994). The environment, hormones, and aggressive behaviour:
A 5-year-study in guinea pigs. *Psychoneuroendocrinology, 19,* 697–707.

Sapolsky, R. M. (1993).The physiology of dominance in stable versus unstable social hierarchies.
In Mason, W. A., & Mendoza, S. P. (Eds.), *Primate social conflict* (pp. 171–204). Albany, NY:
State University of New York Press.

Schecter, M. D., & Calcagntti, D. J. (1993). Trends in place preference conditioning with a cross-
indexed bibliography. *Neuroscience and Biobehavioral Reviews, 17,* 21–41.

Schliebs, R., Kullman, E., & Bigl, V. (1986). Development of glutamate binding sites in the visual
structures of the rat brain: Effect of visual pattern deprivation. *Biomedica Biochimica Acta, 45,*
495–506.

Schopler, E. S., & Mesibov, G. B. (Eds.). (1987). *Neurobiological issues in autism.* New York: Plenum
Press.

84   Jaak Panksepp et al.

Schuurman, T. (1980). Hormonal correlates of agonistic behavior in adult male rats. In P. S. McConnell, G. J. Boer, H. J. Romijin, N. E. van de Poll, & M. A. Corner, (Eds.), *Adaptive capabilities of the nervous system* (pp. 415–420). Amsterdam: Elsevier/North Holland.

Seress, L., & Ribak, C. E. (1988). The development of GABAergic neurons in the rat hippocampal formation: An immunocytochemical study. *Developmental Brain Research, 44*, 197–202.

Sherwin, B. B., & Gelfand, M. (1987). Differential symptom response to parenteral estrogen and/ or androgen administration in the surgical menopause. *American Journal of Obstetrics and Gynecology, 151*, 153–162.

Siegel, A., & Pott, C. B. (1988). Neural substrates of aggression and flight in the cat. *Progress in Neurobiology, 32*, 261–283.

Siviy, S. M., & Panksepp, J. (1987). Juvenile play in the rat: Thalamic and brain stem involvement. *Physiology and Behavior, 41*, 103–114.

Thor, D. H., & Holloway, W. R. (1984). Developmental analyses of social play behavior in juvenile rats. *Bulletin of the Psychonomic Society, 22*, 587–590.

Tsutsui, Y., Shinoda, A., & Kondo, Y. (1994). Facilitation of copulatory behavior by pCPA treatments following stria terminalis transection but not medial amygdala lesion in the male rat. *Physiology and Behavior, 56* 603–608.

Valzelli, L. (1984). Reflections on experimental and human pathology of aggression. *Progress in Neuro-Psychopharmacology and Biological Psychiatry, 8*, 311–325.

van Pelt, J., Corner, M. A., Uylings, H. M. B., & Lopes da Silva, F. H. (Eds.). (1994). *Progress in brain research: Vol. 102. The self-organizing brain: From growth cones to functional networks.* Amsterdam: Elsevier/North Holland.

Winberg, J., & Kjellmer, I. (Eds.). (1994). The neurobiology of infant–parent interaction in the newborn period. *Acta Paediatrica, 83* (Suppl. 397). Oslo: Scandinavian University Press.

Winslow, J. T., Hastings, N., Carter, C. S., Harbaugh, C. R., & Insel, T. R. (1993). A role for central vasopressin in pair bonding in monogamous prairie voles. *Nature, 365*, 544–548.

Winslow, J. T., & Insel, T. R. (1992). Social and environmental determinants of centrally administered oxytocin effects on male squirrel monkey behavior. *Annals of New York Academy of Sciences, 652*, 452–455.

Wise, R. A., & Bozarth, M. A. (1987). A psychomotor stimulant theory of addiction. *Psychological Review, 94*, 469–492.

Zadina, J. E., & Kastin, A. J. (1986). Neonatal peptides affect developing rats: B-endorphin alters nociception and opiate receptors, coricotropin-releasing factor alters corticosterone. *Developmental Brain Research, 29*, 21–29.

Zagon, I. S., Gibo, D. M., & McLaughlin, P. J. (1991). Zeta (z), a growth-related opioid receptor in developing rat cerebellum: Identification and characterization. *Brain Research, 55*, 28–35.

Zagon, I. S., Zagon, E., & McLaughlin, P. J. (1989). Opioids and the developing organism: A comprehensive bibliography. *Neuroscience and Biobehavioral Reviews, 13*, 207–235.

4

Differential Emotions Theory and Emotional Development

Mindful of Modularity

Brian P. Ackerman, Jo Ann A. Abe, and Carroll E. Izard

Differential emotions theory (DET) packs the infant. Infants gain possession of a limited set of discrete emotions in the first months of life, and these emotions are organized as a modular system with a high degree of independent functioning. The number of emotions, their expressive signatures, and their links to one another undergo remarkable change over time, to be sure, as do system organization and articulation. The core processes in emotional development, however, consist of the construction and consolidation of affective–cognitive structures, which mediate intersystem coordination of the emotions, cognitive, and motor systems.

We unpack the infant in this chapter by discussing our constructs of discrete emotions and a modular emotions system. It pays to be mindful of modularity for the infant, because a modular and preadapted emotions system equips the infant to engage the world in a meaningful manner. We then repack the developing child by discussing affective–cognitive structures that mediate intersystem control and coordination. Development consists of

Brian P. Ackerman, Jo Ann A. Abe, and Carroll E. Izard • Department of Psychology, University of Delaware, Newark, Delaware 19716.

What Develops in Emotional Development? edited by Michael F. Mascolo and Sharon Griffin. Plenum Press, New York, 1998.

the breakdown of relatively insular modules in favor of an integrated system of connected and coordinated modules.

DISCRETE EMOTIONS

An emotion is composed of (1) neurochemical processes, (2) expressive behavior, and (3) a subjective experience or feeling state. The neurochemical component variously involves processes in the somatic nervous system that activate and regulate emotion. There are processes in the autonomic nervous system that sustain emotion over time as well as processes in the reticular activating system that amplify and attenuate emotions (Izard, 1977; Izard & Harris, 1995). The central neural substrate, particularly the amygdala (Aggleton & Mishkin, 1986; LeDoux, 1987), evaluates the significance of internal and external stimuli and activates emotion processes leading to the experiential and expressive components. These components have their own neural substrates that are similar to and different from the activating component (LeDoux, 1987).

Expressive behavior involves discrete motor patterns of facial movements and vocalic expressions and more molar postural and gestural movements. Expressive behavior has a cue-value for others in social exchanges, and sensory feedback from expression contributes to the activation and regulation of the internal experience of an emotion.

The subjective experience or feeling state of an emotion derives from the neural and motoric processes of the other two components and has organizational and motivational functions. This subjective experience may or may not be accessible to verbal processes mediating labeling and self-report.

Whereas an *emotional experience* may involve cognition, DET defines *emotion feeling* more narrowly as a quality of consciousness that includes action-tendencies and readiness. The quality thus has nonrandom intentionality directed toward environmental objects and events. When connected to cognitive constructions, a specific emotion feeling recruits particular types of cognitive and motoric correlates. For example, fear recruits cognitive appraisals and attributions that are mediated by representations of previous fear experiences in memory, and the current emotion feeling motivates a specific and limited set of action-tendencies, among them flight and withdrawal. This connection of emotion feeling and cognitive processes constitutes an "affective–cognitive" schema that forms a fundamental building block of mental life and self. Indeed, the self-appraisals that constitute the self-concept clearly have an affective component (cf. Damon & Hart, 1989) and are prime examples of significant affective–cognitive structures.

On the other hand, disconnections of related affective and cognitive processes contribute to maladaptive behaviors and to motivation that may not be available to consciousness. It is important to stress these points, because DET assumes that feeling states are evolutionary distillates and thereby *inherently adaptive*. Maladaptive behavior may thus reflect dysfunctional affective–cognitive connections or disconnections. Inflated and unrealistic self-appraisals that render the individual vulnerable to negative feedback triggering interpersonal aggression exemplify such dysfunctional connections (cf. Baumeister, Smart, & Boden, 1996).

What is unique about DET is that it makes four specific claims about discrete emotions that have developmental implications. These claims represent the core aspects of DET. Our discussion of the core aspects of DET includes recent extensions and refinements in the theory, most notably, a distinction between discrete emotions that represent independent and dependent emotion systems.

Core Aspects of DET

Independent Emotion Systems

The first claim is that a small set of emotions are independent. The independent emotions include joy, interest, sadness, anger, fear, surprise, and disgust. These emotions are "independent" because they do not depend on cognitive development or appraisal processes for their activation. They can achieve consciousness rapidly and automatically, and influence subsequent perception and cognition. The emotion of interest, for example, focuses and sustains attention (Langsdorf, Izard, Rayias, & Hembree, 1983).

The independent emotions also are identifiable by unique facial expressions that are universal across the human species and that appear early in infancy on a predictable timetable. Expressions of interest, joy, sadness, and anger emerge in the first weeks to 2–4 months, for example (Izard, Hembree, & Huebner, 1987; Izard & Malatesta, 1987; Langsdorf et al., 1983), and fear appears between 7 and 9 months. Emergence of these emotion expressions is primarily a function of the maturation of neural circuits and is independent of cognition. Emotions such as guilt and shame, which emerge later in childhood and are dependent on cognitive processes, do not meet these criteria and, therefore, are not independent. We discuss these emotions in greater detail in the section on dependent emotion systems.

The evidence for the presence of an emotion rests on expressive behavior, because the infant's felt experience or feeling state is inaccessible to observers, and the neurophysiological evidence is not yet sufficiently emotion-specific. The inaccessibility of the feeling state has led Campos (Barrett & Campos, 1987; Campos, 1994; Campos, Mumme, Kermoian, & Campos, 1994) and others (cf. Lewis & Michalson, 1983) to argue for "functionalist" theories that do not treat inner emotion states. From the perspective of DET, a problem with this "black box" functionalism is that the same behavior can be motivated by different emotions (e.g., avoidance can be motivated by either fear or disgust). DET also holds that it is reasonable to infer feelings associated with expressions because facial, vocalic, and gestural behaviors are correlated and form coherent affective configurations in young infants (Weinberg & Tronick, 1994). These configurations also are associated with environmental events that have specific affective values for independent observers (cf. Blumberg & Izard, 1991; Weinberg & Tronick, 1994). For example, maternal joy and sadness evoke corresponding infant facial expressions (Termine & Izard, 1988), as does a painful event like an injection in a medical clinic (Izard et al., 1987). Most important, mothers pack their infants with emotion feeling states, just like DET, in that infant facial expressions cue corresponding maternal behaviors.

Discreteness

A second claim is that these independent emotions are *discrete* and *distinguishable*. One criterion for discreteness is that each emotion is associated with a specific neuromuscular pattern of facial movements. Izard (1979) has generated a reliable system for coding these facial movements. A second criterion is that each has a unique adaptive function. For example, interest motivates orienting and exploration, fear motivates avoidance, and anger motivates removal of a goal obstruction.

Developmental researchers have posed two major challenges to the core concept of discreteness. The objections concern the development of emotion expressions per se and are that (1) developmental orthogenesis (cf. Werner, 1948) requires development from a relatively global and undifferentiated state to a more differentiated state (Camras, 1992; Oster, Hegley, & Nagel, 1992), and (2) negative emotion displays are frequently characterized by blends rather than by discrete emotions (cf. Matias & Cohn, 1993).

Izard et al. (1995) directly tested these objections with data from a large longitudinal database that tracked infant emotion expressions from 2.5 months to 9 months. The tasks involved maternal displays of specific emotions in dyadic play interactions with infants. The play situations featured both positive and mild negative stimulation (including still-face maternal expressions in Study 2). Infant facial expression was coded reliably with the microanalytic MAX (Izard, 1979) and Affex (Izard, Dougherty, & Hembree, 1983) systems, which are anatomically based.

The results showed that interest, joy, anger, and sadness accounted for 99% of all emotion expressions and that the frequency was similar across age. For example, in Study 1, the frequency of full-face expressions for *interest* was 49.9% at 2.5 months and 47.2% at 9 months, and the frequency for *joy* was 16.1% and 20.0%, respectively. The mean percentages of anger and sadness across age were 4.7 and 1.9, respectively. In addition, the forms of the expressions were categorized as full-face, partial (or component), and blends. For each emotion except sadness, the frequency of full-face expressions exceeded the frequency of blends. For example, the mean frequency of full-faced expressions of *joy* across age was 18.3%, whereas the mean frequency of joy blends was 0.4%. Similar results occurred in Study 2. These results suggest that discreteness is the game for some basic emotion expressions, at least, and offer little support for the orthogenetic hypothesis and the successive differentiation of discrete expressions across age.

Stability

A third claim of DET is that independent emotions are stable across early development. Certainly the evidence from Izard et al. (1995) shows stability of facial expressions of interest, joy, anger, and sadness from 2.5 months to 9.0 months. Thus, the basic forms of emotion-specific expression components and configurations appeared early in infancy and were constant across early development. The functional importance of stability is that it may facilitate maternal interpretation of infant feelings and needs.

The theoretical motivation for the claim for expression stability is the implication that little postnatal development occurs in the neurological and muscular components of interest, joy, anger, and sadness. Instead, the structural hardware of the expression must be preadapted and present at birth. The neural substrate of other components, of course, may develop over time, and neural maturation probably contributes to the relatively late onset of other emotions. Fear, for example, requires some postnatal maturation of the hippocampus and sympathetic nervous system (cf. Jacobs & Nadel, 1985).

Similarly, a core tenet of DET is that the emotion feeling states associated with discrete expressions also are stable and unchanging over time. Once an infant reliably displays an emotion, the motivational feeling state of the specific emotion is invariant; fear is fear is fear. Thus, a fear expression is always linked with the same motivational state, which energizes the same type of behavior: escape or harm avoidance across development.

Activation Thresholds

Emotion thresholds differ among individuals, as does the intensity of a feeling state when an emotion is activated. Thresholds and intensity contribute to trait emotionality, and these differences contribute to more molar aspects of temperament. Indeed, most temperament theories include emotionality as a core component in addition to activity level and sociability, and the roots of differences in later emotionality may be found in neonates. Stifter and Fox (1990), for instance, found relations between neonatal physiological stress responses and later aspects of emotionality.

Furthermore, Kagan and his associates (Kagan, Reznick, Clarke, Snidman, & Garcia-Coll, 1984; Kagan, Reznick, & Snidman, 1987) have shown that extreme behavioral inhibition in about 10% of toddlers is stable across the early elementary school years. From the perspective of DET, the fear system in this group of toddlers is the major determinant of their inhibition. Thus, what may differentiate inhibited from uninhibited toddlers is different activation thresholds for fear. In this regard, DET is both a normative theory of emotional development and a theory of individual differences and dysfunctional operations of emotions.

What Develops

To this point, we have described discrete phenomena that are relatively age-invariant. These phenomena appear in the first year of life or so but change little thereafter. We review some of these first-year developments next and then describe aspects of emotions that change with increasing voluntary control of expressive behavior and feeling.

Early Development

Independent emotions emerge in a preadapted and predictable timetable. According to DET, emergence is mediated by neural and neuromuscular maturation, as well as by environmental demands. This argument for innateness does not preclude modifiability. Infant experience is a necessary stimulus to genetic unfolding and the development of the brain and nervous system (Schore, 1994), and experience can alter the timetable somewhat. Furthermore, DET predicts that the expressive component of discrete emotions changes through neural maturation and socialization experiences. For example, some early displays of facial expressions are full-face and seemingly stereotypical and instinctive. Over time, these expressions are more likely to become restricted or controlled (i.e., partial or component), and more complex patterns (blends) or emotions emerge (cf. Smith & Scott, 1996).

To date, little systematic research has examined developmental changes in the expressive aspect of discrete emotions. Preliminary findings from an ongoing longitudinal study support the view that infants' facial expressions become more restricted and controlled over time (Abe, Takahashi, Putnam, & Izard, 1995). In this study infants' full-face and component (partial) displays of interest, joy, anger, and sadness were coded during Episode 4 (first separation) to Episode 8 (last reunion) of the Strange Situation. Between 13 and 18 months of age, infants exhibited a significant increase in their component displays of joy, interest, and sadness, and a decrease in their full-face displays of joy, interest, and anger.

A third aspect of emotion expression that undergoes change concerns the concordance of emotion expression with the feeling state or subjective experience of the emotion. Although the fundamental core feeling state of fear is invariant, with development, children learn to control emotion signals for communicative purposes and thus to mask feeling states. The socialization of emotion expression is one mediator of this increasing flexibility.

Dependent Emotion Systems

DET describes a set of dependent emotions that typically emerge in the late-toddler period and early childhood, perhaps as a function of both the maturation of inhibitory mechanisms and of cognitive growth. These emotions include shame, guilt, and contempt. Unlike the independent emotions, these emotion systems are dependent because they involve some interplay between affective and cognitive processes and thus cannot operate without the following: (1) a sense of self, (2) the ability to discriminate self and other, (3) the ability to sense self and other as causal agents, and (4) a cognitive evaluative or appraisal process that enables at least rudimentary forms of comparison and judgment. Furthermore, these dependent emotion systems do not have consistent and discrete signatures in expressive behavior over the life span.

The dependent emotions thus represent a fundamentally different ontogenetic process and dynamic than the independent emotion systems. We mention these dependent emotions here to demonstrate that the set of emotions we consider independent does not exhaust the set that have some ontological status across cultures, and that there are developmental and social processes at work in the articulation and elaboration of subjective emotional experiences.

The emergence of these dependent emotions reveals the role of experience, learning, and socialization in emotional development. Socialization processes also are responsible for the conventionalization of display rules or the flexible use of the variable relation between subjective experience and expressive relations to meet social expectations. DET has little unique to say about these socialization processes, except that they involve emotion–cognition relations and affective–cognitive structures, and do not represent properties of the emotions system alone. We address affective–cognitive structures after we discuss the modularity of the emotions system.

Individual Differences

Even though emotionality emerges as a relatively stable phenomenon in infancy that is capable of objective measurement on the basis of expressive behavior (cf. Seifer, Sameroff, Barrett, & Krafchuk, 1994), emotionality shows discontinuity as well as continuity. Gunnar, Porter, Wolf, Rigatuso, and Larson (1995) found, for example, that greater neonatal stress reactivity to a heelstick blood draw, which could be a function of the anger system, is associated with less distress rather than more distress later in the first year (cf. Izard et al., 1987; Izard, Hembree, Dougherty, & Spizzirri, 1989).

The functional importance of these individual differences in proneness to express discrete emotions is that they render the infant differentially sensitive to particular environmental contingencies (cf. Gandour, 1989), and they often transact with specific emotional attributes of caregivers (cf. Mangelsdorf, Gunnar, Kestenbaum, Lang, & Andreas, 1990) and become transformed into affective–cognitive schemas, like the relationship representations associated with secure and insecure attachment. With exceptions such as extreme inhibition (Reznick et al., 1986), the lasting simple effects of early individual differences in emotionality probably are few. Instead, development is a function of *interactions* with aspects of the infant's emotional environment that transform both the infant and the environment.

Abundant evidence is emerging for this transactional view of emotional differences in the effects of postpartum maternal disposition variables and infant emotionality. Infant negative emotionality contributes to postpartum symptoms and also may mirror that symptomatology in affect-matching processes (cf. Tronick, Ricks, & Cohn, 1982). However, the effects are buffered in middle-class families by the presence of multiple caregivers and the mother's ability to mask depressive affect (Campbell, Cohn, Flanagan, Popper, & Meyers, 1992). In highly stressed families, in contrast, individual differences in emotionality may be sustained by aspects of the continuing mother–infant relationship and even amplified over time (Alpern & Lyons-Ruth, 1993).

SYSTEM MODULARITY

In addition to the discrete emotions construct, another core developmental construct of DET is the idea that the independent emotions are subsystems of a quasi-independent and modular emotions system; that is, the independent emotions interact to form a larger modular system. This section develops this construct.

We are theoretically mindful of system modularity for four reasons. First, the systems idea implies that behavioral and developmental regularities are governed by mechanisms serving inherent emotions functions. Thus, orthogenesis in other developmental systems need not apply to emotions. For instance, assumed qualitative shifts in cognitive systems may have no analogue in the emotions system. Indeed, the contrast between stage-related aspects of cognitive development and the relative developmental invariance of the emotions system provides evidence for the relative independence and modularity of the emotions. Conversely, the emotions system also has discrete and special attributes not characteristic of other systems.

Although modular, the emotions system is highly interactive, and its interaction with cognition in the forming of affective–cognitive structures increases with maturation of the brain, particularly the frontal lobe and hippocampus (Schore, 1994). Emotion–cognition interactions do not *transform* emotion feeling states. They *connect* invariant feelings with changing images and thoughts. Thus, the emotion feeling is the stable component of an affective–cognitive structure or schema.

Second, treating emotions as a system *qua* system focuses attention on emergent properties and patterns that are not predicted by or reducible to the discrete elements alone. Order and complexity emerge out of elements and subsystems, and form the basis of complex behavior. Third, the modularity of the emotions system and its quasi independence of other systems highlights the phylogenetic and ontogenetic primacy of emotions in framing person–environment transactions from infancy and serves to emphasize the causal role of emotions in all behavior. Fourth, the modularity focuses attention on intersystem connections and communication as the proximal zones of development.

Conceptualizing emotions as a modular system thus focuses theoretical attention on the causal and adaptive functions of emotions (cf, Izard & Ackerman, 1995) and locates most developmental processes not in the system per se but in connections with other systems. The heuristic value of this treatment is as an antidote to popular and emerging views of emotions as derivative of other functions. Cognitive models, for instance, center on the "central dogma" that emphasizes cognitive appraisal processes in driving emotions (cf. Lazarus, 1991). From an emotions system perspective, however, emotions are causal in their own right, and system organization and complexity emerge out of stable patterns and interactions of discrete emotions. These patterns are flexibly assembled in response to contextual and environmental demands and action-tendencies, and are not instructed by cognition. Purely "functional" models of emotional development, as espoused by Campos et al. (1994), also emphasize the social, interpersonal, and goal-oriented functions of emotion, but, unlike DET, avoid treatments of the endogenous architecture and mechanisms that mediate function.

From the perspective of DET, the emotions and cognitive systems are highly interactive and show reciprocal causality, but also show a degree of independent functioning, which is greatest in early childhood. The independence stems from the modularity of the emotions system (cf. Fodor, 1983), which means simply that infants and young children are biologically predisposed to detect and respond to input to the emotions system in highly specific and determined ways. Modules centrally concern input processes and the transduction of sensory and perceptual information (cf. Fodor, 1983).

Thus, some of the operating principles of the emotions module are biologically derived, are different from the principles of other modules, and cannot be attributed to some overarching general learning mechanism governing all developing systems. The key properties of modules are (1) encapsulation, (2) hardwiring, (3) fast processing, and (4) vertical organization. These properties are associated with specific adaptive functions in motivating behavior and in mediating organism–environment relations (i.e., caretaker–infant relations), some of which we have already described.

Encapsulation

Encapsulation is the variable and restricted access of one module to another. *Variable access* means that the emotions system is activated by multiple processes that change in influence both moment to moment and over development. As Izard (1993) discusses at length, emotion activation processes include biogenetic, sensorimotor, and cognitive processes as well as intrasystem affective processes. Therefore, emotion activation is mediated by cellular information in enzymes and genes (biogenetic processes, such as hormonal changes), organismic information reflecting physiological drive states and ongoing emotion states (affective processes, such as pain, sex drive), sensory feedback from somatic activity (sensorimotor processes, such as facial feedback), and cognitive representations. On the other side of the equation, the emotions system contributes both constant and variable output to the cognitive system and conscious awareness. The constant output often involves the emotion of interest, which motivates orienting and exploration, and sometimes consists of other emotions such as enjoyment and sadness, which motivate receptivity and approach or slowing of functions and withdrawal, respectively. The variable output reflects both feedback from cognitive appraisal and attribution processes, and the influence of emotions on cognitive representations in implicit memory.

The restricted access centrally involves the lack of association and synchronization of cognitive and emotional processes. Although cognitive and conscious monitoring of emotion feeling and expression develop over time in normal children, there is abundant evidence from children with Down syndrome (Cicchetti, 1990, 1991) and from autistic children (Sacks, 1995) of rather extended autonomous development in modular systems. Indeed, restricted intersystem access may be a major source of developmental problems in these children. In older children and adults, one manifestation of the problem of restricted access may be dissociation, with its attendant clinical and behavioral anomalies (Van der Kolk, 1994; Van der Kolk & Van der Hart, 1994).

Encapsulation, thus, is inconsistent with the "central dogma" of both cognitive theories and certain functionalist theories that cognition and cognitive goals are the primary causes of emotions in children. Encapsulation implies that the information input to the emotions system need not be cognitive or representational, that the input may come from multiple sources, and that the system does not require cognitive interpretation to function. To understand emotion, then, the modular aspects of the system per se must be conceptualized.

Hardwiring

Hardwiring requires that a specific function is associated with dedicated, localized, and innate neural structures. As we described for the independent emotion systems, the result is that specific functions appear early in development and may involve maturational processes but *not* extended experience or learning. Indeed, constraint on inductive processes is a key component of modular systems.

Much of the neural architecture dedicated to specific emotions remains to be determined. However, some researchers (Davis, 1992; LeDoux, 1992) have described dedicated neural circuits that mediate conditioned fear and that can function independently of the neocortex and cortically mediated cognitive processes. One function of the amygdala is to transform sensory stimuli into emotion-eliciting information. The amygdala, then, is the sensory gateway to the emotions and forms a pathway to emotion activation that can function independently of neocortical processes and cognitive pathways (LeDoux, 1987). Other evidence for dedicated emotional hardware and quasi-independent activation comes from developmental studies of normal and autistic children (cf. Cicchetti, 1990; Sacks, 1995).

Whatever the specific neural mechanisms, the evidence for innate or early-developing discrete emotions that are constant across culture and experience (cf. Ekman, 1972; Izard, 1971) implies that the wiring is "hard" and innately specified (cf. Izard, 1977; Izard & Harris, 1995; Izard & Malatesta, 1987). Similarly, a subset of basic emotions seems privileged phylogenetically (cf. Izard, 1971) and may represent evolutionary homologues. The implication is that the innate motivational functions of the emotions have survival value, and that the neural circuitry mediating function has been under pressure of natural selection and other evolutionary processes and is preadapted in humans.

Fast Processing

Hardwiring helps mediate fast processing. Fast processing results because the dedicated neural structures need to consider only a fraction of the available stimulus information to activate a specific type of action-tendency or behavioral response. The fraction concerns sensory information, and the operation that transforms the information is precognitive and at times even preattentive. Thus, the transformation of sensory information into emotion information occurs early in perceptual processing and prior to object recognition and identification processes.

One clear function of fast processing is the enabling of fast responding to sensory patterns that may eventually constitute a survival threat. Precognitive rapid processing of sensory information is characteristic of processes stimulating both stalking and flight and withdrawal in predator–prey interactions. Similarly, a function of the precognitive aspect of hardwired fast processing may be the enabling of interpersonal communication processes in infancy.

Unfortunately, it is difficult to demonstrate fast processing in infants because of their long response latencies. Fast processing has an analogue, however, in dedicated and innately specified processing, and this claim for innately specified processing in infants is supportable. Fernald (1993), for example, found that infants respond differentially to affective qualities of maternal vocalizations (i.e., pitch contours associated with approval, comfort, and prohibition). Similarly, other researchers have found that 10-week-old infants (Haviland & Lelwica, 1987) and 2.5-month-old infants (Izard et al., 1995) respond deferentially to maternal facial expressions of happiness, sadness, and anger in combination with tone of voice. These responses seem precognitive to the extent that they are prerepresentational. Recent research by Balaban (1995) supports this precognitive interpretation by showing that the size of the blink component of the startle responses of 5-month-olds was augmented during the viewing of pictures of angry maternal expressions and was reduced for happy expressions. This affective modulation of startle does not require or involve voluntary motor control or cognitive processes. Instead, potentiated startle seems purely a sensory phenomenon.

Organization

Organization requires discrete elements that function both separately and in combination, and structure that is stable over time. Our construct of independent emotions fits these criteria.

Vertical organization requires developmental articulation across time, the construction of structural properties and patterns that are reducible to elements, and also the emergence of integrative functions that are not reducible to elements without loss of emergent functions. Certainly, late-appearing, dependent emotions and the links of emotions to cognition reflect developmental articulation.

Similarly, Izard (1972, 1992) has shown that each emotion tends to form stable links to other emotions, and that emotions frequently occur in clusters or patterns. In stable patterns, multiple emotions occur simultaneously or cyclically, and the rate of oscillation may vary individually and across time and situation. Organization, pattern, and order thus emerge from local and episodic interactions of elements that are repeated over time. Organization is both self-assembled and rapidly assembled early in development, but the assembly is prepared by evolutionary adaptations that favor certain patterns and interactions (i.e., fear and anger) and the linkage of these patterns to action-tendencies.

Finally, we can make the case that some of these patterns have emergent properties in the sense that they produce complex affective states. A good example may be depression, which reflects emotion patterns composed of sadness, anger, and shame elements (Blumberg & Izard, 1985, 1986; Izard, 1977), and in which the elements lose some discreteness. Anxiety may be another example (cf. Izard & Youngstrom, 1996).

SYSTEM CONNECTIONS

The modularity and the quasi-independent functioning of the emotions system in early development suggest that emotional development in the main consists of increases in intersystem communication and the construction of control mechanisms for monitoring and regulating emotions and for monitoring and regulating cognition. These mechanisms constitute emotion understanding and emotion regulation and reflect the interaction of affective and cognitive processes and thus represent affective–cognitive structures. These structures show remarkable growth, articulation, and consolidation in middle childhood. In this section, we describe aspects of these domains.

Emotion Understanding

Emotion understanding involves the recognition and labeling of discrete emotions, comprehension of the causes and consequences of emotions, comprehension of the social uses of expressive behavior, and knowledge of the full repertoire of coping skills. Central aspects of recognition processes are preadapted for most independent emotions, although recognition certainly becomes more precise and extended with experience. Labeling processes require accurate perceptual recognition of emotion cues as well as a cognitive component attaching verbal concepts (i.e., "fear") to feeling states and expressive displays. In this sense, a label represents an affective–cognitive structure that bridges a conceptual lexicon and a modular system. The evidence is strong that most children by age 4 and 5 have good control of emotion labels appropriate for facial expressions such as joy, sadness, anger, and fear. Less is known about labeling for postural and gestural cues, in part because these cues may have less distinctive expressive signatures, and in part because of lack of relevant research (but see Duclos et al., 1989; Riskind, 1984).

Research on normative development in emotion understanding reveals that children's cognitive attribution and appraisal processes about the causes and consequences of emotions develop rapidly through the late-preschool years and into kindergarten and first grade. Harris (Harris, Johnson, Hutton, Andrews, & Cooke, 1989; Izard & Harris, 1995) has described these skills acquisitions in detail. Development of these forms of emotion understanding certainly reflects emotional experiences inside and outside the family and, to some extent, are tutored by parents (cf. Brown & Dunn, 1992; Dunn, Brown, & Beardsall, 1991; Garner, Jones, & Miner, 1994; Harris, 1994). They also may reflect independent developments in children's theory of mind (Harris, 1994; Wellman, 1990) concerning personal-appraisal processes and the relation between internal representations of emotional experience and objective affective reality (cf. Cermele, Ackerman, Morris, & Izard, 1995; Harris et al., 1989). Problems in understanding the variability in this relation probably contribute to the somewhat later development of understanding of mixed emotions (cf. Peng, Johnson, Pollock, Glasspool, & Harris, 1992) and the intentional use of misleading and "false" expressions.

Some evidence that these normative developments in emotion understanding contribute to intersystem communication and management comes from research on Down children (cf. Cicchetti, 1990). The consequences of quasi-autonomous development of the emotions and cognitive systems in these children suggest that one intrapsychic function of emotion understanding might be to monitor and help regulate emotion feeling states and expressive behavior. Other- or self-labeling of a feeling, for instance, might help bring the feeling more into a child's conscious awareness and clarify exactly what the child is feeling, and might help provide clues about coping and situationally appropriate behavior.

Further evidence that emotion understanding contributes to intersystem communication and construction of control structures comes from research on individual differences in emotion understanding. Research by Dodge and his associates (Strassberg, Dodge, Pettit, & Bates, 1994; Weiss, Dodge, Bates, & Pettit, 1992) and by Campbell and others (Campbell, Pierce, March, & Ewing, 1991; Campbell, Pierce, March, Ewing, & Szumowski, 1994), for example, shows relations between social information processing, emotion regulation, and aggressive behaviors in elementary school children. Similarly, Denham, McKinley, Couchoud, and Holt (1990) and Garner et al. (1994) found that differences in emotion understanding are related to differences in social competence. Finally, research by Eisenberg and her associates (cf. Eisenberg et al., 1993; Fabes, Eisenberg, Karbon, Troyer, & Switzer, 1994) found that knowledge of a full repertoire of coping processes may contribute to emotion regulation.

From the standpoint of DET, the bulk of the existing research on emotion understanding has two major limitations. First, it is dominated by descriptions of products rather than constructive and associative processes. For example, it is relatively easy to determine when a child has a conventional *fear* script and can correctly link fear to specific stimulus situations. We know less about how this script is constructed or about the development of emotion regulation processes in responses to specific fears. Second, the typical self-report measures of emotion knowledge overemphasize the semantic or declarative component of emotion understanding. Descriptive accounts of autistic adults show that a declarative understanding of emotions processes does not necessarily contribute to emotion activation (e.g., Sacks, 1995). As such, the extant research on emotion understanding, unfortunately, provides a limited understanding of the ontogenesis of affective–cognitive links and the breakdown of modularity. A central task confronting researchers is to figure out how emotion understanding is related to a child's *own* emotion feeling and control of his or her expressive behavior.

Much more immediate in a young child's life, and seemingly more important, may be discrete representations of emotional experiences in memory that reflect an amalgam of emotion cues and cognitive interpretations. If the experiences are repeated, they may form generalized affective–cognitive packages that meld and blur the details of individual experiences. Once packaged, these structures may form the building blocks of memory and personality and eventually an abstraction that constitutes emotion understanding. The consolidation of these packages remains to be described. The kinds of processes that Nelson (1986) describes for the construction of generalized event representations (GERs) in concept development may be useful for understanding construction of the GERs for emotion packages and scripts.

Emotion Regulation

Emotion regulation describes processes involved in initiating, motivating, and organizing adaptive behavior and in preventing stressful levels of negative emotions and maladaptive behavior. A modular emotions system regulates itself to some extent, but the developmental correlation between increasing cognitive control functions and increasing emotion modulation suggests that much of the work of emotion regulation is performed by affective–cognitive structures. Although detailed work on emotion regulation in middle childhood is just beginning, the modularity metaphor of DET is useful in framing what develops in emotion regulation. We focus on control mechanisms and functions.

Control Mechanisms

Regulation requires some mechanism that serves to control emotional intensity and coordinate emotion and action. Whatever the nature of control, it must constrain inputs to the emotions system and outputs of the system, and it must translate emotional output into nonrandom and goal-directed or emotion-related action. The inputs concern the separable causes of emotions in neural, sensorimotor, affective, and cognitive processes. The output regulator is likely to reflect and affect feedback cycles of reciprocal cause and effect between the emotions and cognitive systems. The motivated action must reflect goals derived from the motivational force of specific emotions and instrumental (i.e., cognitive) intent.

Research on control mechanisms that involve affective and cognitive components is scarce. A central problem is constructing independent measures of emotionality (i.e., regulation) and cognitive processes. Cognitive measures are abundant and usually focus on attentional and gating processes. One emerging solution for measuring emotionality is to use heart-rate measures to index children's arousal in the context of emotion-eliciting stimuli. For example, Derryberry and Rothbart (1983) found a relation between children's reallocation of attention and regulation of arousal. An interpretation of this relation is that cognitive distraction may serve to regulate stimulus input to the emotions system.

On the output side, Fabes, Eisenberg, Karbon, Troyer et al. (1994) related kindergarten and second-grade children's heart-rate variance associated with the sound of a crying infant to maternal reports of children's coping responses and to prosocial comforting behaviors. The hypothesis was that empathy as a prosocial behavior reflects both sympathy and moderate personal distress (i.e., moderate arousal or emotional intensity). Thus, children who show sympathy and can modulate distress are able to exhibit empathy. This study extends several others (Eisenberg et al., 1993; Fabes, Eisenberg, Karbon, Bernzweig et al., 1994) on children's emotion-focused coping responses that target the output–control function of affective–cognitive structures. From the viewpoint of DET, the central aspect that is missing from this research on mechanisms of emotion regulation is a consideration of discrete and specific emotions.

Perhaps the best examples of affective–cognitive structures that regulate emotions are the constructs of working models of attachment relations and children's self-theories of personality and cognitive competence (Dweck, 1991; Smiley & Dweck, 1994). Working models of attachment reflect generalizations across multiple caregiver–infant affective exchanges and infant emotional experiences, and they clearly represent an interconnection of modular emotions and cognitive systems. According to attachment theorists, the models regulate input to the emotions system both qualitatively (i.e., separation anticipation or experiences stimulate arousal and specific emotions) and quantitatively (i.e., intensity), and coordinate emotion systems output (i.e., separation anxiety) and action in the form of exploratory play and approach–avoidance behaviors. For DET, the working model construct has heuristic value as a way of conceptualizing the internalization of emotion control mechanisms and the interconnection of cognitive and affective elements. Similarly, Dweck (1991) argues that children gradually construct entity or incremental theories of self out of affective–cognitive experiences. One function of these structures is to regulate input to the emotions system in response to performance failures.

These control aspects suggest that problems of emotion regulation are different from problems of emotion dysregulation. Problems of emotion regulation concern weak or absent control structures or structures that are overwhelmed by disabling emotional inputs. When control is absent, emotions may be disorganizing. Because control mechanisms develop in childhood, many problems of emotion regulation in early and middle childhood may predominately reflect the weak influence of regulatory processes. A failure to inhibit behavior, for example, reflects weak or nonexistent emotion–action links.

In contrast, dysregulation involves existing control structures (inappropriate links) that operate in a maladaptive manner and direct emotion toward inappropriate (i.e., unconventional) goals. For example, most externalizing and internalizing problems in later childhood reflect the linking of emotions to deviant cognitive and action strategies. These kinds of problems show the power of emotions in motivating deviant behavior as well as adaptive behavior.

Functions

This description of control mechanisms also suggests certain key functions that constitute control. The control essentially represents intersystem communication that facilitates conscious awareness of feelings, desires, impulses, expressive behavior, and perhaps coping options. Thus, the control mechanisms promote *monitoring* of input to and output from the emotions system. Given access to feelings, the monitoring then promotes *modification* of emotional inputs and outputs and of the coordination of emotion and action. The emerging research on children's emotional coping responses directly concerns the modification function.

The processes of emotions system modification remain to be fully described or understood. At the least, modification includes processes that (1) attenuate or deactivate a current emotion, (2) amplify an emotion, (3) activate a specific emotion, and (4) mask an emotion feeling state. Diverting attention, for example, is one way to attenuate or deactivate an undesired emotion. On the other hand, activating and amplifying interest and enjoyment may serve to maintain task behavior in the context of environmental distraction or even weaken the effects of negative emotions arising from failure and loss. Kobak and Cole (1994) provide a specific example in describing possible deactivating attachment strategies by adolescents. Working models of attachment may dampen undesired emotions, such as sadness and anger, in response to separation by diverting attention from attachment needs and cues.

CONCLUSION

We have argued in this chapter that the emotions system in early childhood is modular in important respects and that the proximal zone of much emotional development concerns the construction of affective–cognitive structures and schemas that serve intersystem communication and regulation. Modularity is revealed in a core set of independent emotions that show discrete and stable expressive signatures and that have predictable activation thresholds in infancy that differ among individuals. These independent emotions constitute a modular system to the extent that functioning is encapsulated, is served by dedicated and hardwired neural structures, is fast, and emerges out of complex interactions among the independent emotions. Dependent emotions emerge from this modular functioning, as well as developments in the cognitive system, as affective–cognitive structures.

The construct of modularity provides a theoretical framework for understanding emotional development from the perspective of differential emotions theory. From this perspective, the breakdown of modularity is the core component of normative emotional development. Similarly, failures to interrelate the emotions and cognitive systems and maladaptive interconnections constitute core processes that mediate deviant development such as externalizing and internalizing behaviors in children. Thus, it pays to be mindful of modularity in understanding emotions in children.

REFERENCES

Abe, J. A., Takahashi, M., Putnam, P. H., & Izard, C. E. (1995). Developmental changes in 13- to 18-month-old infants' expressive behavior and their implications for socioemotional competence in toddlerhood and early preschool years. Unpublished manuscript, University of Delaware, Newark, DE.

Aggleton, J. P., & Mishkin, M. (1986). The amygdala in emotion. In R. Plutchik & H. Kellerman (Eds.), *Emotion: Theory, research, and experience* (Vol. 3, pp. 281–299). San Diego: Academic Press.

Alpern, L., & Lyons-Ruth, K. (1993). Preschool children at social risk. *Development and Psychopathology, 4,* 29–48.

Balaban, M. T. (1995). Affective influences on startle in five-month-old infants: Reactions to facial expressions of emotion. *Child Development, 66,* 28–36.

Barrett, K. C., & Campos, J. J. (1987). Perspectives on emotional development II: A functionalist approach to emotions. In J. D. Osofsky (Ed.), *Handbook of infant development* (pp. 555–578). New York: Wiley.

Blumberg, S. H., & Izard, C. E. (1985). Affective and cognitive characteristics of depression in 10- and 11-year-old children. *Journal of Personality and Social Psychology, 49*, 194–202.

Blumberg, S. H., & Izard, C. E. (1986). Discriminating patterns of emotions in 10- and 11-year-old children's anxiety and depression. *Journal of Personality and Social Psychology, 51*, 852–857.

Blumberg, S. H., & Izard, C. E. (1991). Patterns of emotion experiences as predictors of facial expression of emotion. *Merrill–Palmer Quarterly, 37*, 183–197.

Brown, J. R., & Dunn, J. (1992). Talk with your mother or sibling? Developmental changes in early family conversations about feelings. *Child Development, 63*, 336–349.

Campbell, S. B., Cohn, J. F., Flanagan, C., Popper, S., Meyers, T. (1992). Course and correlates of postpartum depression during the transition to parenthood. *Development and Psychopathology, 4*, 29–48.

Campbell, S. B., Pierce, E. W., March, C. L., & Ewing, L. J. (1991). Noncompliant behavior, overactivity, and family stresses as predictors of negative maternal control with preschool children. *Development and Psychopathology, 3*, 175–190.

Campbell, S. B., Pierce, E. W., March, C. L., Ewing, L. J., & Szumowski, E. K. (1994). Hard-to-manage preschool boys: Symptomatic behavior across contexts and time. *Child Development, 65*, 836–851.

Campos, J. J. (1994, Spring). The new functionalism in emotion. *SRCD Newsletter*, pp. 9–11.

Campos, J. J., Mumme, D. L., Kermoian, R., & Campos, R. G. (1994). A functionalist perspective on the nature of emotion. *Monographs for the Society for Research in Child Development, 59*, 284–303. (1, Serial No. 240).

Camras, L. A. (1992). Expressive development and basic emotions. *Cognition and Emotion, 6*, 269–283.

Cermele, J. A., Ackerman, B. P., Morris, A., & Izard, C. E. (1995). Children's understanding of the relation between emotion evidence and emotion experiences. Unpublished manuscript, University of Delaware, Newark, DE.

Cicchetti, D. (1990). The organization and coherence of socioemotional, cognitive, and representational development: Illustrations through a developmental psychopathology perspective on Down syndrome and child maltreatment. In R. Thompson (Ed.), *Nebraska Symposium on Motivation: Vol. 36. Socioemotional development* (pp. 259–366). Lincoln: University of Nebraska Press.

Cicchetti, D. (1991). Fractures in the crystal: Developmental psychopathology and the emergence of self. *Developmental Review, 11*, 271–287.

Davis, M. (1992). The role of the amygdala in fear and anxiety. *Annual Review of Neuroscience, 15*, 353–375.

Denham, S. A., McKinley, M., Couchoud, E. A., & Holt, R. (1990). Emotional and behavioral predictors of preschool peer ratings. *Child Development, 61*, 1145–1152.

Derryberry, D., & Rothbart, M. (1983). Emotion, attention and temperament. In C. E. Izard, J. Kagan, & R. Zajonc (Eds.), *Emotions, cognition and behavior* (pp. 132–166). New York: Cambridge University Press.

Duclos, S. E., Laird, J. D., Schneider, E., Sexter, M., Stern, L., & Van Lighten, O. (1989). Emotion-specific effects of facial expressions and postures on emotional experience. *Journal of Personality and Social Psychology, 57*, 100–108.

Dunn, J., Brown, J., & Beardsall, L. (1991). Family talk about feeling states and children's later understanding of others' emotions. *Developmental Psychology, 27*, 448–455.

Dweck, C. A. (1991). Self-theories and goals: Their role in motivation, personality, and development. In R. Dienstbier (Ed.), *Nebraska Symposium on Motivation, Vol. 38: Perspectives on motivation* (pp. 199–234). Lincoln: University of Nebraska Press.

Eisenberg, N., Fabes, R. A., Bernzweig, J., Karbon, M., Poulin, R., & Hanish, L. (1993). The relations of emotionality and regulation to preschoolers' social skills and sociometric status. *Child Development, 64*, 1418–1438.

Ekman, P. (1972). Universality and cultural differences in facial expressions. In J. R. Cole (Ed.),

Nebraska Symposium on Motivation (Vol. 19, pp. 207–283). Lincoln: University of Nebraska Press.

Fabes, R. A., Eisenberg, N., Karbon, M., Bernzweig, J., Speer, A. L., & Carlo, G. (1994). Socialization of children's vicarious emotional responding and prosocial behavior: Relations with mothers' perceptions of children's emotional reactivity. *Developmental Psychology, 30*, 44–55.

Fabes, R. A., Eisenberg, N., Karbon, M., Troyer, D., & Switzer, G. (1994). The relations of children's emotion regulation to their vicarious emotional responses and comforting behaviors. *Child Development, 65*, 1678–1693.

Fernald, A. (1992). Human maternal vocalizations to infants as biologically relevant signals: An evolutionary perspective. In J. H. Barkow, L. Cosmides, & J. Tooby (Eds.), *The adapted mind: Evolutionary psychology and the generation of culture* (pp. 391–428). Oxford, UK: Oxford University Press.

Fodor, J. (1983). *The modularity of mind: An essay on faculty psychology.* Cambridge, MA: MIT Press.

Gandour, M. J. (1989). Activity level as a dimension of temperament in toddlers. *Child Development, 60*, 1092–1098.

Garner, P. W., Jones, D. C., & Miner, J. L. (1994). Social competence among low-income preschoolers: Emotion socialization practices and social cognitive correlates. *Child Development, 65*, 622–637.

Gunnar, M. R., Porter, F. L., Wolf, C. M., Rigatuso, J., & Larson, M. C. (1995). Neonatal stress reactivity: Predictions to later emotional temperament. *Child Development, 66*, 1–13.

Harris, P. L. (1994). The child's understanding of emotion: Developmental change and the family environment. *Journal of Child Psychology and Psychiatry and Allied Disciplines, 35*, 3–28.

Harris, P. L., Johnson, C. N., Hutton, D., Andrews, G., & Cooke, T. (1989). Young children's theory of mind and emotion. In C. E. Izard (Ed.), *Development of emotion–cognition relations, 3*, 379–400.

Haviland, J. J., & Lelwica, M. (1987). The induced affect response: 10-week-old infants' responses to three emotion expressions. *Developmental Psychology, 23*, 97–104.

Izard, C. E. (1971). *The face of emotion.* New York: Appleton–Century–Crofts.

Izard, C. E. (1972). *Patterns of emotions.* San Diego: Academic Press.

Izard, C. E. (1977). *Human emotions.* New York: Plenum Press.

Izard, C. E. (1979). Emotions as motivations: An evolutionary-developmental perspective. In R. A. Dienstbier (Ed.), *Nebraska Symposium on Motivation* (Vol. 26, pp. 163–200). Lincoln: University of Nebraska Press.

Izard, C. E. (1992). Basic emotions, relations among emotions, and emotion-cognition relations. *Psychological Review, 99*, 561–565.

Izard, C. E. (1993). Four systems for emotion activation: Cognitive and noncognitive processes. *Psychological Review, 100*, 68–90.

Izard, C. E., & Ackerman, B. (1995, Winter). What's new in the new functionalism? What's missing? *SRCD Newsletter*, pp. 1–2, 8, 10.

Izard, C. E., Dougherty, L. M., & Hembree, E. A. (1983). *A system for identifying affect expressions by holistic judgments (Affex).* Newark: University of Delaware, Computer Network Services and University Media Services.

Izard, C. E., Fantauzzo, C. A., Castle, J. M., Haynes, O. M., Rayias, M. F., & Putnam, P. H. (1995). The ontogeny and significance of infants' facial expressions in the first nine months of life. *Developmental Psychology, 31*, 997–1013.

Izard, C. E., Hembree, E. A., Dougherty, L. M., & Spizzirri, C. C. (1983). Changes in facial expressions of 2- to 19-month-old infants following acute pain. *Developmental Psychology, 19*, 418–426.

Izard, C. E., & Harris, P. (1995). Emotional development and developmental psychopathology. In D. Cicchetti & D. J. Cohen (Eds.), *Manual of developmental psychopathology: Vol. 1. Theory and methods* (pp. 467–503). New York: Wiley.

Izard, C. E., Hembree, E. A., & Huebner, R. R. (1987). Infants' emotion expressions to acute pain: Developmental change and stability of individual differences. *Developmental Psychology, 23*, 105–113.

Izard, C. E., & Malatesta, C. Z. (1987). Perspectives on emotional development I: Differential emotions theory of early emotional development. In J. D. Osofsky (Ed.), *Handbook of infant development* (2nd ed., pp. 494–554). New York: Wiley Interscience.

Izard, C. E., & Youngstrom, E. A. (1996). The activation and regulation of fear and anxiety. In D. A. Hope (Ed.), *Nebraska Symposium on Motivation: Vol. 43. Perspectives on anxiety, panic, and fear.* Lincoln: University of Nebraska Press.

Jacobs, W. J., & Nadel, L. (1985). Stress-induced recovery of fears and phobias. *Psychological Review, 92*, 512–531.

Kagan, J., Reznick, J. S., Clarke, C., Snidman, N., & Garcia-Coll, C. (1984). Behavioral inhibition to the unfamiliar. *Child Development, 55*, 2212–2225.

Kagan, J., Reznick, J. S., & Snidman, N. (1987). The physiology and psychology of behavioral inhibition in children. *Child Development, 58*, 1459–1473.

Kobak, R., & Cole, H. (1994). Attachment and metamonitoring: Implications for adolescent autonomy and psychopathology. In D. Cicchetti & S. L. Toth (Eds.), *Rochester Symposium on Developmental Psychopathology, Vol. 5. Disorders and dysfunctions of the self* (pp. 267–298). Rochester, NY: University of Rochester Press.

Langsdorf, P., Izard, C. E., Rayias, M., & Hembree, E. A. (1983). Interest expression, visual fixation, and heart rate changes in 2- to 8-month-old infants. *Developmental Psychology, 19*, 375–386.

Lazarus, R. S. (1991). Cognition and motivation in emotion. *American Psychologist, 46*, 352–367.

LeDoux, J. E. (1987). Emotion. In F. Plum (Ed.), *Handbook of physiology, Section 1. The nervous system: Higher functions of the brain* (pp. 419–459). Bethesda, MD: American Physiological Society.

LeDoux, J. E. (1992). Brain systems and emotion memory. In K. T. Strongman (Ed.), *International review of studies on emotion* (Vol. 2, pp. 23–29). Chichester, UK: Wiley.

Lewis, M., & Michalson, L. (1983). *Children's emotions and moods: Developmental theory and measurement.* New York: Plenum Press.

Mangelsdorf, S., Gunnar, M., Kestenbaum, R., Lang, S., & Andreas, D. (1990). Infant proneness-to-distress temperament, maternal personality, and mother–infant attachment. *Child Development, 61*, 820–831.

Matias, R., & Cohn, J. F. (1993). Are Max-specified infant facial expressions during face-to-face interaction consistent with differential emotions theory? *Developmental Psychology, 29*, 524–531.

Nelson, K. (1986). *Event knowledge: Structure and function in development.* Hillsdale, NJ: Erlbaum.

Oster, H., Hegley, D., & Nagel, L. (1992). Adult judgments and fine-grained analysis of infant facial expressions: Testing the validity of a priori coding formulas. *Developmental Psychology, 28*, 1115–1131.

Peng, C., Johnson, C. N., Pollock, L. J., Glasspool, E., & Harris, P. L. (1992). Training young children to acknowledge mixed emotions. *Cognition and Emotion, 6*, 387–401.

Reznick, J. S., Kagan, J., Snidman, N., Gersten, N., Baak, K., & Rosenberg, A. (1986). Inhibited and uninhibited behavior: A follow-up study. *Child Development, 51*, 660–680.

Riskind, J. H. (1984). They stoop to conquer: Guiding and self-regulatory functions of physical posture after success and failure. *Journal of Personality and Social Psychology, 47*, 479–493.

Sacks, O. (1995). *An anthropologist on Mars: Seven paradoxical tales.* New York: Knopf.

Schore, A. N. (1994). *Affect regulation and the origin of the self: The neurobiology of emotional development.* Hillsdale, NJ: Erlbaum.

Seifer, R., Sameroff, A. J., Barrett, L. C., & Krafchuk, E. (1994). Infant temperament measured by multiple observations and mother report. *Child Development, 65*, 1428–1490.

Smiley, P. A., & Dweck, C. S. (1994). Individual differences in achievement goals among young children. *Child Development, 65*, 1723–1743.

Smith, C. A, & Scott, H. S. (1996). A componential approach to the meaning of facial expressions. In J. A. Russell & J. M. Fernandez Dols (Eds.), *The psychology of facial expression* (pp. 229–254). New York: Cambridge University Press.

Stifter, C., & Fox, N. A. (1990). Infant reactivity: Physiological correlates of newborn and 5-month temperament. *Developmental Psychology, 26,* 582–588.

Strassberg, Z., Dodge, K. A., Pettit, G. S., & Bates, J. S. (1994). Spanking in the home and children's subsequent aggression toward kindergarten peers. *Development and Psychopathology, 6,* 445–462.

Termine, N. T., & Izard, C. E. (1988). Infants' responses to their mothers' expressions of joy and sadness. *Developmental Psychology, 24,* 223–229.

Tronick, E., Ricks, M., & Cohn, J. (1982). Maternal and infant affective exchange: Patterns of adaptation. In T. Field, & A. Fogel (Eds.), *Emotion and early interaction* (pp. 83–100). Hillsdale, NJ: Erlbaum.

Van der Kolk, B. A. (1994). The body keeps the score: Memory and the evolving psychobiology of posttraumatic stress. *Harvard Review of Psychiatry, 1,* 253–265.

Van der Kolk, B. A., & Van der Hart, O. (1994). The intrusive past: The flexibility of memory and engraving of trauma. *American Imago, 48,* 425–454.

Weinberg, M. K., & Tronick, E. Z. (1994). Beyond the face: An empirical study of infant affective configurations of facial, vocal, gestural, and regulatory behaviors. *Child Development, 65,* 1503–1515.

Weiss, B., Dodge, K. A., Bates, J. E., & Pettit, G. S. (1992). Some consequences of early harsh discipline. *Child Development, 63,* 1321–1335.

Wellman, H. M. (1990). *The child's theory of mind.* Cambridge, MA: MIT Press.

Werner, H. (1948). *The comparative psychology of mental development.* New York: International Universities Press.

III

Functionalist Perspectives

5

A Functionalist Perspective to the Development of Emotions

Karen Caplovitz Barrett

In this chapter, I address the three questions to which the editors have asked me to respond: (1) What is an emotion? (2) What about emotions undergoes developmental change, and, more specifically, what developmental changes occur in one or two specific emotion families? (I will examine shame and pride). (3) What are the functions of these emotions for the child? I address questions 1 and 2 in turn, and, in doing so, I will address question 3.

WHAT IS (AN) EMOTION?

The first and most basic question I was asked to address is "What is (an) emotion?" According to the present approach, emotions are not entities that reside in brain or behavior; they are processes that *evolve* from the interdigitating impact of organism and environment on each other, as appreciated (appraised) by the organism. These processes may or may not be felt; when they are felt, the feeling is an important part of the process. These processes may or may not be associated with overt behavior, but they almost always are associated with an *inclination* toward a type of action. Again, whether or not overt behavior takes place, and, if so, what specific form of behavior

Karen Caplovitz Barrett • Department of Human Development and Family Studies, Colorado State University, Fort Collins, Colorado 80523.

What Develops in Emotional Development? edited by Michael F. Mascolo and Sharon Griffin. Plenum Press, New York, 1998.

occurs are important features of the emotion process. Thus, emotions are not specific "expressive" or other behaviors, not specific cognitions, or specific feelings; each of these elements is *a part* of the emotion process. Overt behaviors, feelings, and thoughts help shape and define each ongoing emotion. The emotion process does not spring forth, fully formed, from a program in the brain, nor is it created completely anew on each occasion. Rather, the particular family member is created in response to the organism's involvement with the environment, but the type or "family" of emotion that is displayed is defined by the *set* of functions that this type of process serves. Each new occasion of emotion is a new member of an emotion family, although certain "subtypes" may be distinguished in particular languages (e.g., embarrassment as a type of shame; frustration, rage, and wrath as types of anger).

Typically, the emotion process begins when the experiencing individual appreciates the significance of a particular type of relationship with the environment; in fact, knowing the appreciations that are associated with each emotion can help one in determining which person–event–context combinations are most likely to be associated with each emotion family. However, it is possible for the process to be initiated by other means (e.g., emotion communication), and appreciations need not be conscious or contemplative but may be "prewired" and immediate. In order for a behavioral process to be emotional, it must involve an ongoing relationship between organism and (internal or external) environment that is *significant*—that has implications for the organism's adaptation to that environment. Most of the activities in which we engage at least *involve* some emotion. However, it seems possible to distinguish "emotion processes" or "emotions" on the one hand, from "emotion-impacted processes" on the other. In the ensuing paragraphs, I do so.

Emotion Processes (Emotions)

Some organism–environment processes primarily involve a significant relationship between organism and environment, and behaviors that serve the functions invoked or implied by that relationship. Such processes can be termed emotion processes or emotions, and typically can be described using ordinary emotion terms such as *shame* or *fear*. There are important similarities among certain emotion processes, across contexts and ages of respondents, that have led language users to devise words for categories of emotions, such as *joy*, *pride*, *fear*, and *anger*. Many of these emotion terms do seem to categorize families of related emotion processes.

For example, persons in the United States use the term *fear* to describe their reactions to being faced by a rabid dog, to almost falling off a cliff, or even to having a mental image of their child out by himself at night long after he is expected home. Clearly, these situations are not identical, nor would responses to these situations be identical. One would be unlikely to display a "fear face" when thinking about the absent child, but one might show one when almost falling from a cliff. One would be unlikely to run away quickly after almost falling from a cliff, but one might well do so when faced with a rabid dog. Yet there are important similarities among these three situations and responses to them. All involve a potential danger—to the self or a part or extension of the self. All of the "fears" would be likely to motivate attempts to avoid the harmful consequences of the danger. One might back away from the cliff edge, run away from the dog, and either avoid thinking about the dangers facing the child, call to make sure the child has avoided harm, or try to find the child and thus help him avoid harm. Many emotion terms, when analyzed, can be found to include a set of behavior processes that share the three types of functions. When this is true, such terms can be used to refer to the relevant emotion family (see also Barrett, 1995; Barrett & Campos, 1987).

A particular emotion "family" is defined by the three adaptive functions it promotes. Each family is associated with a particular behavior-regulatory function, a particular social-regulatory (interpersonal communication) function, and a particular internal-regulatory (intrapersonal) function. For example, the behavior-regulatory function of fear is avoiding danger/harm; the social-regulatory function is warning others of potential danger; the internal-regulatory function is to focus attention on the impending threat and how to avoid it. These functions are not specific behaviors; they are what any of many potential behaviors *do for the organism in the context of its ongoing relationship with the environment.* The individual who is involved in (experiencing) the emotion process is moved by the emotion to behave in a manner that fulfills the relevant functions. Moreover, an observer usually can see evidence that the set of functions that pertains to a particular emotion family is being realized by noting the organism's behaviors or reported thoughts and feelings, and/or by noting the responses of others observing the emoting individual. Furthermore, "behavior-regulatory" functions may involve cognitive "acts" as well as overt behavior. For example, the inclination to avoid the dangerous situation in fear may be instantiated by the individual's effort to avoid *thinking* of a psychological danger, or the inclination to spend time with a loved one may lead to thinking about the person a lot when physical proximity is not possible or desirable. Note that avoiding thinking about a danger by no means fulfills fear's internal-regulatory function of focusing attention on the impending threat; in contrast, it distances one from a psychological threat. To the extent that this makes the threat "go away," however, there is no longer the need to focus attention on it. Table 1 presents the three functions and appreciations (appraisals) associated with several emotion families.

Table 1. Characteristics of Some Emotion Families

Family	Behavior-regulatory functions	Social-regulatory functions	Internal-regulatory functions	Apprec re: self	Apprec re: other	Action-tendency
Shame	Distance self from evaluating others; reduce "exposure"	Communicate deference/submission; communicate self as "small" or inadequate	Highlight rules, standards, goals; aid in acquisition of self as object and, to some extent, self as agent; reduce arousal	I am bad	Someone thinks I am bad; everyone is looking at me	Withdrawal; avoidance of others; hiding of self
Pride	Decrease distance from evaluating others	Show others one has achieved standard, rule, or goal; show dominance/superiority	Highlight standards, rules, and goals; aid in acquisition of knowledge of self as object and agent	I am good	Someone/everyone thinks (or will think) I am good	Outward movement; inclination to tell or show others
Sadness	Cease attempting to gain unrealizable goal, object, or relationship	Communicate loss, defeat, and/or helplessness; communicate need for help/succorance	Conserve energy and resources in the face of unattainable outcome	I cannot obtain it; it/he/she is lost to me		Passive withdrawal; cessation of activity
Joy	Continue ongoing activities	Communicate to others that ongoing activities are enjoyable	Expand available positive or creative thoughts; motivate one to continue successful activities	I like this person, event, activity, or object; I can have/obtain this		Outward movement; active interaction; relationship building

Note. Apprec = Appreciation

The functions of emotions can and must be *inferred* from behaviors in context, report of behaviors and thoughts in context, or both. Thus, functions are one step removed from what can actually be observed. However, unlike appreciations (see Barrett & Campos, 1987), they allow for direct predictions of the types of behaviors that would be a part of the relevant emotion process, and they *can* be inferred directly from ongoing behaviors. Moreover, the emoting individual need not be aware of the functions being served by his or her behavior (much less be *trying* to fulfill those functions), or of feeling the ongoing emotion(s).

The strongest inferences can be made when overt behavior fulfilling both the behavior-regulatory and social-regulatory functions is present, in context. However, although all three of the functions are essential in defining emotion families as a whole, one or more of the functions may not be observable for a particular family member. For example, a person may control facial, vocal, and behavioral responses sufficiently well that social and/or behavior-regulatory functions are not observable. Moreover, as mentioned, behavior-regulatory functions may be served by thought processes. Because of such factors, some ongoing emotion processes may not be reliably detected or may be detected via self-report but not overt behavior, or overt behavior but not self-report. It is highly desirable to use multiple methods to assess multiple functions, when possible, to maximize the likelihood of detecting emotion processes that are present. It also is highly desirable to use multiple variables to assess each function, in that there is no single response or even any invariant set of responses that indicates that "the true emotion" is present, independent of context (see also Barrett, 1993).

Not all emotion terms describe different emotion families, moreover, and the boundaries around families are not rigid. Given that emotions are processes that evolve in context, the functions served may change over time as the situation and the individual's relationship with it changes. Thus, in a given context, more than one emotion process may occur, and several emotion processes may overlap or co-occur. The utility of the concept of emotion families is twofold: (1) its ability to highlight the important similarities in functions across different sets of responses, thus enabling one to make predictions as to what emotion process should or could occur under a particular set of circumstances; and (2) its ability to suggest a set of responses that could be considered indicative of a particular emotion family because it fulfills a particular function in a particular context.

Emotion-Impacted Processes

In order to define emotion, it is necessary to distinguish it from other behavior-regulating (behavioral) processes. As alluded to earlier, according to this approach, there are very few behavioral processes that do not involve emotion. A behavioral process would be unemotional only if no ongoing relationship between the person and environment is significant. Such a situation might occasionally occur if one is, for example, driving to work "automatically" and nothing is sensed to be relevant to one's adaptation. Automatic driving itself often would not elicit emotion, because in order to react emotionally, one must, at some level (not necessarily consciously), react to a person–environment relation as relevant to one's adaptation, and one is not likely to react this way when driving automatically. Usually, however, something else would attract one's attention (such that interest would be elicited), or one would be thinking about something significant and emotion would become involved in the process.

Nevertheless, according to the present approach, some processes that involve emotion still would not be considered "emotion processes" (or emotions). Such "emotion-impacted" behavioral processes are affected by an emotion process but do not directly address the functions implied by the significant relationship. Such processes may be termed *emotion-impacted processes*. For example, a woman who is studying may read something that reminds her of a boyfriend whom she loves and for whom she feels lonely. Her resultant thoughts of how and when she can see him again may interfere with her concentration while studying, so studying has been *affected* by the emotion process of loving/longing for her boyfriend. In that sense, studying can be viewed as an emotion-impacted process. However, unless studying itself is responsive to or inductive of the significant relationship, it is not a part of an emotion process. For example, if the woman found the material very meaningful and "capturing," she would be likely to become involved in an interest-family emotion process involving studying, and concentration on studying would likely be enhanced by this emotion process. In that case, studying behavior would be a part of the emotion process. *Much of the time, when emotions are viewed as "dysregulating," the focus is on an emotion-impacted process rather than an emotion process.* By directing attention, energy, and behavior toward the person–environment relationship about which it is concerned, emotion processes often both regulate behavior that is *relevant* to that relationship and dysregulate behavior that is *irrelevant or in opposition* to that relationship (see also Barrett & Campos, 1991).

WHAT DOES AND DOES NOT DEVELOP IN EMOTIONAL DEVELOPMENT?

Before I discuss the changes that take place as the child develops, it is important to indicate what I mean by *emotional development*. Emotional development is defined as changes in emotion processes and/or emotion families associated with experiences and/or maturational changes that take place as the person grows older. Development is not restricted to cognitive or structural change but includes any age-related change that affects emotion processes. Given this broad view of development, emotional development is necessarily complex, with most inputs into each process changing. Nevertheless, the set of three general functions that define each emotion family is not believed to change with development. However, one may use emotion displays for purposes beyond those central to the emotion family, and these "extra" purposes (e.g., display of angry voice and face in order to get a repair person to service your appliance more quickly) should increase in number with development.

The many changes that do take place with development, however, affect both measurement and emotion itself. Both socialization pressures to control and ability to control emotional responses increase as the child grows older, making overt behaviors less reliable indicators of emotion-relevant functions as the child grows older. On the other hand, development would be expected to have complex effects on the utility of self-report in assessing emotion. Babies and young toddlers are unable to provide consistent, reliable self-reports due to language (and possibly cognitive) limitations. However, socialization pressures may adversely affect the reliability of self-reports by children, adolescents, and adults. This suggests that self-reports should be supplemented with observed responses whenever possible. Changes in the relation between display and feeling, other behaviors, and/or appreciations change the nature of the emotion processes and increase the number and quality of emotion family members possible.

Development does not just affect the relations among observable and unobservable aspects of emotion, however; it affects every aspect of the emotion process itself except for the functions served. With development, the organism becomes aware of more different relationships with the environment; thus, more situations and aspects of situations become capable of eliciting emotion. With development, the organism's repertoire for emotional responses (including "coping" behavior) increases dramatically. With development, emotional responses become highly socialized. All of these changes make possible new subtypes of family members of most emotion families, changing the very nature of these families. For example, fear that no one will find one's theory compelling is a fear-family member that would not be possible during infancy and is in almost every way different from infantile fear of heights. One would be unlikely to show even part of the facial pattern associated with fear in the former type of fear; one might show at least "fearful eyes" with the latter. One would have at most a modest increase in heart rate in the former case but would likely have a substantial increase in the latter type of fear. One would most likely engage in cognitive distancing in the former type of fear and physical distancing or freezing in the latter type of fear. The cognitive processes involved in the former type of fear would be quite complicated and conscious; they would be brief and often outside of consciousness in the latter. These developmental changes in emotion, which occur as a function of cognitive development, social development, personality development, motor development, and socialization experiences, are cumulative and gradual, but they do result in qualitative change; few would suggest that these two forms of fear are the same.

In addition, with development, certain emotion *families* that are highly dependent on socialization, such as shame, guilt, and pride, may become evident for the first time. Nevertheless, the entire set of family members does not emerge at a particular age; different family members become possible at different ages, and the age of appearance of new families is dependent on individual experience.

The changes in emotions that occur with development have important implications for the child's adaptive functioning—both *inter*personally (socially) and *intra*personally (psychologically). The child is appropriately (or inappropriately) responsive to a wider and more complex array of situations, and his/her responses communicate this to others. The social emotions, which become possible largely as a function of socialization experiences, have important implications for the child's self-regulatory, moral, and achievement-related behaviors, as well as for the development of self. In the remainder of this chapter, I elaborate on specific developmental changes in and personal- and interpersonal-regulatory implications of these changes in the shame and pride families of emotion processes.

THE DEVELOPMENT OF SHAME AND PRIDE

What Are Shame and Pride?

Just how shame and pride are defined has important implications for when and how these emotions are said to develop. According to the present approach, shame and pride are "social emotions," and therefore are (1) socially constructed, (2) invariably connected with (real or imagined) social interaction, (3) endowed with significance by social communication and/or relevance to desired ends (see below), and (4) associated with appreciations (appraisals) regarding others as well as the self. Table 1 presents the appreciations associated with shame and pride.

The shame emotion family is extremely closely related to the sadness emotion family, and the pride emotion family is extremely closely related to the joy emotion family, as Table 1 suggests. There are three important differences between joy and sadness on the one hand, and pride and shame on the other: (1) Joy and sadness concern themselves with having or possessing anything, including a goal or end after which one is striving, but also including a person or object, whereas pride and shame concern themselves with meeting standards, obtaining goals, or following rules appropriately; (2) joy and sadness do not require even rudimentary evaluation of oneself or one's abilities, whereas pride and shame do; (3) joy and sadness do not necessarily involve approaching or avoiding other people, whereas pride involves an inclination to approach and/or display oneself or one's achievement to others, and shame involves an inclination to withdraw from or avoid others. Pride and shame are socially constructed in that they evolve in the context of relationship formation; if one does not care what others think, one will not display pride or shame. This is not necessarily true for joy and sadness.

Most researchers and theorists who write about shame and pride agree that these emotions occur when one evaluates one's behavior vis-à-vis some standard, rule, or goal (e.g., see Barrett, 1995; Heckhausen, 1984; Lewis, Sullivan, Stanger, & Weiss, 1989; Stipek, 1995). According to such approaches, the requirement that behavior be *evaluated* in relation to a standard or goal sets pride and shame apart from emotions such as joy or pleasure and sadness or frustration/anger. One cannot simply be excited about a stimulus display or upset that the stimulus display is not available; one must be excited about *one's accomplishment*, or upset about *one's failure*.

Given this emphasis on self-evaluation in relation to standards, rules, and/or goals, many researchers and theorists assume that these emotions cannot develop until children can recognize themselves as objects (so that they can evaluate themselves), have developed standards, rules, and/or goals, and can compare their performance to those standards (e.g., Heckhausen, 1984; Lewis et al., 1989; Stipek, 1995). However, although it is quite logical to suggest these abilities as prerequisites to shame and pride, the *level of awareness or understanding* that is needed for each of these is unclear. To the extent that the level of awareness needed is one that is present from early infancy, cognitive capacities should not place a constraint on the onset of these emotions.

Most research on the development of self-awareness utilizes one, well-researched paradigm. Although the literature indicates rather clearly when children "have self-recognition" using this paradigm, it is not clear that having this type and level of self-awareness is necessary for all members of the pride and shame families. Moreover, evidence supporting the proposition that pride and shame emerge at a particular point in development when standards are understood in relation to performance is even weaker. In contrast, evidence seems to support progressive development of shame, pride, and related abilities and responses, beginning in earliest infancy. I first present evidence on these cognitive prerequisites suggested by well respected theorist/researchers. Then, I present my own, alternative view regarding the development of shame and pride.

Cognitive Prerequisites for Shame and Pride?

Self-Recognition

The most widely utilized measure of self-recognition during toddler-hood is one in which children's noses are marked with rouge and children are placed in front of a mirror (Amsterdam, 1968). In order to be viewed as recognizing themselves, children need to touch the marked nose (rather than touching the mirror) upon seeing themselves in the mirror. Studies of this measure suggest that toddlers first are able to recognize themselves in a mirror some time between about 15 and 24 months of age (e.g., see Lewis & Brooks-Gunn, 1979). If self-recognition is a prerequisite for shame and pride (as Lewis et al., 1989, and Stipek, 1995, suggest), then one would expect that all children who show shame or pride also demonstrate self-recognition.

Lewis and his colleagues (1989), as well as Pipp, Robinson, Bridges, and Bartholomew (1997) have found an association between mirror self-recognition and embarrassed or coy behavior in middle-class samples (but see Schneider-Rosen & Cicchetti, 1991, for contrary findings with a working-class sample); however, I know of no studies examining the relation between pride or shame and mirror self-recognition (except to the extent that one considers embarrassment a form of shame, which Lewis does not). Moreover, some children in these studies showed embarrassed/coy behavior but did not touch their nose. Of course, any measure of any construct can be expected to have some measurement error, so these imperfect findings can be explained in this fashion. However, simple measurement error cannot explain Schneider-Rosen and Cicchetti's contrary findings. The probable reason why the rouge–mirror paradigm has not been used in association with Lewis and colleagues' studies of shame and pride is that children in the shame–pride studies were older, making the mirror paradigm of questionable utility. Nevertheless, until shame and pride are studied at younger ages, and studied in relation to the mirror situation and other indexes of self-recognition, it is hard to know whether self-recognition is a prerequisite for the first observable members of the shame and pride families, and, if so, what level of self-recognition is needed.

Evaluating Behavior vis-à-vis Standards

The age at which children are first capable of evaluating their behavior vis-à-vis a standard, rule, or goal, as well as whether this capacity is necessary for pride and shame, are also quite unclear. Kagan (1981) placed the emer-gence of this ability at around the middle of the second year of life, based on observations of toddlers' "anxiety" when they could not follow a model's pretense actions and on their excessive concern about flawed objects (which Kagan interpreted as stemming from concern about who broke the objects).

However, virtually no research has been conducted to determine whether sensitivity to behavior standards is present at younger ages, and how it relates to the development of shame and pride.

To my knowledge, only one study has examined standard sensitivity in relation to shame-relevant behavior (Kochanska, Casey, & Fukumoto, 1995), and one in relation to pride-relevant behavior (Bullock & Lutkenhaus, 1988). Kochanska and her colleagues' (1995) distress/withdrawal variable involves primarily shame-like, not guilt-like responses (i.e., high distress/withdrawal, infrequency of commenting about the mishap after harming an experimenter's possession, and low reparation). This variable (along with two guilt-relevant variables) was correlated with 2- to 3½-year-old children's verbal and physical concern about flawed objects and preference for and positive comments about unflawed objects. Results indicated that boys who made more positive comments about unflawed objects showed more shame-like responses when they thought they harmed the experimenter's possessions. On the other hand, girls who showed more verbal and physical concern about flawed objects were more likely to show shame-like behavior when they thought they had harmed the experimenter's possessions. Unfortunately, given that the youngest children in this study were 26 months of age, this study does not address whether and how sensitivity to standards might be related to shame at younger ages, or whether standard sensitivity is a prerequisite for shame. Moreover, because pride was not addressed in this study, the study provides no information regarding the relation between sensitivity to standard violations and pride. Finally, sensitivity to physical flaws in objects does not clearly indicate sensitivity to behavioral standards.

Bullock and Lutkenhaus's (1988) study of 15- to 35-month-olds revealed that although adherence to socially sanctioned standards for achievement increased with age during toddlerhood, only 15- to 18-month-olds displayed greater attention to standards (as evidenced by having a simple standard, stopping when one meets the standard, taking care to align tower pieces, and making corrections) on tasks on which they displayed pride-relevant responses. It is possible that a ceiling effect on adherence to standards compromised results for older children. However, this study does suggest that even 15-month-olds adhere to some simple behavioral standards, and that the extent to which they do is related to their tendency to show pride-like reactions. Again, younger children did not participate in the study, so determination of age of onset of attention to standards or of the effect of such attention on pride behaviors is not available. Moreover, again, the study did not address whether at least some awareness of standards is prerequisite to pride.

It should also be pointed out that Bullock and Lutkenhaus (1988) did not label their affective responses "pride," nor did Kochanska et al. (1995) label their responses "shame." The responses simply are comparable to those labeled as such in other investigations. Thus, many unanswered questions remain.

However, other relevant studies even less clearly address sensitivity to behavioral standards. Evaluation with respect to such standards is so central to the definition of shame and pride that the capacity often is inferred from shame- and/or pride-relevant responses. Heckhausen (1984), for example, suggested that "a sense of personal competence" does not develop until after 3 years of age, based on his observation of children's pride- and shame-relevant responses to success or failure on a competitive task (making a tower *more quickly than* someone else can make one). However, when the goal was obvious and intrinsic to the task, rather than being competitive, Stipek, Recchia, and McClintic (1992) found that children showed apparent pride and shame much earlier, which they too interpreted as meaning that evaluation with respect to standards was possible.

Stipek and her colleagues (1992) found that even infants as young as 13 months of age smiled and looked up at the experimenter after they accomplished an unambiguous goal. At all ages, from 13 to 39 months of age, some toddlers were more likely to look up at the experimenter if they accomplished the goal than if the experimenter accomplished the goal; however, the difference in amount of looking up at the experimenter for their own versus the experimenter's accomplishments only was significant for toddlers who were in the 22 months or older groups. In free play, children who were 13 or 15 months old were as likely as older toddlers to smile, exclaim, and/or clap after accomplishing something; however, with age, more children were likely to call others' attention to their accomplishments (although some children of all age groups did so). Moreover by 24 months of age (the youngest age tested in the follow-up study addressing shame), Stipek and her colleagues found that children smiled and had an open posture more when they succeeded and avoided eye contact and had a closed posture more when they failed.

Both Haekhausen (1984) and Stipek et al. (1992) interpreted their findings as indicating that children could evaluate their accomplishments vis-à-vis goals, given that such an ability was deemed prerequisite to these emotions. However, there was no independent evidence that children could do so, and no children under 13 months were studied, leaving the question of the development of this ability unanswered.

In my own ongoing work, I have found that children as young as 11 months of age react more positively to success than failure, even when their parent is not reacting more positively to success than failure (Barrett, Mac-Phee, & Sullivan, 1992). These were reactions to outcomes, rather than process, which is one criterion that Stipek and colleagues (1992) give to distinguish pride responses from mastery pleasure; however, some researchers still might suggest that these responses did not necessarily involve "true pride" (e.g., see Stipek, 1995).

There is some evidence from other labs, however, that by 11 or 12 months of age, infants begin to distinguish between tasks in terms of how difficult tasks are for them (see Morgan & Maslin-Cole, Study 3, in Barrett, Morgan, & Maslin-Cole, 1993; Redding, Morgan, & Harmon, 1988). Knowing that something is too difficult for one suggests that one has some "sense of personal competence" on that task and some rudimentary standard of achievement (e.g., putting the puzzle pieces in the right place). Infants as young as 12 months of age persist longer at tasks at which they are at least moderately successful than at those that are extremely difficult (Redding et al., 1988), suggesting that they appreciate more than just whether or not they are causing an interesting event; they seem to be able to tell that a task is hard or easy for them.

Moreover, by the middle of the second year of life, there is evidence of differential affectivity to easier versus harder tasks and success versus failure. At 17 months of age (the youngest age studied), toddlers react with more Duchenne smiles (Ekman & Friesen's, 1982, "felt" smiles) when they are working on a task that is moderate in difficulty, and more non-Duchenne smiles (Ekman & Friesen's, 1982, false or miserable smiles) when they are working on a task that is too difficult or too easy for them (Nelson & Barrett, 1995).

Taken together, these findings suggest that as early as the end of the first or beginning of the second year of life, toddlers are beginning to be able to evaluate their own actions vis-à-vis at least some very obvious goals and standards for success, and that by the middle of the second year, such evaluation affects relevant emotional responses.

This by no means indicates that infants of 11 or 12 months of age appreciate very many goals or standards and display pride and/or shame across a wide array of contexts. There is some reason to believe, for example, that infants do not have a clear notion that they are supposed to *complete* a multipart task until the middle of the second year of life, and their awareness of other standards is first observable at even later ages (e.g., see Barrett & Morgan, 1995; Bullock & Lutkenhaus, 1988; Jennings, 1991; Morgan & Harmon, 1984). However, extant data at least indicate that evaluation with respect to some standards may be possible by the end of the first year of life. Much more research is needed regarding these phenomena during infancy.

The Origins of Shame and Pride: A Functionalist Approach

When Are Shame and Pride Present?

The preceding review is rather unsatisfying if one's goal is to determine when, in development, shame and pride "emerge." However, according to the present functionalist approach, a better question is "Under what condi-

tions are members of the shame and pride families observable at which ages?"
*To the extent that the functions of shame or pride are served by the ongoing behavior,
in an appropriate context, a member of those families is considered to be present.*

Thus, to the extent that children act to decrease their (physical or psychological) distance from evaluating other(s), and show positive, open, dominant, behaviors that communicate (or would communicate if others saw
them) positivity and self-worth or dominance to others after achieving a
behavioral standard, they are showing pride-family behavior. They do not
need to *understand fully* themselves or the goals and/or standards they are
meeting or failing to meet in order to become involved in these emotion
processes. Nor do the standards need to be those that others would have
devised for them, especially early in development.

Learning Social Standards

In fact, shame and pride help children learn societal standards by involving evaluating others in the emotion process; to the extent that children's
behavior violates socialization agents' rules and standards, the socialization
agents will intervene, changing the emotion process. Rather than a positive
experience, in which, for example, the toddler gets to play with the beautiful
china figure or the interesting electronics equipment, the encounter becomes
a negative one in which the child cannot play with the interesting object and is
grabbed way from it, yelled at, and/or punished. Under the proper conditions, such experiences may elicit shame and transform the child's inclination
to interact with the forbidden object to an inclination to avoid it. The child
learns that it is not okay not play with that type of object in part because of his
or her negative experiences associated with approaching and/or handling the
object. Moreover, pride and shame not only help children acquire standards
but also they help children learn about themselves—what they can and
cannot achieve, whether they behave appropriately, and whether others
evaluate them positively (see Barrett, 1995, for an extended discussion of
this topic).

Developmental Stages?

So, according to the present theoretical approach, shame and pride do not
emerge as a whole at a particular age, and these emotions facilitate the
development of the standards and self-understanding that are so closely
linked to these emotions. The next question that many would ask is, if shame
and pride are not entities that emerge at particular ages, and if these emotions
develop in part through a bidirectional process of development of self- and
standard-understanding, what shame and pride family members are present
at various ages?

Several theorists have suggested developmental stages or steps for the shame and pride families (e.g., see Mascolo & Fischer, 1995; Stipek, 1995); however, according to my approach, it is not meaningful to describe specific stages or even steps in the development of shame and pride, or to give names to specific developmental levels of each of these families. The reason that one cannot meaningfully describe stages and names is that each situation in which a child attains or fails to attain a standard or goal—when this attainment or failure has significance to the child—could elicit pride or shame. Moreover, each of these emotion processes is a somewhat different family member, and the differences are due to *many* variables and not just to one variable, such as cognitive development, for which stages or steps might be determined. Furthermore, even if the standard's attainment or violation was not significant when the child first enacted the relevant behavior, it may become significant before the behavioral process is over because of others' reactions, so what begins as a shame- or pride-*irrelevant* situation becomes a part of a shame or pride emotion process.

Thus, one does not have one particular type of shame or pride that becomes possible at, say, 18 months; one has a multitude of family members that become possible at *around* that age, depending greatly on the particular socialization and other experiences that that particular child has had, as well as individual differences in temperament and cognitive ability. Although one can narrow the domain to a specific type of task and examine steps in the development of family members relating to this task, it seems more useful to determine the types of contexts in which these emotions arise at different ages, the types of socialization experience associated with individual differences in response to these contexts, and the implications of these emotion families for children's becoming "members of society" and coping with their worlds.

Endowing Significance

Socialization is viewed as crucial to the development of shame and pride; if one does not care about standards and rules, and about other people's evaluation of one's behavior, shame and pride should not be manifested, given that key elements of both shame and pride are displays to others and evaluation with respect to standards. One essential element in the development of shame and pride is learning to care about a wide array of standards and rules, and about others' evaluation of one's performance relative to them (i.e., endowing the relevant person–environment relationships with significance). A common experience of babies that has the potential for endowing standards or rules with significance is emotional communication around standards, rules, and achievement/mastery. For example, a parent might react with anger and grab a child when he or she starts to touch an electrical outlet, or may react with joy and applause when the child completes a tower, or when the child smiles after completing the tower.

Very little direct information exists regarding the effects of such communication, however. Stipek and colleagues (1992) found that although toddlers showed pride-like behavior even when parents did not praise them (in fact, toddlers were more likely to show pride-relevant behavior when they initiated the activity, and parents were more likely to praise success on parent-initiated activities), greater parental praise for children's achievement was associated with more frequent positive reactions to achievement. Alessandri and Lewis (1993) did not replicate this finding, but did find that children's shame responses were associated with parents' increased negative evaluations and decreased positive evaluations. Much more research is needed regarding the role of emotion communication and shame and pride development.

Moreover, emotion communication occurs in the context of a relationship between the communicator and the recipient of the communication. To the extent that the communicator and recipient have no relationship, the recipient should be less inclined to heed the communication and draw from it implications about the significance of the event. Even a relationship of "She is an adult–I am a child" may be sufficient to cause a child to heed the communication and to endow the standard with significance. However, a strong positive relationship, in which the child cares deeply about the communicator (e.g., a parent) and trusts the communicator, would seem more likely to induce the child to endow significance to the events on a long-term basis. Simply stated, if children care about a parent and trust that parent to keep them safe, then they are more likely to accept the parent's communication indicating that the standard is significant (affects their adaptation to the environment).

In the literature on child rearing, a consistent finding is that a warm, reciprocal relationship, in which children and parents seem to "meet minds" and interact harmoniously, is associated with long-term adherence to externally imposed or internalized standards and rules (e.g., Kochanska & Aksan, 1995; Londerville & Main, 1981; Maccoby & Martin, 1983; Parpal & Maccoby, 1985; Rocissano, Slade, & Lynch, 1987; Silverman & Ragusa, 1990). It seems quite possible that one reason why children from such harmonious relationships adhere to parental standards is that such adherence has become significant to them because they care what their parents think. Adhering to parental standards becomes significant via a significant relationship with the parents. Much more research is needed, however, to determine whether emotion communication around standards and achievement is related to these harmonious relationships and to the development of standards, shame, and pride.

Developmental Changes in Shame and Pride

Although specific stages of the development of shame and pride cannot be specified in connection with the present theory, developmental progression and sources of such changes can be specified. These emotion families originate in goal-oriented behavior. Babies are oriented toward attaining desired ends which they may or may not attain. One reason a baby does not attain the goal is inability. Typically, situations in which the child attains a significant goal after exerting some effort, and attainment ends the process, or the child fails to attain the goal because of inability, would be framed as mastery or achievement situations.

Interestingly, the other type of situation in which shame and pride are likely, namely, those involving socially imposed "moral" or behavior standards, also can be construed as conditions requiring mastery. Delaying gratification and urinating in the toilet, like building a tower, require self-control and practice or experience. Both types of achievements might result in external reward (although "moral" or social standard attainment typically would be less intrinsically rewarding, at least at young ages). Similarly, failure to adhere to behavioral or moral standards is in many ways similar to failure in a mastery situation. In both cases, one often seeks to attain a desired end. In the moral or social standards case, failure to attain some goals that the child desires may result from the goal's *inconsistency* with *social standards*; that is, one reason that children fail to attain a goal such as taking away their brother's toy is because the behavior is prohibited and someone intervenes to prevent attainment. Given the close connection between mastery/achievement situations and the types of situations in which shame and pride are likely to occur, my discussion of the early development of shame and pride will draw primarily upon the literature on mastery motivation.

As Stipek (1995) noted, responses to mastery are exceedingly difficult to distinguish from responses construed as pride. She believes that shame responses are more easily distinguished from responses to unsuccessful mastery; however, I would submit that shame responses are quite difficult to distinguish from sad responses to failed goal attainment. According to my own approach, the specific behaviors manifested are less important than the functions they serve and the conditions under which they occur. To the extent that goals are positively socially sanctioned and/or are viewed as having implications for self- (and other-) evaluation, our language classifies the attainment emotion as pride and nonattainment emotion as shame (or guilt), and I maintain that distinction. However, the distinction between mastery joy and pride is somewhat arbitrary, as is the distinction between sadness at nonattainment of a goal and shame. In some cases, I may discuss responses as pride-relevant when others might view them as mastery pleasure. To the extent that the relevant functions are observable, however, the important phenomena are being investigated, and the terminology used to describe the phenomena is of lesser importance. In the sections that follow, I describe seven factors that affect the development of shame and pride, and describe some relevant ideas and empirical findings on the early development of these emotions in relation to these seven factors.

FACTORS AFFECTING THE DEVELOPMENT OF SHAME AND PRIDE

At least seven major factors act to change the incidence and complexity of shame- and pride-family emotions as the child develops: (1) the development of an increasing number and complexity of standards, rules, and goals as a product of socialization and cognitive development; (2) the endowment of an increasing number and complexity of standards, rules, and goals with significance as a result of socialization and other experiences; (3) increased understanding of self as agent; (4) increased understanding of self as object; (5) significant relationships with an expanding network of people; (6) an expanded repertoire of behaviors; and (7) exposure to an expanded array of situations.

The Development of an Increased Number and Complexity of Standards, Rules, and Goals

As indicated earlier, research on the early development of standards, rules, and goals is scant; however, that which exists strongly supports the idea that children begin life with only the most rudimentary goals (which might better be labeled "concerns," see Fridja, 1994), and then progressively add more goals, standards, and rules to their repertoire as they get older. Moreover, as they develop, the standards that they develop come increasingly under social control, such that they more and more come to reflect the standards of the society in which they are reared (e.g., Bullock & Lutkenhaus, 1988; Stipek et al., 1992). Elsewhere, Morgan and I have suggested that, from birth onward, behaviors directed at obtaining some end can be observed. It is beyond the scope of this chapter to reiterate all of that information here (see Barrett & Morgan, 1995); however, I will review some relevant information.

First, there is evidence that even neonates will suck differentially so as to turn on a preferred stimulus, and that they can learn that they are unable to control the presentation of the preferred stimulus. In fact, there is evidence of a "learned helplessness" effect when the preferred stimulus is presented noncontingently with respect to newborns' actions (DeCasper & Carstens, 1981). These findings and others from the same laboratory suggest some rudimentary goal orientation, in that the neonate will behave in a particular fashion so as to obtain a particular goal (hearing the preferred stimulus). Moreover, although it is extremely unlikely that these neonates *understand* that they are successful or unsuccessful in turning on the preferred stimulus, they must have some sense that their sucking pattern controls or fails to control the stimulus, or else they would not continue the appropriate sucking pattern when successful (achieve the goal) and discontinue when unsuccessful (fail to obtain goal). These findings also demonstrate that from birth, infants may begin building a repertoire of experiences in which they are or are not successful, and that, from the beginning, success may be associated with positive outcomes and failure with negative outcomes.

Thus, even neonates have some primitive sense of what they are and are not able to do, and are presented with more positive outcomes when they can than when they cannot do things. According to my approach, a full understanding is not necessary for the elicitation of emotion, so these findings are very important. However, the goal for the neonates is not a socially valued behavior standard, but rather a familiar sound. Moreover, neonates in such situations seem unlikely to have, at any level, a sense of standards for mastery or other behaviors. It is extremely unlikely that young infants have a sense of *how good* they are at turning on the stimulus (or any other mastery situation). It is highly improbable that they concern themselves with how long it took them to learn the behavior or how accurately they perform the sucking response. In fact, a large mastery motivation literature suggests that it is not until around 9 months of age that the average baby even has an *a priori* sense of which actions to perform to achieve which goals (a very primitive form of rule), and not until 11 or 12 months of age that they have a sense of which tasks are more or less difficult for them. All of these ages, moreover, should be considered very rough guidelines; the age at which children display these senses is probably highly dependent on task requirements, experience with similar tasks, and other contextual factors.

Gradually and progressively, as a function of their experiences, infants come to learn the rules and standards of society. As Stipek et al. (1992), Bullock and Lutkenhaus (1988), Jennings (1991), and Barrett and Morgan (1995) have observed, young toddlers do not always follow adults' expectations when "pursuing a goal." The parent or experimenter may assume that the goal of a ring stacker is to stack rings in order, so that all fit on the ring; a young toddler may simply try to put rings on and remove them, with little concern about order, and little concern about whether all rings are on the stand. Similarly, a young toddler may put in and remove the same puzzle piece repeatedly, never trying to put the other pieces in. Such children are not following the societal standard of task completion, but they are oriented toward and successful at achieving an end. Later, toddlers will try to put all of the puzzle pieces in place, all of the rings on in order, or all of the shapes in the position that matches a picture. Competitive standards seem to be attempted at a later age than do simpler and more concrete standards that are intrinsic to the task (Stipek et al., 1992). Depending on the complexity of the standard and their exposure to that standard (i.e., feedback indicating what the goal of the task "should be"), the standard will be acquired at an earlier or later age. Thus, the contexts in which shame and pride are likely to occur greatly expand as the child grows older and become more closely linked to societal standards (and, thus, more clearly and prototypically the type of contexts viewed as shame- and pride-relevant).

All of the foregoing situations concern mastery situations. There is very little research on the early development of moral or other social/conventional standards. An ongoing study of mine suggests that 17-month-olds already have some awareness of such standards (e.g., Barrett, 1995). This type of standard *must* be socialized; thus, neonates should not have developed awareness of it. Most likely, such awareness develops progressively through-out life, just as is true for other standards. However, much more research is needed on this topic.

Endowment of Significance to More Different Standards, Rules, and Goals

Simply knowing standards is not sufficient to induce emotion when standards are violated according to the present approach (but see Kagan, 1981, for an alternative position). Emotion requires *significance*: The organism–environment relationship needs to be seen as relevant to the organism's well-being or adaptation. The process of endowing attainment of standards with significance via emotional communication and relationship development has already been discussed. This process is viewed as one of the most important means of establishing significance of standards, rules, and goals during early development. However, of course, nonsocial outcomes, such as painful shocks or burns, interesting visual displays, and so on, may help establish the significant of goals as well. Moreover, the significance of some goals probably is established innately. Perhaps familiar voices and smells are significant goals for the neonate, because biology has equipped the baby with such inclinations so as to promote proximity and attachment. Of course, this is very speculative and difficult to test. However, it would explain how neonates only hours old will work to hear a familiar voice. The point is that most individuals *know* of many standards, even of their own culture, that they have no inclination or desire to achieve and for which nonattainment fosters no shame. Simple, "cold" cognitions cannot induce emotion; significance is essential.

Increased Understanding of Self as Agent

Although cognitive development is not sufficient to create emotion fami-lies, and high-level cognitions are not necessary to emotion, cognitive devel-opment strongly affects which family members are possible. Although much has been said about the role of self-as-object (self-recognition) to the develop-ment and shame and pride, surprisingly little has been said about self-as-agent (the self that makes things happen; see Pipp et al., 1997). The develop-ment of both shame and pride affect and are affected by the development of self as agent (as well as self as object). All of the aforementioned research related to goal orientation during infancy and toddlerhood also is relevant to the development of self-as-agent. Even rudimentary goal- and concern-directed behavior suggests some, albeit low-level, awareness of one's power to affect events, and, as awareness of one's ability and inability to achieve various ends improves, more members of the shame and pride family can occur.

Moreover, shame and pride affect the development of self-as-agent. As I have indicated before (Barrett, 1995), *guilt* is likely to influence the development of self-as-agent, even more than self-as-object, whereas, shame is more influential on the development of self-as-object than on the development of self-as-agent. To the extent that *guilt* rather than shame is more frequently experienced in the context of standard violations, the focus should be on the harmful *act* (and the child's responsibility for that act), rather than on a globally bad self. Thus, the child's power to harm others should be highlighted and, to the extent that reparation occurs and leads to positive outcomes, the power of the child to help others should be highlighted as well. Still, in mastery situations, shame may highlight *inability* to accomplish goals or meet standards, thus playing some role in the development of self-as-agent. Moreover, pride should highlight successful actions as agent, playing an even stronger role in the development of self-as-agent.

Increased Understanding of Self-as-Object

I already have discussed the role of self-as-object in the development of shame and pride in conjunction with the "cognitive prerequisite" of self-recognition. Moreover, shame and pride are not only affected by the development of self-as-object but they also are crucial influences on such development.

Shame and pride experiences highlight the self as others see one (or as one must appear to others), causing the person to step back from the self-as-agent and evaluate that self and, thus, elaborate and/or modify one's view of self. Moreover, as affective experiences, they highlight the *significance* of the experiences. I have elsewhere provided more details about how shame affects the development of a sense of self-as-object by providing conflict between a working model of loved ones as need- and wish-gratifiers and ongoing information indicating that those loved ones are preventing one from gratifying one's desires (e.g., possession of a china figure; see Barrett, 1995). Pride, too, may highlight self-as-object by showing that others notice and care about one's accomplishments and others provide feedback about when one performs well, according to their standards.

Significant Relationships with an Expanding Network of People

Shame and pride develop as a function of increasing numbers and complexity of standards (and, especially, increasing awareness of social standards), endowment of significance to that burgeoning array of standards, and the development of self-awareness and evaluation, and *all* of these developments occur primarily in the context of interpersonal relationships. One learns social standards form others and endows those standards with significance because one cares what those others think. The young baby is likely to be influenced primarily by caregivers when learning standards. However, as the child's social world expands, the child is exposed to the standards of increasingly different people. To the extent that these standards are the same as those of other people, the standards are underscored as important, or as moral givens, the *"everyone"* should follow (see Shweder, Mahapatra, & Miller, 1987). To the extent that they conflict, the person may reevaluate his or her standards, act differently in different social contexts, and/or decide which standards he or she values more. Thus, events that may have elicited shame or pride before may cease to do so, or those that did not elicit these emotions may come to do so as the person's network increases.

An Expanded Repertoire of Behaviors

It is obvious that one's ability to achieve standards is in part dependent on one's behavioral capacities. Thus, tasks that were too difficult at an earlier point in development can be accomplished, leading to new pride experiences. However, as abilities improve, standards often increase as well, such that a simple task from which one derived pride at one point in development may no longer induce pride (because it is expected), but may induce shame (when it is *not* accomplished). For example, urinating in the toilet properly is unlikely to elicit pride in a 7-year-old, but *failing* to do so (urinating in pants or bed) may elicit shame. Lewis, Alessandri, and colleagues (e.g., Lewis, Alessandri, & Sullivan, 1992) have demonstrated that even young children are more likely to display shame-relevant behavior when they fail on an easy task than when they fail on a difficult task, and that they are more likely to display pride-relevant behavior when they succeed on a difficult task than when they succeed on an easy one.

Not only are accomplishments and standards affected by the development of behavioral skills but also the responses that can be part of the emotion process are affected. For example, once babies can walk, they can more easily go over to their parents to display their success or get away from their parents when they have done something wrong. This greatly expands the range of family members that are possible.

Exposure to an Expanded Array of Situations

This factor is obvious as well; as children are engaged in more different encounters with the social and inanimate world, they have more experiences upon which to base standards. Those children who are exposed to a wider array of situations will develop standards in relation to a wider array of situations. Although this is obvious, it is important. Children who have been exposed to only a narrow spectrum of experiences may have difficulty "being appropriate" in other situations and may seem "uncultured," or "rude" when in those environments. They may not experience shame (or pride) when others believe they should, because they are completely unaware of the relevant standards.

CONCLUDING COMMENTS

Shame and pride, like other emotion families, promote adaptive responses to relevant aspects of the environment, but may interfere with adaptive responses to other aspects of the environment. According to the functionalist perspective espoused herein, the origins of these emotions can be seen in earliest infancy. Extant research is incapable of indicating when, in development, the entire set of functions that represents each of these emotions is first observable. Moreover, there are so many family members for each of these emotion families that it would not be fruitful to try to establish names for each of those variants of the emotions. Developmental research should be aimed at determining (1) what kinds of contexts give rise to these emotions at different points in development; (2) whether and when individual differences in these emotions arise, and how stable such differences are across situations and development; (3) the developmental antecedents of typical and atypical levels of shame and pride, especially antecedents involving relationships and socialization; and (4) the bidirectional relationship between self-development and the development of shame and pride. Much of this chapter has been quite speculative given the paucity of available data. It is hoped that this chapter will help stimulate research aimed at remedying this deficit.

REFERENCES

Alessandri, S. M., & Lewis, M. (1993). Parental evaluation and its relation to shame and pride in young children. *Sex Roles, 29,* 335–343.

Amsterdam, B. K. (1968). *Mirror behavior in children under two years of age.* Unpublished doctoral dissertation, University of North Carolina, Chapel Hill.

Barrett, K. C. (1993). The development of nonverbal communication of emotion: A functionalist perspective. *Journal of Nonverbal Behavior, 17,* 145–169.

Barrett, K. C. (1995). A functionalist approach to shame and guilt. In J. P. Tangney & K. W. Fischer (Eds.), *Self-conscious emotions* (pp. 25–63). New York: Guilford.

Barrett, K. C., & Campos, J. J. (1987). Perspectives on emotional development: II. A functionalist approach to emotions. In J. Osofsky (Ed.), *Handbook of infant development* (2nd ed., pp. 555–578). New York: Wiley.

Barrett, K. C., & Campos, J. J. (1991). A diacritical function approach to emotions and coping. In

E. M. Cummings, A. L. Greene, & K. H. Karraker (Eds.), *Life-span developmental psychology: Perspectives on stress and coping* (pp. 21–41). Hillsdale, NJ: Erlbaum.

Barrett, K. C., MacPhee, D., & Sullivan, S. (1992, May). *Development of social emotions and self-regulation.* Paper presented at meeting of the International Society for Infant Studies, Miami, FL.

Barrett, K. C., & Morgan, G. A. (1995). Continuities and discontinuities in mastery motivation during infancy and toddlerhood: A perspective and review. In R. MacTurk, E. Hrncir, & G. Morgan (Eds.), *Mastery motivation: Origins, conceptualizations, and applications* (pp. 57–93). Norwood, NJ: Ablex.

Barrett, K. C., Morgan, G. A., & Maslin-Cole, C. (1993). Three studies on the development of mastery motivation during infancy and toddlerhood. In D. Messer (Ed.), *Mastery motivation in early childhood: Development, measurement, and social processes* (pp. 83–108). London: Routledge.

Bullock, M., & Lutkenhaus, P. (1988). The development of volitional behavior in the toddler years. *Child Development, 59,* 664–674.

DeCasper, A. J., & Carstens, A. A. (1981). Contingencies of stimulation: Effects on learning and emotion in neonates. *Infant Behavior and Development, 4,* 19–35.

Ekman, P., & Friesen, W. V. (1982). Felt, false, and miserable smiles. *Journal of Nonverbal Behavior, 6,* 238–252.

Frijda, N. H. (1994). Emotions are functional, most of the time. In P. Ekman & R. J. Davidson (Eds.), *The nature of emotion* (pp. 112–122). New York: Oxford University Press.

Heckhausen, H. (1984). Emergent achievement behavior: Some early developments. In J. Nicholls (Ed.), *Advances in motivation and achievement: Vol. 3. The development of achievement motivation* (pp. 1–32). Greenwich, CT: JAI Press.

Jennings, K. D. (1991). Early development of mastery motivation and its relation to the self-concept. In M. Bullock (Ed.), *The development of intentional action: Cognitive, motivational, and interactive processes* (pp. 1–13). Basel, Switzerland: Karger.

Kagan, J. (1981). *The second year: The emergence of self-awareness.* Cambridge, MA: Harvard University Press.

Kochanska, G., & Aksan, N. (1995). Mother–child mutually positive affect, the quality of child compliance to requests and prohibitions, and maternal control as correlates of early internalization. *Child Development, 66,* 236–254.

Kochanska, G., Casey, R. J., & Fukumoto, A. (1995). Toddlers' sensitivity to standard violations. *Child Development, 66,* 643–656.

Lewis, M., Alessandri, S., & Sullivan, M. (1992). Differences in shame and pride as a function of children's gender and task difficulty. *Child Development, 63,* 630–638.

Lewis, M., & Brooks-Gunn, J. (1979). *Social cognition and the acquisition of self.* New York: Plenum Press.

Lewis, M., Sullivan, M., Stanger, C., & Weiss, M. (1989). Self development and self-conscious emotions. *Child Development, 60,* 146–156.

Londerville, S., & Main, M. (1981). Security of attachment, compliance, and maternal training methods in the second year of life. *Developmental Psychology, 17,* 289–299.

Maccoby, E., & Martin, J. (1983). Socialization in the context of the family: Parent–child interaction. In P. Mussen (Ed.), *Handbook of child psychology: Vol. 4, Socialization, personality, and social development* (pp. 1–102). New York: Wiley.

Mascolo, M. F., & Fischer, K. W. (1995). Developmental transformations in appraisals for pride, shame and guilt. In J. P. Tangney & K. W. Fischer (Eds.), *Self-conscious emotions: The psychology of shame, guilt, embarrassment and pride* (pp. 64–113). New York: Guilford.

Morgan, G. A., & Harmon, R. J. (1984). Developmental transformations in mastery motivation: Measurement and validation. In R. Emde & R. Harmon (Eds.), *Continuities and discontinuities in development* (pp. 263–292). New York: Plenum Press.

Nelson, G. C., & Barrett, K. C. (1995, April). *Toddler smiling in the context of parent–child tasks.* Paper presented at the Society for Research in Child Development meetings. Indianapolis, IN.

Parpal, M., & Maccoby, E. E. (1985). Maternal responsiveness and subsequent child compliance. *Child Development, 56,* 1326–1334.

Pipp, S., Robinson, J. L., Bridges, D., & Bartholomew, S. (1997). Sources of individual differences in infant social cognition: Cognitive and affective aspects of self and other. In R. J. Sternberg & E. L. Grigorenko (Eds.), *Intelligence: Heredity and environment.* New York: Cambridge University Press.

Redding, R. E., Morgan, G. A., & Harmon, R. J. (1988). Mastery motivation in infants and toddlers: Is it greatest when tasks are moderately challenging? *Infant Behavior and Development, 11,* 419–430.

Rocissano, L., Slade, A., & Lynch, V. (1987). Dyadic synchrony and toddler compliance. *Developmental Psychology, 23,* 698–704.

Schneider-Rosen, K., & Cicchetti, D. (1991). Early self-knowledge and emotional development: Visual self-recognition and affective reactions to mirror self-images in maltreated and nonmaltreated toddlers. *Developmental Psychology, 27,* 471–478.

Shweder, R., Mahapatra, M., & Miller, J. (1987). Culture and moral development. In J. Kagan & S. Lamb (Eds.), *The emergence of morality in young children* (pp. 1–82). Chicago: University of Chicago Press.

Silverman, I. W., & Ragusa, D. M. (1990). Child and maternal correlates of impulse control in 24-month-old children. *Genetic, Social, and General Psychology Monographs, 116,* 435–473.

Stipek, D. (1995). The development of pride and shame in toddlers. In J. P. Tangney & K. W. Fischer (Eds.), *Self-conscious emotions* (pp. 237–252). New York: Guilford.

Stipek, D. J., Recchia, S., & McClintic, S. (1992). Self-evaluation in young children. *Monographs of Society for Research in Child Development, 57* (1, Serial No. 226).

Tangney, J. P., Wagner, P., & Fletcher, C. (1992). Shamed into anger? The relation of shame and guilt to anger and self-reported aggression. *Journal of Personality and Social Psychology, 62,* 669–675.

Tangney, J. P., Wagner, P., & Gramzow, R. (1992). Proneness to shame, proneness to guilt, and psychopathology. *Journal of Abnormal Psychology, 101,* 469–478.

6

Emotion and the Possibility of Psychologists Entering into Heaven

Terrance Brown and Arnold Kozak

> When all men formed a single unit and began their wanderings over the earth they arrived at the Plain of Shinar and conceived the idea of a structure which would enable them to reach Heaven. The gods were alarmed at this suggested intrusion and, descending to the earth, struck terror to the hearts of men by confounding their speech so that no man could understand his neighbour.... The site of the tower is now but a hole in the ground.
>
> *Encyclopaedia Britannica*, 1959, p. 839—after Genesis XI

Since Babel, the idea of constructing a tower of stones as a means of entering into heaven has given way to the idea of constructing a tower of understanding. Philosophers since the ancient Greeks and psychologists for at least 100 years have tried to reach the paradise of everlasting epistemological bliss by unlocking the secrets of the mind. In that struggle and despite the vicissitudes of psychological fashion, the study of emotion has played an essential, if not always explicit, role. In virtually every text we have examined, emotion is

Terrance Brown • 3530 North Lake Shore Drive, 12-A, Chicago, Illinois 60657. **Arnold Kozak** • RR1, Box 1276, Cambridge, Vermont 05444.

What Develops in Emotional Development? edited by Michael F. Mascolo and Sharon Griffin. Plenum Press, New York, 1998.

assumed, mistakenly and unscientifically, to be a term that is mutually understood (cf. Quine, 1960) or, attempting to foil the gods much space is devoted to the problem of definition. That is where our story starts.

Perhaps the best example of just how bad the situation is comes from the lexicon of our new scientific psychiatry. Feeling and emotion are not listed in the glossary of that discipline's frequently rewritten bible, the fourth edition of the *Diagnostic and Statistical Manual of Mental Disorders* (DSM-IV; American Psychiatric Association, 1994), but they are characterized to some extent in the entries on affect and mood. *Affect*, for example, is specified as observable behavior by which emotion or mood is expressed and, in the same entry, *emotion* is said to be "a subjectively experienced feeling state" (p. 763). Under the entry on *mood*, one further learns that emotion is a temporary state ("the weather"), whereas *mood* is a pervasive and sustained emotion ("the climate") that "colors the perception of the world" (p. 768). Any emotion could, therefore, be either just a passing condition or a manifestation of a mood, but neither is observable and must be inferred from affect. Common examples of *affect* mentioned are sadness, elation, and anger; common examples of *mood* mentioned are depression, elation, anger, and anxiety. Throughout, *sadness* and *depression* are used interchangeably (cf. discussion of "Episode Features," p. 320). *Affects*, which are behaviors, have the same names as emotions, which are subjectively experienced feeling states, making sadness, elation, and anger both observable and unobservable.[1]

Once definitions of such precision and clarity are in place, it of course follows that there are neither emotional disturbances nor emotional disorders (at least such entities are not mentioned in the book), that there are affective disturbances, but they do not constitute disorders, and that there are mood disturbances that do constitute disorders, but only for two moods (i.e., depression and elation). By sleight of definition, *anxiety*, an emotion which when sustained gives rise to a mood, does not when disordered constitute a Mood Disorder but rather an Anxiety Disorder. The exception to this comes, of course, when the defining emotion is focused on physical signs or symptoms, in which case disordered anxiety is neither a Mood Disorder nor an Anxiety Disorder but is, rather, a Somatoform Disorder. Further insight and epistemic comfort are provided when one observes that several of humankind's most troubling passions (e.g., anger, guilt, and shame) are not associated with disorders at all (Brown, 1991).

With some justice, one might object that there are more lucid discussions of emotion than psychiatry's official account. The sad fact is, however, that it is biological psychiatry's conception that rules popular understanding and

---

[1]This sort of polysemy encourages signifiers to be mistaken for what they signify and, indeed, in one of the earlier versions of the psychiatric bible (DSM-III; American Psychiatric Association, 1980), what are now referred to as Mood Disorders were called Affective Disorders.

public policy (Ross & Pam, 1995). It is its conception that underlies the idea that Mood Disorders can be explained as "chemical imbalances in the brain" (e.g., Coyle, 1988) and legitimates a multibillion dollar industry peddling psychoactive drugs. Alongside social phenomena of that magnitude, scholarly interpretations pale.

WHAT IS EMOTION?

We do not have space nor would it prove fruitful to enter into every definitional boondoggle brought up by the term *emotion*. Nor can we examine every theoretical issue raised by affective and emotional phenomena. We shall, therefore, limit our discussion to three areas that we believe are important to emotion theory today. The first of these has to do with repeated attempts to reduce psychology (and along with it, emotion) to biology. The second has to do with a highly selected history of emotion concepts in the twentieth century leading to the empirical bottom-up approach favored by a majority of psychologists over the last 10 years. The third has to do with a functional analysis of emotion that we believe might provide a framework for interpreting existing empirical studies and that might stimulate interesting research.

Can Emotion Be Reduced to Biology?

With regard to attempts to interpret emotion as a purely biological phenomenon, people have long been aware that subjective experiences of emotion are coincident with somatic events and have wondered what causes what. Thinkers like Herbart and Freud were quite explicit about their belief that the psychological phenomena of emotion produce the somatic effects of emotion. At the turn of the twentieth century, James and Lange reversed that causal hypothesis (and wasted 20 years of psychologists' time) with their claim that the peripheral physical events that occur during emotional reactions cause the psychological experience of emotion. In experiments gruesome beyond description, Cannon (1915, 1927a, 1927b) and others demonstrated the impossibility of that interpretation, and psychology went on to other follies. Now, in our much vaunted "decade of the brain," the James–Lange hypothesis (James, 1884; Lange, 1895) has resurfaced in new and virulent form. Seduced by modern technologies of nonintrusive study and the more tawdry charms of pharmaceutical and governmental gold, most psychiatrists, many psychologists, and even a few philosophers have convinced themselves that exhaustive study of brain biology will yield up the secrets of the soul. With regard to emotion, a burgeoning new molecular phrenology has replaced James and Lange's crude invocations of peripheral autonomic

effects so that, sadness, for instance, is reduced to an epiphenomenal elaboration of norepinephrine or serotonin depletion in specific areas of the brain
(Coyle, 1988; Drevets & Raichle, 1995; an example follows). Despite its many
superficial adherents and its many outrageous applications, this point of view
merits consideration in competent hands. It should be noted that this discussion does not address the generally accepted idea that biological effects
accompany or are part of emotional reactions. That concept will be discussed
later. The notion examined here is the notion that emotion can be reduced to—
is nothing more than—neurophysiology.

One of the more prominent spokespersons for the idea of reducing
psychological theory, theories of emotion included, to neurophysiological
theory is P. S. Churchland. In *Neurophilosophy: Toward a Unified Science of the
Mind/Brain*, Churchland (1986) argues that, although it is obvious that no truly
psychological phenomenon has yet been reduced to neurophysiology, there is
no principled reason why "neuroscience will never reduce psychology in
such a way that subjective experience can be identified with states of the
brain" (p. 327).

However, it is significant (and somewhat characteristic of the neuroscientific literature) that almost all of the examples of reduction that Churchland
uses are drawn from physics. She provides no psychological examples. All
she includes relative to psychology is a list of five phenomena whose reduction to neurophysiology she does not believe to be contentious (p. 296). All
relate to low-level, unintentional perceptual, conditioning, or discriminatory
responses. Contended reductionist propositions, for Churchland, fall into two
main categories. The first has to do with what she disdains as folk-psychology
concepts, which many hold to be indispensable to a theory of psychology, and
which, such thinkers insist, will prove irreducible to neurophysiology. Examples include subjective experience, consciousness, and reasoning (p. 315). The
second has to do with functionalist concepts that encompass certain of the
folk-psychology concepts just mentioned as well as intentional states and
logical processes "essential to the psychological level of description [that] will
not reduce to categories at the neurobiological level of description" (p. 350).
Churchland provides extensive, although not particularly convincing, ratio-
nales as to why she believes that these objections to reduction do not hold.
Space permitting, we would enter that discussion. As it is, it seems more
important to address what we think are the essential problems with Churchland's framing of the issues.

It is clear that Churchland, like everyone else, wants to know what the
mind is for and how mental functions are realized physically. What is prob-
lematic with Churchland's manner of going about things is that she believes
that the way to get at the problem is through reduction, and she erroneously
assumes a linear explanatory relation among the sciences. Put bluntly,
Churchland believes that psychology reduces to biology, biology reduces to
chemistry, and chemistry reduces to physics, thereby providing knowledge in

its most satisfying form. She does not provide room for the possibility that physics itself reduces to another discipline. Regarding that possibility, Piaget contended that all forms of knowledge arise from cyclic interactions between subjective and objective aspects of experience, and that this "circle" of knowledge is the "fundamental structure of the sciences themselves" (1950, pp. 42–49). This "circle of science" suggests that physics reduces to mathematics, and mathematics to logic, and logic to psychology and sociology, thus closing an epistemological circle unconsidered in Churchland's philosophy. Not having included Piaget in her bibliography, she is free to argue that concepts associated with the higher mental functions will be replaced by as yet unspecified neurophysiological concepts much in the same way that Aristotle's principle of antiperistasis was replaced by Newton's principle of inertia.

Adding to the confusion, Churchland's framing of the reductionist relation between mind and brain leads her to conflate explanations with causes, concepts of different logical levels (Cellérier, 1976/1983). Explanation is a concept of higher order than cause. It has to do with how causes have come together—with how they happen to have occurred in whatever combination they do occur. As far as inorganic phenomena are concerned, the causal mechanisms involved have come to interact by chance (aleatoric morphogenesis); in organic phenomena, they have come to interact with teleonomic control, either biological, psychological, or social (teleonomic morphogenesis). Explanation rests, therefore, on the morphogenesis of causal systems, not on the causal mechanisms themselves. To provide a concrete illustration, consider the story of David and Goliath. The cause of Goliath's untimely death may have been an injury to his brain, but its explanation was David's ethnically and politically motivated hatred. Biological analysis, however detailed, of just how the rock from David's slingshot fatally disrupted Goliath's neurons provides no additional meaning to the explanation of Goliath's death.

If we insist at length on the importance of this confusion, it is because it has had, and continues to have, grave social consequences. When people mistake teleonomic for aleatoric explanations of causal events, one arrives at horrors such as those described by Lévy-Bruhl (1976) in *La Mentalité Primitive*. In the societies that he studied, people tended to make mistakes of this order. For example, six men living in a village in the Congo were drowned when their canoe was caught in a whirlpool. According to tribal wisdom, the tragedy could not have been accidental; it had to have resulted from the work of witches. Because punishments were required, 18 persons identified as witches were executed (p. 46). In our own time, thinking of the very same kind leads misguided moralists to look on AIDS as a punishment for evil rather than as a viral illness. Churchland's error is, however, the mirror image of this mistake. Whereas Lévy-Bruhl's subjects and religious zealots mistake intentional organizations of causes for aleatoric or biological organizations of causes (reduction of the lower to the higher), Churchland mistakes or wants to mistake biologically organized causes for intentionally organized causes (reduction of the higher to the lower). Lest one think that this does not have consequences equal in their horror to the examples from Lévy-Bruhl or religious zealotism, consider the following case, in no way fictional, recently considered in a class on medical ethics taught by one of the authors. An elderly man in poor health and with no other family lost his wife. Nothing left to justify living, he shot himself through the roof of the mouth. By unhappy chance, the bullet was deflected by the bony structures of his skull, leaving him alive but blind. After regaining consciousness, he requested that no treatment be given and that he be allowed to return home. Asked what he intended to do, he answered candidly, "Kill myself." It was at this point that Churchland's mind–brain philosophy stepped in. Under the definitions cited previously, the patient was ruled to have "major depression" and, therefore, a "chemical imbalance in his brain." He was involuntarily committed to a psychiatric ward and given antidepressant medication on the reductionistic rationale that suicidal intent could not be normatively entailed by old age, failing health, loss of wife, blindness, and the absence of family or friends. Instead, the idea that maybe there was nothing left to live for was reduced to the idea that the patient was suffering from norepinephrine and/or serotonin depletion in certain parts of his brain and that his will to live could be chemically restored. Mind, after all, is only brain. Happily for the patient, aleatoric causal events undid both the teleonomy of his body's biology and his physicians' psychology, and he died of a coronary thrombosis—caused, perhaps, by antidepressant drugs.

To conclude this part of our discussion, let us simply state that Churchland's confidence in the inevitable reduction of mind to brain notwithstanding, there is nothing more scientific about neurology than psychology. If we must speak of neuroscience, we must also speak of psychoscience. Understanding neurology will not explain the functions of psychology, although it might possibly demonstrate how psychological regulations are causally achieved. By contrast, psychology, being of higher organizational level than neurology, will eventually help us understand why neurons have the properties they have, and why they are organized in the ways they are. In other words, function explains mechanism. At this point in our knowledge, however, loose talk of eliminatory reduction or massive application of somatic treatments for psychological events is unwarranted (Brown, 1991; Ross & Pam, 1995). And, in any case, physical cause explains nothing about function; only the morphogenetic composition of causes explains at that level.

Contemporary Attempts to Construct a Tower

If, then, we reject the idea that functional explanations of emotion or any other psychological phenomenon can be developed by studying the brain, we are left with the extremely difficult task of trying to understand emotion psychologically and socially. Rather than attempt an exhaustive examination of definitions and theories, we shall consider three older texts that had begun to point, piecemeal and variously, toward a conception of affective processes and emotion that we believe remains the proper conceptual foundation for theories of emotion. Then, we shall consider two recent anthologies indicating where emotion theory stands today.

In one of the finest works ever published on the affective life, Pierre Janet (1928) points out that phenomena brought together under the rubric of "feelings" (*les sentiments*) have always had an important place in the study of the mind. The ancients distinguished the passions from the reason, and classical philosophical psychology placed affection after cognition and before conation in its hierarchical specification of mental faculties. Janet discusses briefly the problems of definition and moves on to condemn the philosophical psychology of feelings as well as the peripheral theory of feelings in a passage that seems strangely pertinent to contemporary discussions of emotion.

> The peripheral theories of feelings, exactly like the philosophical theories which they resemble more than one would like to think, come under the influence of a philosophical doctrine important in our time, the doctrine of parallelism. In both theories, feeling itself is without importance but, instead, expresses something which is outside of feeling. In philosophical theory, feeling is the expression of what is happening in the soul, facilitated or hindered in its aspirations. In the peripheral theory, feeling is the reflection of what is happening in the viscera, but it is still only an image in a mirror and has no function. This conception of the affective life is quite false.... The psychological fact is neither spiritual nor corporal ... [it is] no more in the soul than in the stomach. It is a change in the whole of conduct. A local phenomenon, a change in the heartbeat, only becomes a psychological fact if it contributes to modifying conduct as a whole. It is, then, this modification of conduct that one must study under the name of feeling. (Janet, 1928, pp. 35–36, authors' translation)

Janet rejects, therefore, the doctrine of parallelism and insists that both feeling and its physiological components be understood from the point of view of the role they play in regulating conduct as a whole. In doing so, he lays the cornerstone for a new tower of psychological understanding. But Janet did not stop there. He placed at least two more important stones in this foundation. On the one hand, he differentiated *cognitive*—what he called "primary"—regulations from *affective*—what he called "secondary"—regulations. The latter acted on the former, determining their activation, energy modulation, and termination, and thus played an important role in motivation. On the other, he differentiated the everyday feelings of secondary regulation from emotion. The feelings associated with secondary regulation are universally present in normal people and play a constant role in ordinary life.

> But there are [other kinds of feelings] that are much less clear in consciousness. These do not correspond to well-regulated conduct but rather determine great

disorder. Without always being specifically pathological, they verge upon illness, to which they often give birth, and they are not a completely normal element in people's conduct. We must, therefore, add these abnormal forms, the principal forms of which are the emotions, to our study of feelings in general. (Janet, 1928, p. 449, author's translation)

Some 30 years later, these foundations of emotion theory are found still standing in P. T. Young's (1961) classic book, *Motivation and Emotion*. Young revisits the definitional turmoil that surrounds the term *emotion* and concludes that it arises because emotion is confused with other affective processes. Like Janet, Young insists that emotion cannot be conceived in terms of a mind separate from the body, that its behavioral, experiential, and physiological components must be conceived as a single event relating to the organism as a whole (p. 359), and that the key to emotion is disorganization.

If it were not for the fact of disorganization, psychologists could dispense with the concept of emotion entirely. There are plenty of concepts within motivational psychology to describe well-integrated, goal-directed, purposive forms of behavior. It is because disorganization exists as a fact of nature, and for no other reason, that we need the concept of emotional disturbance (Young, 1961, p. 355).

Then, in one of the better articles on emotion written in the last 50 years (appearing only 2 years after Young's book), Fraisse (1963/1968) reaffirms Janet's and Young's theses and extends them. Elaborating on Janet, Fraisse makes the important point that Dewey's functionalist approach, foreshadowed in Darwin, went a long way toward avoiding the dualism inherent in the philosophical and peripheral approaches. According to Fraisse, Dewey accomplished this by admitting the functional importance of both mental and physiological events and refusing to consider the primacy of either in the study of emotion. In line with Janet and Young, Dewey moved psychology toward a conception of emotion as behavior that "occurs only when instinctive, normal, or voluntary action is thwarted" (Fraisse, p. 107).

A second theme present in the works of his predecessors, but magnified by Fraisse, has to do with the notion of energy level. Cannon's (1927a) physiological studies in reaction to the James–Lange hypothesis led him to posit a theory of emergency reaction in which the physiological concomitants of emotion mobilize the physical energy needed to cope with fear, anger, or pain. It was subsequently discovered that "by progressively stimulating the reticular formation it is possible to follow the different states which succeed each other in the animal, through the range of levels of consciousness from deepest sleep to rage or fear" (p. 110). Physiologically oriented students of emotion immediately interpreted this as evidence that emotion, with all of its messy qualitative diversity, could be reduced to the simpler quantitative notion of activation or arousal (Lindsley, 1951). That idea eventually foundered on the fact that the reactions produced by stimulating the reticular system are psychologically meaningless unless they are contextualized with respect to specific situations and to specific behavioral reactions (Fraisse, 1963/1968, p. 110).

A third important issue developed by Fraisse had to do with the relation of emotion to motivation. Above the level of reflexive reactions, motivation has to do with the habitual or intentional regulation of behavior. Because it is a tenet of many people's intuitive psychology that emotion causes people to do the things they do, they often equate emotion with motivation. Motivation, Fraisse argues, cannot be identified with emotion for the simple and obvious reason that emotion only results when a person's motives are thwarted—when maladaptation to a given goal occurs.[2] Properly interpreted, this idea can be seen to be inherent in Darwin's theory of emotion and continues throughout all functionalist thought. Fraisse, however, (as Young did also) gives it particular empirical meaning. Basing himself on the Yerkes–Dodson law. Fraisse cites evidence showing that as the intensity of motivation increases, performance improves only up to a certain point. After that, emotion takes over and performance falls off. Emotional reactions are, therefore, identified with what happens when performance disorganizes, not with motivation itself. Insofar as emotion serves a function, it is to restore order, even if only order of a lower sort, once the goal–means structures set up by motivation has been destroyed. That being the case, Fraisse states bluntly (and, in our view, correctly) that "[i]t is incorrect to speak of emotion as synonymous with feeling, as in the expression 'an aesthetic emotion' or to use it whenever a subject is 'moved'" (authors' translation, p. V-112).

The Gods Strike Back

Looking at this little piece of history, it appears that earlier in this century thinkers such as Janet, Young, and Fraisse had begun to build a tower of understanding. However slowly, a theory of emotion that avoided dualism, that distinguished emotion from other affective phenomena, and that began to envision emotional reactions as having a specific function in psycho-social–physiological adaptation had started to rise above the ground. Ever-

---

[2]It is sometimes objected that this could not be true for positive emotions such as love or happiness. This objection arises from the very terminological confusion we are attempting to clear up. Recall that feeling, by itself, does not constitute emotion. Because positive feelings are generally experienced when things are going well, they often are not accompanied by the other components of emotional reactions. There is, therefore, relatively less positive than negative emotion. But this does not mean that positive emotional reactions never occur. An example might be a reunion after long separation, where joy is so intense that instrumental action is disturbed (e.g., the person affected cannot button clothes, spills the champagne he or she is trying to pour, etc.). There is high arousal, powerful feeling, autonomic discharge, emotional expression (sometimes paradoxical, such as weeping), and defenses in the form of stopping trying to do anything until the emotion has subsided, taking measures to calm down, and so on.

vigilant, the gods discovered this new menace, and employing the ingenious strategy of diverting attention from the study of emotion, moved to ensure that the tower being constructed would be neglected and fall to ruin. Evidence of their mischief can be found in the Introduction to a compendium of articles on *Emotions, Cognition, and Behavior* (Izard, Kagan, & Zajonc, 1984) published 21 years after Fraisse's article. In that text, three of today's most distinguished students of emotion wonder at the reemergence of interest in the subject when "[f]or most of the last two decades learning theory and cognitive psychology in general, as well as social-psychological and personality theory, [have been] largely devoid of emotion concepts" (p. 7).

Predictably, 20 years of neglect has led many scholars to forget what Janet and his followers had constructed. Emotion is no longer differentiated from affect; physiology is frequently opposed to or substituted for psychology, and there is no longer any suggestion that emotion relates to disorganization or disturbance. Regarding the issue of definition, the claims in Izard et al.'s book vary from the idea that defining emotion is not useful to the Queen-of-Hearts' contention that emotion means whatever one wants it to mean to the Churchland-taunting notion that people's naive or intuitive ideas of emotion are about all we have and are somewhere near the truth. We provide examples of each argument.

Defining Emotion Is Not Useful

When knowledge is lacking, formal definitions may sometimes do more harm than good.... Although definitions that subsume one concept to the other may be appealing as part of the superstructure of a general systems theory or a systems theory approach, we do not believe that such definitions are the most fruitful for guiding empirical research. (Izard et al., 1984, pp. 5–6)

Emotion is a superordinate term representing the varied relations among external incentives, thoughts, and detected changes in feeling states, as weather is a superordinate term for the relations among wind velocity, humidity, temperature, barometric pressure, and form of precipitation. We do not ask what weather means but determine, instead, the relations among the measurable phenomena and name the discrete coherences. Similarly, it may not be useful to debate the meaning of emotion. (Kagan, 1984, pp. 40–41).

Emotion Is Whatever People Say It Is

Given the range of perspectives and productive research efforts concerning emotion, a unifying theoretical definition of emotion need not assume broad importance.... For our purposes, no formal definition of 'emotion' is required other than an assertion that it is a shared concept among children and adults in a given society. Indeed, in one sense the definition of emotion *is* the variable under study, emotion as it is operationally defined ... by the beliefs and expectancies of persons. (Masters & Carlson, 1984, p. 439; emphasis in original)

Naive Theories of Emotion Are Somewhere Near the Truth

> Understanding emotion appears to require that children and adults have and use
> naive theories about emotions. It may be the case that these naive theories are not
> very different in their simplest forms from the sophisticated theories of those who
> study emotions. (Schwartz & Trabasso, 1984, p. 410).

To further evaluate the neglect of the foundation laid by Janet, Young, and Fraisse, two more recent, although no less representative, texts were reviewed: Ekman and Davidson's (1994), *The Nature of Emotion: Fundamental Questions*, and Gazzaniga's (1995) *The Cognitive Neurosciences*. In the first volume, the editors' goals are to move the field forward by "focusing attention on some of the most important questions about the nature of emotion that confront research and theory alike" (p. 3). This volume is organized around a series of questions. The first asks, "Are there basic emotions?" In the commentary on the contributions by such noted authors as Averil, Ekman, Panksepp, Scherer, and Shweder, they conclude that "although everyone agrees that more data are needed, they disagree about how much reliable data are now available, and what kind of data will be most useful in furthering our understanding of the emotions" (Ekman & Davidson, 1994, p. 47). Although we do not agree with his emphasis on reducing emotions to their underlying neural circuitry, Panksepp (1994), in contrast to his colleagues, offers a definition of emotion that includes a differential functional taxonomy. He laments, as we do, that when it comes to differentiating the functions that come under the rubric "emotion," a general lack of understanding still prevails in the field.

> Emotional systems also generate characteristic internal feeling states (which may
> have been the most efficient neurosymbolic way to encode incoming information
> with values). Without internal biological values, I doubt if any credible model of
> behavior could ever be generated, and it is *long overdue for disciplines concerned with
> the objective behavior of animals to take such issues seriously.* (Panksepp, 1994, p. 24,
> emphasis added)

The second question that Ekman and Davidson pose is "How are emotions distinguished from moods, temperament, and other related affective constructs?" In the commentary on this section of the book, which includes contributions from such luminaries in the field as Frijda, Goldsmith, Kagan, Lazarus, and Panksepp, they conclude that all of the contributors make a distinction between various components on the basis of such issues as temporality, antecedents, and consequences (pp. 94–96). Still missing is the distinction, considered crucial in this chapter, that emotions are not synonymous either functionally or componentially with feelings.

In the second text cited, a long section on emotion begins with a chapter by LeDoux (1995):

> Unfortunately, when we attempt to relate emotion to brain we quickly run into a
> problem. There is no universally agreed upon definition or theory of emotion that
> delimits emotional phenomena in a way that is useful for relating those phenomena
> to neural systems. If we cannot define emotion, how can we hope to identify the
> emotion system or systems in the brain? (p. 1049).

The second chapter in this section (Bloom, 1995) "examines the mechanism of intercellular communication pertinent to the neuroscience of emotion" without defining emotion in any way. The third chapter (Weinberger,
1995) studies fear as a kind of emotion state while leaving the concepts of fear
and emotion unanalyzed. The fourth chapter (Rolls, 1995) harks back to a
Behaviorism we thought defunct. The fifth chapter in this section labeled
emotion (Brothers, 1995) discusses the "cognitions" necessary for social adaptation and informs us that "the cognition in question takes the form of a sort of
dictionary to innate social 'feelings'" (p. 1108). In the ensuing discussion,
feelings and emotions are considered to be equivalent. The sixth chapter
(McEwen, 1995) begins with a statement that not only does not distinguish
emotions from feelings but also applies equally to cognitions:

> Emotions are the product of an individual's own processing of occurrences on the
> basis of his or her own prior history and biology, and an emotional response
> activates neural and neuroendocrine effector systems and leads to a variety of short
> and long-term consequences that may or may not result in disease. (p. 1117).

Terms such as *fear* and *anxiety* are used but not defined.

Space does not permit us to continue, but these examples suffice to
illustrate our general thesis. In current practice, what is taken as emotion—or
at least as some part of emotion—is so variable and relies so heavily on
intuitive psychologies of various sorts that we are led back to LeDoux's
question: "If we cannot define emotion, how can we hope to identify the
emotion system or systems in the brain?"

From our reviews of representative texts on emotion, we conclude that
none of them are really books about emotion, according to the definition of
emotion offered here. Either they are books about the neurophysiological
basis of folk psychology or they are books about affective processes in general.
When they are the first, they make the mistake of assuming that mind can be
discovered by studying brain; when they are the second, they conflate affects
and emotions. This conflation neglects the specific functional roles that affectivity (explicated later) and emotion perform. By missing the function of
affectivity, the enterprise of affects in general is set against cognition in
general, in what then becomes a spurious separation (Brown, 1996). Were
space available, we would illustrate the substitution of reductionism for
dualism, and the loss of any true understanding of the functional necessity of
emotion in the same manner.

In summary, although it is the case that a collection of empirical bricks has been brought to the building site, there is little evidence of a plan for a tower. What is needed to construct an edifice of that sort is an architect of Darwinian, Einsteinian, or Piagetian order to give theoretical meaning to what is only a disorganized heap of empirical data. Admitting fully that neither singly nor in consort are we synthesists of that order and that, moreover, synthetic theories are currently out of academic fashion, we would nevertheless like to take a stab at a top-down functionalist approach.

A Functional Approach to Affectivity and Emotion

Only three topics can be considered in this very brief exposition. The first has to do with the functional nature of mind; the second has to do with the functional contribution of feelings to mental adaptation; and the third has to do with the functional nature of emotion within mental processes in general.

The Functional Nature of Mind

Although the idea is very old (Campbell, 1987), by far the most powerful and influential theory of mind as mentally realized extension of biological adaptation is that of Piaget (Brown, 1994). On Piaget's view, behavioral schemes, classifications, propositions, theories, value systems—mental structures of any kind—are adaptive organs just as much as mitochondria, ligaments, and retinae are. As a system regulating the use of the physical organs, in particular the musculoskeletal system, the mind plays a central role not only in biopsychosocial homeostasis but also in biopsychosocial evolution. That role is to create adaptations in the form of knowledge structures. In contradistinction to historical—particularly scholastic—usage, knowledge is not, strictly speaking, a purely cognitive affair. It can neither be invented nor can it function without affective and conative control.

As adaptation, knowledge evolves through some version of Darwin–Wallace variation, selection, and transmission. Piaget's particular version of that story is a theory of how both material and mental structures are constructed through functional perturbation and optimizing equilibration (Piaget, 1967/1971; Piaget, 1974/1980). It is the only extant theory explaining how Kant's "categories of reason" are constructed (Brown, 1996). It is also the only extant theory that deals convincingly with the emergence of the objective values of logicomathematical necessity and empirical truth (Brown, 1996). The problem is that, as written, Piaget's theory of equilibration is wrong (Brown, 1994). This is not because equilibration–stabilization is not the cogent explanatory principle[3] but because Piaget believed that equilibrium could be sought directly. Between ignorance and objectivity, however, a system of subjective probability must be interposed. This system is what people rely on for estimating the adaptive value of actions, choices, and so on. Piaget glimpsed, but only dimly, that the need for this system of subjective probability is why people have feelings. He only suspected intermittently that that is what affectivity is for (Brown, 1996; Piaget, 1950; Piaget, 1953–1954/1981; Piaget 1965/1971).

The Functional Nature of Feelings

More clearly than anyone else, Pugh (1977) has seen that the nature of so-called *cognitive appraisal* is an affective affair. Cognition, as understood epistemologically, has to do with how objectivity and relative certainty are achieved. Hence, in attempting to deal cognitively with psychological phenomena, we have to wade through interminable statistical analyses determining how certain we can be of just how uncertain we are. That this approach is optimal for academic psychologists dealing with highly simplified questions is, perhaps, arguable. That it is optimal for real people dealing with real situations is not even remotely possible. The level of certainty required by most psychological journals is, without any doubt, practically unachievable in daily life, where decisions of far greater importance than those focused on by academics must be made. Real people, among whom we do not include the statistical subject of experimental psychology or Piaget's epistemic subject, have to decide quickly and without much knowledge whether to do things such as sell their stocks, buy earthquake insurance, divorce their spouse, proceed with a dangerous cancer treatment, punish or praise their children, lie to the IRS, or vote for Pat Buchanan. Even if it were possible in principle to make such decisions with absolute certainty, which it is not, real people could not wait around for certainty to be attained. They have to act, and they do so on the basis of their feelings. Cognitively, they may be able to rule out relatively small numbers of simple courses of actions or establish the probability of relatively simple events, but in the end, all of the great human decisions

[3]For Piaget (1972/1985), equilibration was the principle upon which organization rested. Piaget's conception of equilibration is biological, not physical. It involves active compensation of change. For example, a movement from right to left can be compensated by a movement from left to right; the assertion p can be compensated by the assertion $\neg p$, and so on. An equilibrated—and therefore, stable—structure is one in which there are inverse and/or reciprocal compensations for every transformation. To avoid terminological confusion, it should be pointed out that in nonequilibrial thermodynamics, equilibration is the principle underlying entropic *disorganization*, whereas stabilization is the principle underlying negentropic *organization*. For reasons of history and tradition, we use Piaget's term, while at the same time recognizing that this discrepancy exists (cf. Inhelder, Garcia, & Vonèche, 1976).

involve so many degrees of freedom that objectivity and certainty are un-achievable. In such cases, feelings decide. For that reason, Pugh interpreted human intelligence as a value-driven system in which feelings play both deciding and motivating roles. More specifically, affectivity constitutes a complex system of evaluative heuristics that function as a surrogate for the evaluations effected by natural selection in biological evolution. This system is used to make adaptive decisions under the difficult conditions of too little knowledge, too little time, and too little processing capacity. Feelings, in Pugh's conception, are simply the conscious manifestation of these affective evaluative activities. Although presented here in very abbreviated fashion, these ideas have been extensively worked out in Brown and Weiss (1987) and Brown (1990, 1994, 1996).

The Functional Nature of Emotion

It must be obvious that, up to this point, nothing has been said about emotion. That is because we believe that the conceptual progress made by Janet, Young, and Fraisse was real. Emotion is not synonymous with feeling, nor is it just another name for affective processes in general. Rather, it is a particular form of reaction that occurs only in conjunction with adaptive malfunction. Emotional reactions have six main characteristics. First and most important, they occur either when a person's adaptive capacities are over-taxed or when a person, for various reasons, chooses to react emotionally rather than to react adaptively to a situation. For example, asked to add another errand to a list that is already too long, a person may become angry because it simply is impossible to accomplish everything on the list or be-cause, although not impossible, it is another in a long list of impositions by an inconsiderate acquaintance. In the first case, it is impossible for the person to see how everything can be done. In the second case, it appears impossible to stop repeated intrusions by the imposer. In either case, there is disorganiza-tion of the subject's original goal–means structure; there is disparity between what is being demanded and what the person either can or wants to do. The second characteristic of emotional reactions—correlative to the first—relates to the motivational role of affectivity. All goal-directed and goal-corrected behaviors involve affective evaluation of both goals and means. What one wants or feels obligated to do and how one wants or has to do it are affectively determined. When impediments arise and disorganization threatens, adapta-tion, in part, requires reevaluation of both goal and means. In emotional reactions, such reevaluation is not undertaken; the intensity of the original values is simply reinforced and other systems of regulation, described later, are activated. This means that emotional reactions always involve intense feeling, but it does not mean that feelings and emotion are equivalent, as modern theorists would have it. The two phenomena are, in fact, functionally distinct. Feelings, as the conscious manifestation of evaluative activity, serve the function of estimating adaptive value and are present in all behavior above the instinctive level. In contrast, emotional reactions, not just limited to intense feeling, serve the function of restoring adaptive order, even if only of a lower level, when adaptation fails. Emotions occur only when implementation of a given goal–means structure is impeded. As restorative responses to failed adaptation, emotional reactions involve several kinds of regulation that provide four more characteristics of an emotional reaction. To begin with, they instigate both central and peripheral biological changes that are nonspecific but that aid the organism in carrying out its basic strategies of reequilibration (e.g., fight or flight). These central and peripheral biological changes constitute the third and fourth characteristics of emotional reaction. The fifth characteristic of emotional reactions consists of stereotyped involuntary behaviors, in particular facial expressions, that allow the emotional state of the subject to be "read" by others. This makes it possible for others to take the subject's emotional state into account in their dealings with him or her. The sixth and final characteristic of emotional reactions is that they activate generic, nonspecific equilibration strategies or defenses. These may either be sensorimotor actions such as fight or flight, or they may be semiotic–operational maneuvers aimed at readapting meaning, for example, Piaget's (1974) idea of cognitive repression or Anna Freud's (1946) ego defenses. If all goes well in our example, the emotional reaction of anger might, for a person in the first case, lead to the adaptive outcome of prioritizing, planning, and perhaps giving up certain goals that he or she wanted to accomplish. In the second case, anger might lead to the adaptive outcome of refusal, confrontation, and renegotiation of the friendship.

DOES EMOTION DEVELOP?

Even under the narrow functional definition advocated here, which holds emotion separate from mental adaptation in general and from affectivity in particular, there is no question that the experience and expression of emotions changes as a function of development. It is widely accepted that when development, in general, goes well, both the frequency and the intensity of emotional reactions decrease. If, as is the case in certain personality disorders, an individual reaches adulthood without achieving the expected diminution in the frequency and intensity of emotional reactions, he or she is considered maladapted or sick. For the parent, teacher, friend, or clinician who has to deal with people having the emotional constitution of a 3-year-old and the executive powers of an adult, the experience can be overwhelming. However, the mechanisms of emotional development remain obscure. We shall examine them from the point of view of the characteristics of emotion that we identified earlier (i.e., disadaptation, intense affectivity, and defensive activities).

Disadaptation

Perhaps Fraisse (1963/1968, p. 173–181) speaks most directly to the issue of disadaptation. Fraisse remarks that, as children develop, it is clear that their emotions become differentiated, but that the most essential developmental feature is a decrease in the absolute frequency of emotional reactions. He relates this to two of the factors central to our concept of emotion. On the one hand, the frequency of emotional reactions seen in infants has to do with the fact that the infant knows relatively little and, for that reason, cannot adapt to many situations. As knowledge grows, the child meets fewer and fewer situations that he or she cannot handle and emotional reactions become less common. So one important reason for emotional development is increased psychological adaptation or, in other words, increased knowledge. The other factor Fraisse makes responsible for emotional development is increasing control over emotional expression, so that even though emotion may be experienced, it is not necessarily exhibited. This also plays into the decrease in the absolute frequency of emotional reactions as children grow up. We will discuss it further later on.

Affectivity

Because affectivity and emotion are so constantly conflated in recent discussions of emotion, it is difficult to find a really full account of what effect affective development (i.e., the development of value structures) has on the frequency and intensity of emotional reactions. Young and Fraisse make clear that feelings are motivating and that there is an optimal level of motivation beyond which performance deteriorates and the subject reacts emotionally. How then does affective development contribute to emotional development? It does so in two main ways.

To begin with, affective development has to do with the construction of value structures. Babies are born with rudimentary feelings that orient them to or avert them from activities and situations that will prove important in how they develop. We cite as examples preferences for certain tastes, tactile stimulations, and levels of familiarity and stimulation (Stern, 1985). There are many others. Out of these rudimentary value structures, elaborate systems of secondary values will be developed (Pugh, 1977). As we have said before, these value structures are surrogates for natural selection in mental evolution and are, therefore, important instruments in mental adaptation. As such, they decrease emotionality in inverse proportion to the degree of which they help the child adapt to a broader range of situations. As increasingly complex value structures more frequently guide children in the right direction, performance more often succeeds and emotional reactions do not occur.

Affective decentration is the second major way in which affective development aids children in maintaining adaptive equilibrium and avoiding emotional reactions. As the reader may recall, cognitive decentration is a major feature of Piaget's account of mental adaptation. It is much less known that Piaget (1953–1954/1981; 1932/1965) also made affective decentration an important element in his theory of interpersonal exchanges, in his theory of how children move from retributive to distributive morality, and in his theory of the will. In essence, affective decentration means that when things go wrong and children do not know what to do to make them go right, they may change the value scale by which action is evaluated. In this way, affective equilibrium is restored. Although disagreement has arisen concerning the age at which children can decenter in various domains, few doubt its importance.

The problem with the recent literature on the affective aspect of this issue is not only that it conflates affectivity with emotion (e.g., Schwartz & Trabasso, 1984; Harris, 1989), but that it fails to appreciate the ubiquity of decentration as a developmental event in all domains and at every level (Montangero & Maurice-Naville, 1994, pp. 122–128). Were space available, we would attempt to undo all of the confusion. Constraints being what they are, we simply assert that affective decentration constitutes one of the major affective strategies that children (and adults) use to control and contain emotionality. The more they appreciate that a given goal or task can be evaluated from different points of view, the more they are able to substitute one mode of evaluation for another as a way of avoiding disorganization and emotional reactions. For example, if not letting little sister have a turn means that no one will be permitted to play Ninja Turtles, the whole axiology of letting little sister play takes on new value. "Playing now" becomes subordinate to "playing at all."

Defensive Activity

Finally, defensive activity concerns the activation of generic, nonspecific reequilibration strategies or defenses. Young (1961) stresses the importance of the outcome of defensive maneuvers for the development of emotionality in general. On the one hand, when the defensive strategies employed during emotional reactions fail to work, one witnesses the organization of chronic states of maladaptation corresponding to complexes, neuroses, and self-concept problems of every kind. On the other hand, when the defensive strategies do work, emotional experience can be the source of profound positive change in a person's values, interests, and motivations. He cites as an example Lincoln's resolution to try to do something about slavery after he attended a slave auction in New Orleans and reacted with repulsion and despair. Similarly, a little Cajun girl handed the wife of one of the authors a baby nutria during a visit to a Louisiana swamp. As it happened, the wife owned a nutria coat. Reduced to tears, she renounced her oft-repeated claim that she needed a fur coat for warmth, disposed of the furs she owned, and has since refused to touch an article trimmed with fur. She also began donating large quantities of money to animal protection programs. In both instances, emotional experiences changed the affected person's axiology and led to new adaptations rather than to chronic maladaptation and emotionality.

WHAT IS THE FUNCTION OF EMOTIONAL DEVELOPMENT?

Paradoxically, the function of emotional development is to eliminate emotional reactions insofar as possible and, otherwise, to contain them, to control them, and to learn from them. This follows from the fact that emotional reactions occur only in cases where adaptation fails and that their general function is to restore adaptive functioning. What one sees, then, in emotional development is a general decrease in emotional behavior due to a vast increase in adaptive capacity, better control of excessive levels of arousal, richer and more refined feeling occasioned by the construction of new value systems, less autonomic nervous system activity associated with "stress," as well as more specific, more effective, and less costly defensive behavior.

We are unfortunately forced to conclude that Janet, Young, Fraisse, and others were beginning to make functional sense of emotional phenomena, but with the rise of cognitivism, their insights have been lost. Current thinking encumbers the problem of emotion with definitional confusion, functional bewilderment, and a fervor for reduction. Despite numerous experimental studies of various aspects of what now passes for emotion—an admixture of neurophysiological, affective, and cognitive entities—we feel that little progress is being made. What is needed is a guiding synthesis that can keep classes of phenomena straight and create a coherent functional narrative. Without that, as at Shinar, current work on emotion appears to be little more than a hole in the ground. In consequence, there is, today, little chance of psychologists entering into heaven.

REFERENCES

American Psychiatric Association. (1980). *Diagnostic and statistical manual of mental disorders* (3rd ed.). Washington, DC: Author.
American Psychiatric Association. (1994). *Diagnostic and statistical manual of mental disorders* (4th ed.). Washington, DC: Author.
Bloom, F. E. (1995). Cellular mechanisms active in emotion. In M. S. Gazzaniga (Ed.), *The cognitive neurosciences* (pp. 1063–1070). Cambridge, MA: MIT Press.

Brothers, L. (1995). Neurophysiology of the perception of intentions by primates. In M. S. Gazzaniga (Ed.), *The cognitive neurosciences* (pp. 1107–1115). Cambridge, MA: MIT Press.

Brown, T. (1990). The biological significance of affectivity. In N. L. Stein, B. Leventhal, & T. Trabasso (Eds.), *Psychological and biological approaches to emotion* (pp. 405–434). Hillsdale, NJ: Erlbaum.

Brown, T. (1991). Psychiatry's unholy marriage: Psychoanalysis and neuroscience. In D. Offer & M. Sabshin (Eds.), *The diversity of normal behavior* (pp. 305–355). New York: Basic Books.

Brown, T. (1994). Affective dimensions of meaning. In W. F. Overton & D. S. Palermo (Eds.), *The nature and ontogenesis of meaning* (pp. 167–190). Hillsdale, NJ: Erlbaum.

Brown, T. (1996). Values, knowledge, and Piaget. In E. Reed, E. Turiel, & T. Brown (Eds.), *Values and knowledge* (pp. 137–170). Hillsdale, NJ: Erlbaum. (An abbreviated version of this paper will also appear in L. Smith (Ed.). (In press). *Jean Piaget: Critical assessments* (2nd ed.). London: Routledge.)

Brown, T., & Weiss, L. (1987). Structures, procedures, heuristics, and affectivity. *Archives de Psychologie* (Geneva), *55*, 59–94.

Campbell, D. T. (1987). Evolutionary epistemology. In G. Radnitzky & W. W. Bartley III (Eds.), *Evolutionary epistemology, theory of rationality, and the sociology of knowledge* (pp. 48–89). LaSalle, IL: Open Court.

Cannon, W. B. (1915). *Bodily changes in pain, hunger, fear, and rage: An account of recent researches into the function of emotional excitement.* New York: Appleton-Century.

Cannon, W. B. (1927a). The James–Lange theory of emotions: A critical examination and an alternative theory. *American Journal of Psychology, 39,* 106–124.

Cannon, W. B. (1927b). Neural organization for emotional expression. In M. L. Reymert (Ed.), *Feelings and emotions* (pp. 257–269). New York: McGraw–Hill.

Cellérier, G. (1983). The historical genesis of cybernetics: Is teleonomy a category of understanding? (T. Brown, trans.). *Nature and System, 5,* 211–225. (Original published 1976)

Churchland, P. S. (1986). *Neurophilosophy: Toward a unified science of mind/brain.* Cambridge, MA: MIT Press.

Coyle, J. P. (1988). Neuroscience and psychiatry. In J. A. Talbott, R. E. Hales, & S. C. Yudofsky (Eds.), *The American Psychiatric Press textbook of psychiatry* (pp. 3–32). Washington, DC: American Psychiatric Press.

Drevets, W. C., & Raichle, M. E. (1995). Positron emission tomographic imaging studies of human emotional disorders. In M. S. Gazzaniga (Ed.), *The cognitive neurosciences* (pp. 1153–1164). Cambridge, MA: MIT Press.

Ekman, P., & Davidson, R. J. (1994). *The nature of emotion: Fundamental questions.* New York: Oxford University Press.

Encyclopaedia Britannica. (1959). Vol. 2, p. 839—after Genesis XI.

Fraisse, P. (1963). Les emotions. In P. Fraisse & J. Piaget (Eds.), *Traite de psychologie experimentale, tome V: Motivation, emotion et personalitie,* pp. V-97–V-181. Paris: Presses Universitaires de France.

Fraisse, P. (1968). The emotions. In P. Fraisse & J. Piaget (Eds.), *Experimental psychology: Its scope and method. V. Motivation, emotion, and personality* (A. Spillmann, Trans.). New York: Basic Books. (Original published 1963)

Freud, A. (1946). *The ego and the mechanisms of defence.* New York: International Universities Press. (Original published 1936)

Gazzaniga, M. S. (Ed.). (1995). *The cognitive neurosciences.* Cambridge, MA: MIT Press.

Harris, P. H. (1989). *Children and emotion: The development of psychological understanding.* Oxford, UK: Basil Blackwell.

Inhelder, B., Garcia, R., & Vonèche, J. (Eds.). (1976). *Epistémologie Génétique et Equilibration.* Paris: Delachaux et Niestlé.

Izard, C. E., Kagan, J., & Zajonc, R. B. (1984). Introduction. In C. E. Izard, J. Kagan, & R. B. Zajonc (Eds.), *Emotions, cognition, and behavior* (pp. 1–14). Cambridge, UK: Cambridge University Press.

James, W. (1884). What is emotion? *Mind, 9*, 188–205.

Janet, P. (1928). *De l'Angoisse à l'Extase. II. Les Sentiments Fondamentaux.* Paris: Librairie Félix Alcan.

Kagan, J. (1984). *The idea of emotion in human development.* In C. E. Izard, J. Kagan, & R. B. Zajonc (Eds.), *Emotions, cognition, and behavior* (pp. 38–72). Cambridge, UK: Cambridge University Press.

Lange, C. (1895). *Les èmotions* (G. Dumas, trans.). Paris: Alcan.

LeDoux, J. E. (1995). In search of an emotional system in the brain: Leaping from fear to emotion and consciousness. In M. S. Gazzaniga (Ed.), *The cognitive neurosciences* (pp. 1049–1061). Cambridge, MA: MIT Press.

Lévy-Bruhl, L. (1976). *La Mentalité Primitive.* Paris: Retz.

Lindsley, D. B. (1951). Emotion. In S. S. Stevens (Ed.), *Handbook of experimental psychology* (pp. 473–516). New York: Wiley.

Masters, J. C., & Carlson, C. R. (1984). Children's and adults' understanding of the causes and consequences of emotional states. In C. E. Izard, J. Kagan, & R. B. Zajonc (Eds.), *Emotions, cognition, and behavior* (pp. 438–463). Cambridge, UK: Cambridge University Press.

McEwen, B. S. (1995). Stressful experience, brain, and emotions: Developmental, genetic, and hormonal influences. In M. S. Gazzaniga (Ed.), *The cognitive neurosciences* (pp. 1117–1135). Cambridge, MA: MIT Press.

Montangero, J., & Maurice-Naville, D. (1994). *Piaget ou l'intelligence en marche.* Liège, Belgium: Mardaga.

Panksepp, J. (1994). The basics of basic emotion. In P. Ekman & R. J. Davidson (Eds.), *The nature of emotion: Fundamental questions* (pp. 20–24). New York: Oxford University Press.

Piaget, J. (1950). *Introduction a l'epistémologie génétique. I: La pensée mathématique.* Paris: Presses Universitaires de France.

Piaget, J. (1965). *The moral judgment of the child* (M. Gabain, trans.). New York: Free Press. (Original published 1932)

Piaget, J. (1972). *Insights and illusions of philosophy* (W. Mays, trans.). New York: World. (Original published 1965)

Piaget, J. (1971). *Biology and knowledge* (B. Walsh, trans.). Chicago: University of Chicago Press. (Original published 1967)

Piaget, J. (1974). *La Prise de Conscience.* Paris: Universitaires de France.

Piaget, J. (1980). *Adaptation and intelligence: Organic selection and phenocopy* (S. Eames, trans.). Chicago: University of Chicago Press. (Original published 1974)

Piaget, J. (1981). *Intelligence and affectivity: Their relationship during child development* (T. A. Brown & C. E. Kaegi, trans. & eds.). Palo Alto, CA: Annual Reviews. (Original published 1953–1954)

Piaget, J. (1985). *The equilibration of cognitive structures* (T. Brown & K. J. Thampy, trans.). Chicago: University of Chicago Press. (Original published 1972)

Pugh, G. E. (1977). *The biological origins of human values.* New York: Basic Books.

Quine, W. van O. (1960). *Word and object.* Cambridge, MA: MIT Press.

Rolls, E. T. (1995). A theory of emotion and consciousness, and its application to understanding the neural basis of emotion. In M. S. Gazzaniga (Ed.), *The cognitive neurosciences* (pp. 1091–1106). Cambridge, MA: MIT Press.

Ross, C. A., & Pam, A. (1995). *Pseudoscience in biological psychiatry: Blaming the person.* New York: Wiley.

Schwartz, R. M., & Trabasso, T. (1984). *Children's understanding of emotion.* In C. E. Izard, J. Kagan, & R. B. Zajonc (Eds.), *Emotions, cognition, and behavior* (pp. 409–437). Cambridge, UK: Cambridge University Press.

Stern, D. N. (1985). *The interpersonal world of the infant.* New York: Basic Books.

Weinberger, N. M. (1995). Returning the brain by fear conditioning. In M. S. Gazzaniga (Ed.), *The cognitive neurosciences* (pp. 1071–1089). Cambridge, MA: MIT Press.

Young, P. T. (1961). *Motivation and emotion.* New York: Wiley.

IV

Systems Perspectives

7

A Dynamic Systems Approach to Cognition–Emotion Interactions in Development

Marc D. Lewis and Lori Douglas

There is a good deal of debate about what develops in emotional development. Theorists have examined the acquisition of new and more complex emotions, changes in the cognitive concomitants of emotions, and the consolidation of regulatory strategies, social skills, and personality traits. Yet most theorists agree that what develops is a set of new acquisitions added to (or supplanting) a repertoire of existing ones.

This view is common to developmentalists in most fields. Yet it is the product of a set of scientific practices we take for granted. Psychologists tend to round off the immense variability in real behavior, extract a generalized description, and then show the universality of that description for particular ages and/or conditions by testing groups of subjects. The behavior of these subjects, as any researcher knows, includes much that is unexpected. However, by controlling context effects and comparing average scores, while treating unpredicted variance as noise, we often do manage to find verification for our descriptions across samples. This verification serves as evidence that something is or is not acquired by a certain age or under certain conditions.

Marc D. Lewis and Lori Douglas • Ontario Institute for Studies in Education, University of Toronto, Toronto, Ontario M5S 1V6, Canada.

What Develops in Emotional Development? edited by Michael F. Mascolo and Sharon Griffin. Plenum Press, New York, 1998.

Such practices result in a particular bias: a tendency to overlook variability and indeterminacy in behavior. That this is true of normative approaches is already recognized (Kagan, 1984). However, even accounts of individual differences anchor individuality to general conditions, such as gender or early experience, and to enduring structures such as traits or working models. Yet it is clear from common experience as well as scientific study that behavior is highly plastic, sensitive, and difficult to predict, even when observed over brief time periods. This is nowhere more evident than in the case of emotional behavior (Higgins, 1987; Magai & Hunziker, 1993; Wright & Mischel, 1987). A shy 10-year-old may become confident or belligerent in a new social group, with playmates of a different age, or simply after winning a game. Context and prior events are critical influences on what emotions come into play and how they become interwoven with cognition and behavior. What picture of emotional development could encompass this variability?

Dynamic systems approaches to development emphasize that system behavior is always constituted in the moment, through the assembly of system components in potentially novel ways on each lived occasion. Particularly in the last 5 years, work by Fogel, Smith, Thelen, van Geert, and others has brought these approaches to the attention of mainstream developmentalists, leading to increasing interest in what they have to offer. According to dynamic models, human development expresses the inclination for complex systems to converge to coherent states, without determination by some prespecified plan or higher control function. This process is called *self-organization*—the emergence and consolidation of order from the spontaneous coordination of lower-level elements. From this perspective, macroscopic acquisitions, or developmental structures, are conceptualized as real-time processes of self-organization, by which elements can assemble in a variety of ways on any occasion under the influence of contextual forces. At the same time, the patterned, continuous nature of development is conceptualized as self-organization on a larger temporal scale—that of developmental time itself. Developmental self-organization consists of the emergence and consolidation of new possibilities and tendencies for behavior to coalesce in real time.

The importance of real-time emergence puts a unique spin on the question asked by this book. What develops in emotional development, from our perspective, are *tendencies* for system elements to cohere in particular ways in real time. As with many other accounts of emotional development, the elements we specify are cognitive and emotional constituents, and we begin our discussion with a rationale for looking at cognition and emotion as partially independent systems. We then introduce (nonmathematical) dynamic systems terms for *describing* developmental outcomes as a landscape of tendencies. Next, we attempt to *explain* these outcomes by modeling emotional development as a sequence of self-organizing interactions between emotions and cognitions. We then demonstrate how idiosyncratic experiences as well as normative forces influence these outcomes at developmental junctures. Finally, we present some preliminary data showing self-organizing configurations of attention and distress in infant emotional development.

EMOTION, COGNITION, AND SELF-ORGANIZATION

The developing tendencies discussed in this chapter are cognition–emotion interactions. But before proceeding, we need to determine the value of looking at emotion and cognition as different systems and provide a definition of emotion that permits this differentiation. According to Izard (1993), cognition and emotion differ with respect to their phenomenology, function, mode of operation, and neural substrates, and the advantage of demarcating this difference theoretically is to evaluate the action of each system as a function of the action of the other. Yet there are many challenges to this notion of independent systems (Kagan, 1978; Lazarus, 1984; Ortony & Turner, 1990), and some of these challenges have now been reframed by dynamic systems theorists themselves. These theorists view human behavior as the coassembly of many components, none of which can be ignored in any coherent human act. Fogel et al. (1992) claim that emotions themselves are self-organizing systems that necessarily incorporate cognitive and social-contextual processes. They propose that emotional development always reflects variations in the interaction of these components, all of which emerge through reciprocal constraints on one another. Camras (1992) similarly claims that basic emotions do not express a pregiven program, but rather knit together into predictable constellations over varying time frames for individual children. How can the separation of cognition and emotion be reconciled with this dynamic systems "party line"?

Our solution is to view cognition and emotion as subsystems that become progressively integrated over development, in a unique fashion for each individual, through self-organizing processes. We thus require a definition of emotions as primitives, along the lines of basic or discrete emotions. We define emotions as global, nonreducible affective states (1) that are recognized by a specific feeling tone but are nonspecific as to semantic content (Izard, 1984), (2) that are similar physiologically and phenomenologically across individuals and cultures (Ekman, 1984), (3) each of which is elicited by a specific class of situations related to the organism's goals (Oatley & Johnson-Laird, 1987), through perceptual or cognitive activities that correspond with these situations, and (4) each of which motivates a class of behavioral responses to these situations and facilitates cognitive activities that support these responses (Frijda, 1986). All of these features imply an adaptive biological function, and emotions are therefore considered to be phylogenetically specified and unlearned (Izard & Malatesta, 1987). Yet, although many emotions, thus defined, have distinct expressive features, all need not, because the signaling requirements of different emotions may vary. Thus, our definition differs from some discrete emotions definitions, and includes desire, shame, and anxiety.

What of the relationship between cognition and emotion? We agree with Izard that emotion can be triggered independently of cognition (though it rarely is), yet at sufficient intensity emotion *always* induces cognitive activity (or change in cognitive activity) as its effect. Central to our position is the means by which this effect comes about. Emotion seems to function as a field that influences a wide spectrum of activity in the cognitive system (Oatley & Johnson-Laird, 1987). Yet, in our view, this effect has a very specific mechanism: Emotion promotes coupling or linking up among conceptual elements, catalyzing their integration into larger wholes that are semantically meaningful. Emotion is thus the condition or control parameter for cognitive self-organization. The macroscopic, self-organized forms that result are termed *emotional interpretations* (EIs), because they include both an emotional state (one or more discrete emotions activated for some period of time) and the conceptual (interpretive) concomitant of that state. These macroscopic forms are similar to Izard's affective–cognitive structures and Tomkins's ideoaffective structures. Following these authors, we believe that emotions and their cognitive concomitants become linked over development, such that specific emotional interpretations come to characterize the developing personality. It is this convergence that we attempt to explain in the language of self-organization.

Thus, rather than view cognition and emotion as undifferentiable aspects of the same system, we construe them as separate, partially independent systems that become coordinated *through* self-organization. To answer the question posed by this book, then, we would say that what develops in emotional development are (1) links between the emotional and cognitive systems, favoring the recurrence of specific emotional interpretations, and (2) links within the cognitive system, favoring the semantic coherence that underlies these interpretations.

EMOTIONAL DEVELOPMENT AS A CHANGING LANDSCAPE

Much recent debate has been concerned with the role of dynamic systems (DS) modeling in developmental psychology. Do DS terms, such as attractors, phase transitions, and so forth, provide new explanations or merely new descriptions of well-studied phenomena? On this issue, we agree with Fogel (1993), van der Maas (1995), and van Geert (1994), who see DS language as a redescription, not an explanation. However, we believe that this redescription, even at the verbal (nonmathematical) level, encourages new explanatory models or at least powerful revisions of existing models, because of its novel treatment of variability, stability, and transitional phenomena. In the present section, DS terms are used to *describe* emotional behavior and development with an emphasis on individual variability. In the next section, an *explanatory* model, based on emotion theory and developmental theory, is used to make sense of this description.

Because they view human behavior as stochastic and self-organizing, DS theorists attempt to describe it in terms of tendencies or possibilities, not rules. This is why a state-space map or "landscape" provides a useful and appealing metaphor. A state-space map is a model of all possible states a dynamic system can attain. The tendencies of a given system, such as a developing child, may be thought of as topographical features on the map's surface. These features represent the accessibility, durability, and patterning of system states. One of these features is the *attractor*, representing a state toward which the system gravitates from one or more other states. An attractor can be portrayed as a well or valley in a flat surface, such that a ball rolling around on that surface tends to roll in. Once "in" the attractor, the system is relatively stable. The region surrounding the attractor, known as its basin, includes the set of states from which the system can gravitate to the attractor, like a sloping surface surrounding a well. The depth of the attractor represents its durability or resilience (its resistance to perturbations), whereas its breadth can represent its comprehensiveness (Killeen, 1989; Thelen & Smith, 1994). Criteria for determining the presence of an attractor are that (1) the same pattern is observed over occasions, (2) stemming from a range of other states, (3) with a concomitant reduction of overall variability, and (4) which resists perturbations or restabilizes immediately following perturbations (Thelen & Smith, 1994; van der Maas & Molenaar, 1992). These criteria are taken up again later.

Thelen and her colleagues (Thelen, 1989; Thelen & Ulrich, 1991; Thelen & Smith, 1994) have demonstrated the value in viewing developmental forms as attractors. Stable, recurrent behavioral forms, such as walking, smiling, or searching for lost objects, are depicted as attractors to which behavior gravitates, as system elements (e.g., perceptual and motor constituents) self-organize in real time, and in which behavior remains despite small changes or perturbations. However, these forms can coexist with other stable forms that utilize the same elements in different configurations. Thus, walking and crawling are coexisting attractors for toddlers, and either may attract behavior within a given situation. Human behavior is characterized by multi-stability, the coexistence of several attractors for the same set of constituents (Kelso, 1990, 1995), and behavioral change can be seen as a trajectory through a field of attractors (Killeen, 1989). Thelen defines development as the stabilization and destabilization of attractors over developmental time. This conception assumes the two time scales of human self-organization noted earlier: Emergence and change in attractors over months or years constitute developmental self-organization, whereas the convergence of behavior to attractors over seconds or minutes constitutes self-organization in real time (Thelen & Ulrich, 1991). We use the terms *macrodevelopment* and *microdevelopment* to distinguish these scales (Lewis, 1995).

We refer to observable patterns in emotional development as emotional interpretations (EIs), and these patterns are hypothetically comprised of particular interactions among cognitive and emotional constituents. EIs are stable patterns that recur with some degree of likelihood, converge from a variety of other patterns, and resist perturbations once formed: They can therefore be described as attractors. Some EIs, such as prolonged sadness in self-pity, are static and can be modeled as fixed-point attractors. Others, such as cycling between aggression and anxiety, are periodic and can be represented by cyclical attractors called limit cycles or by two linked attractors (called saddles) each giving way to the other. Many EIs, including humiliation, pride, suspicion, cheerfulness, resentment, or love, are normative attractors: They cohere in roughly similar ways for most, if not all, individuals. Presumably, this normativity taps an underlying repertoire of discrete emotions as well as shared cultural constraints. Relations among these attractors may be normative as well, telling us something about their mechanism. For example, pride, shame, and embarrassment attractors may generally be in close proximity, with partially overlapping basins, because they share particular constituents such as attention to the self (see Lewis, 1992).

Yet many cognitive–emotional attractors exist for some individuals and not others. These may include "pathological" states, such as masochism and paranoia, or simply emotional traits such as depression or anxiety. Moreover, even normative attractors vary across individuals in their intensity, resilience, duration, frequency of occurrence, and accessibility from other states. This variability may be due to temperamental differences, but also, particularly important in our treatment, to diversity in the cognitive constituents of emotional interpretations, reflecting each individual's specific learning history. For example, thoughts that correspond with shame include much that is idiosyncratic: conceptions of need, attitudes to authority, assumptions about competencies, attractiveness, and so forth. In "The Shipping News" by E. A. Proulx (1993), a man with a protruding chin, teased by his family throughout his childhood, unconsciously puts his hand over his chin whenever he becomes nervous in the presence of others. This anxiety-shame-hide-chin pattern is a deep attractor that includes idiosyncratic as well as normative features. Thus, a sensitive portrait of emotional development necessitates an attractor landscape that is uniquely configured for each individual. On this landscape, the totality of attractors and basins, denoting emotional biases, moods, inhibitions, and defenses, portrays much that is significant about an individual personality.

Many other state-space features exist (see Abraham & Shaw, 1987), but we will describe only one of particular importance. A *repellor* is a state that a system tends to move away from. It can be portrayed as a hill rising off a surface: The ball representing the state of the system tends to roll quickly away. Thus, repellors are unstable or transient states, easily perturbed and difficult to access. Repellors in emotional development can represent rare or transient socioemotional/behavioral constellations. For example, the anxious child may rarely achieve intimacy or trust, and guilt is rarely experienced by individuals who characteristically blame others. Emotional repellors may also represent states that are consistently avoided for defensive reasons. Thus, shame may be so painful for the shame-prone, narcissistic individual that it is rarely if ever experienced (Lewis, 1992). When in the vicinity of shame, the system might, instead, move to nearby attractors such as grandiosity or solicitousness. In the present account, individual emotional landscapes are viewed as constellations of attractors and repellors, describing tendencies toward and away from cognitive–emotional coherences. A sketch of such a landscape is show in Figure 1. This odd-looking vista is explained in more detail later.

Dynamic systems theory uses additional constructs for describing change. One kind of change is movement from one attractor to another when both attractors are available concurrently (i.e., at the same value of some control parameter), like switching hands while stirring a pot. But a more dramatic sort of change is movement through a *phase shift*, where the state space actually changes its topography, and attractors or repellors that were previously inaccessible suddenly influence behavior. At these points, the system rapidly becomes unstable and sensitive to fluctuations, then restabilizes in a new configuration (Haken, 1977). To the observer, this may appear as a sudden qualitative shift in behavior, such as the switching of a horse's gait from trot to gallop (Kelso, 1995). Abrupt changes in motor behavior (Kelso,

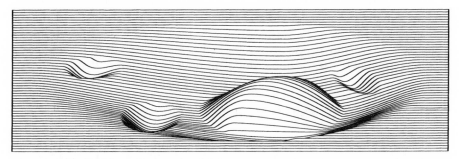

Figure 1. Sketch of the topography of a complex dynamic system. In this region of the landscape, a large basin contains three attractors, where system behavior settles, and one repellor, from which it migrates.

1995; Thelen & Ulrich, 1991) and cortical activity (Freeman, 1995) have been described as phase transitions, but it remains unclear how to identify them in real-time psychological activity. From our perspective, the sudden onset or transition of an EI conveys a qualitative change in the psychological system, thus fitting the description of a phase shift. At a different scale, DS theorists describe abrupt changes in development, including the acquisition of new abilities at cognitive-developmental transitions, as phase shifts (van der Maas & Molenaar, 1992; van Geert, 1991). In emotional development, the reshuffling of emotional habits or personality traits at developmental junctures (e.g., the defiance of the 2-year-old, the petulance of the young adolescent) appear to be qualitative changes of the same sort. Thus, we describe global, discontinuous changes in cognition–emotion as phase shifts in microdevelopment, and global, discontinuous changes in emotional development as phase shifts in macrodevelopment.

Finally, chaotic activity, identified as unpredictable yet nonrandom fluctuation in behavior, may be a necessary prerequisite for self-organization. Chaotic patterns precede the self-organization of coherent structures in living systems, as observed in neural and perceptual processes both in real time (Skarda & Freeman, 1987) and in development (Thelen & Smith, 1994). In a related vein, Fogel (1993) views indeterminacy as the precondition for real-time self-organization, with novel "information" arising out of diminishing variability as systems coalesce. These observations fit Prigogine's characterization of self-organization as "order out of chaos" (Prigogine & Stengers, 1984). More specifically, when a dynamic system is unmoored from its attractor at a phase shift, behavior becomes unpredictable or chaotic before it restabilizes in some novel configuration (van Geert, 1994). Thus, chaotic junctures appear to be sandwiched between stable regimes in self-organization. The role of fluctuations at phase transitions has been a major focus of attention for developmentalists such as Thelen and her colleagues, following work by Haken (1977) and Kelso (1984), and van der Maas and Molenaar (1992), following Thom's (1975) catastrophe theory. In this chapter, we describe chaotic junctures in emotion–cognition self-organization, both in microdevelopment, as emotions and cognitions fluctuate before converging to coherent forms, and in macrodevelopment, as emotional and personality patterns fluctuate at transitional nodes in developmental paths.

SELF-ORGANIZING EMOTIONAL INTERPRETATIONS

A recent model of self-organization in emotional and personality development identifies *positive feedback* and *coupling* as two complementary constructs (Lewis, 1995, 1996, 1997). These terms are somewhat of a convenience, because feedback, both positive and negative, exists at every level of psychological activity, and "coupling" loosely describes feedback relations that have stabilized. However, it seems helpful to continue to use this dualistic terminology, with positive feedback denoting the generative, self-enhancing force in self-organization, and coupling denoting the mechanism of preservation and coherence. *Positive feedback* is defined as a recursive process whose inputs are a positive function of its outputs. Positive feedback cycles, like autocatalytic processes in chemistry, start off small and grow, fueling themselves over time, and they include riots and revolutions, as well as friendships and love affairs. *Coupling* is defined as the entrainment, cooperation, or coordination of system elements that continually adjust to each other as feedback ensues. These elements, like participants in a revolution or people in love, may be viewed as whole structures or systems at a more microscopic level, but their coordination with each other permits them to work together as constituents of a larger, macroscopic whole (see Maturana & Varela, 1980).

Positive feedback in cognition–emotion interactions expresses the idea of reciprocal causation between cognitive appraisal and emotion. This idea is an extension of some fundamental tenets of emotion theory. Cognitive appraisal gives rise to emotion when it denotes a class of situations relevant to the self and its goals (e.g., Lazarus, 1966; Stein & Trabasso, 1992). Emotion, in turn, directs perceptual and cognitive activity to possibilities for influencing those situations (e.g., attention to an obstacle, threat, or loss) through adaptive behavior (Frijda, 1986; Isen, 1984; Izard & Malatesta, 1987). As argued by Frijda (1993b), these cognitive activities *following* emotion can be regarded as an additional appraisal process, more complex and comprehensive than the initial appraisal because it incorporates more aspects of the present situation. Related concepts of secondary appraisal have been proposed by other theorists (Fischer, Shaver, & Carnochan, 1990; Kagan, 1978; Lazarus, 1966). However, in our view, cognitive appraisal before and after emotion constitutes a continuous process, as does emotion itself. Emotion is continuously enhanced or modified by changes in appraisal, whereas appraisal is progressively updated by cognitive adjustments resulting from emotion. As shown in Figure 2, this constitutes a feedback cycle. As emotional states arise, positive feedback permits cognitive and emotional activities to fuel each other through an emerging appraisal of a particular situation. Cognition–emotion interaction feeds on itself, growing from a rudimentary response to a full-blown interpretation and complementary emotional state. As noted earlier, we call this emergent form an EI, because it includes complementary emotional and interpretive processes in a coherent macroscopic relation.

The emergence and stabilization of an EI requires coherence within the cognitive system. In our view, this coherence depends on the coupling of microscopic cognitive elements or subsystems—including images, associations, propositional forms, script elements, and concepts—within a meaningful appraisal. Such appraisals may include past ("mood-congruent") memo-

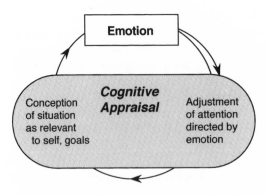

Figure 2. Cognition–emotion feedback loop. Positive feedback between emotion and appraisal fuels the emergence of a coherent interpretation of a given situation.

ries as well as novel assemblies created on the fly. But how do they arise and cohere in an emotional episode? We postulate that an emotion serves to catalyze links among cognitive elements by favoring combinations that fit the general class of situations related to that emotion. In anger, for example, goal frustration and reduced personal agency are templates for cognitive coupling—common denominators of emergent appraisals. Cognitive elements couple in ways that are consonant with these themes because, in doing so, they participate in the energy flow of the feedback cycle. At the same time, this coupling produces a coherent interpretation of the present situation, concatenated with immediate perceptual and attentional processes. Coherence serves to enhance and perpetuate the activation of the emotional state, closing the autocatalytic loop. The end result of this coherence is the stabilization of cognition–emotion feedback—or, coupling on a macroscopic level between an emotion and a cognitive interpretation—to form an EI.

Thus, while an incipient emotional response can be triggered by a variety of perceptual or cognitive events, an emotional interpretation keeps cognition and emotion resonating with each other for a period of minutes or hours. For example, a curt reply from a colleague may elicit a first trace of anger because of a fragmentary association with a parent or sibling. This anger may in turn, highlight images of social powerlessness, such as seeing oneself as unappreciated as the colleague rushes off to a meeting. These elements converge to a script for being dismissed by a valued other, augmenting the anger: Where does he think he's going? Who does he think he is?! The theme of rejection may also pull in imagery about the unavailability of needed others, evoking sadness as well as anger, while sadness heightens awareness of cues related to loss. Thus, a "reasonable" interpretation crystallizes and maintains one's angry–sad emotional state, while other potential interpretations (e.g., he may be rushing off because he doesn't want to be late) become less accessible. At the microscopic level, coupling among cognitive elements holds together inferences about personal powerlessness, thwarted needs for intimacy, and so forth. At the macroscopic level, feedback stabilizes between a comprehensive interpretation of the present situation and an elaborated emotional state.

Self-organizing EIs help explain the coherence and duration of cognition–emotion assemblies. According to Ekman (1984), emotions are brief responses to events, generally lasting only a matter of seconds. Yet, as noted by Frijda (1993a), individuals often report "instances" of an emotion lasting over an hour, with a median of 3–6 hours in one study. Ekman (1984) believes that long-lasting emotions result from enduring elicitors or from summation over several brief emotion episodes. Yet this explanation implies a passive role for the individual, living in a world of objectively-defined events of varying frequencies and durations. Instead, we regard the individual as creating the events which perpetuate his or her emotions. Appraisals are enduring elicitors in their own right, bringing the world into focus in a particular way. Like Frijda, Mesquita, Sonnemans, and van Goozen (1991), we see typical emotion episodes as processes rather than states (though they include states): specifically, self-organizing processes that supply their own coherence and relevance. A challenge for our model is to find a theoretical formalism to predict why some EIs do not endure despite their coherence.

Two DS terms can now be reintroduced. First, as noted earlier, EIs that stabilize repeatedly for a particular individual can be described as attractors on an emotional landscape. These attractors may be more or less accessible at given times, depending on mood, present circumstances, and so forth. On each occasion, movement to one of several attractors representing a range of conceivable interpretations defines the "choices" for microdevelopment. In the example given, one might have become solicitous, aloof, scornful, or sympathetic when faced with an experience of social abruptness. The presence of particular attractors tells us which elements become coupled in which ways, providing insight into an individual's current personality functioning and, as shown in the next section, its history and development as well. Second, the rapid consolidation of an EI within a situation may be described as a phase shift in (real-time) emotional self-organization. The emotional landscape buckles and shifts (or one's activity shifts to a new region of that landscape) as attractors capture emotional behavior or repellors disperse it. At the moment of the phase shift, many possibilities are briefly available, until components couple and stabilize again. An example is the classic plight of the preschooler who falls down, dusts himself off, and retains his equilibrium until he spies his mother, then bursts into tears. In this situation, the sudden shift between appraisals from "I'm alright" to "I'm *not* alright!" accompanies a crescendo of emotion, while this emotion is not proportional to external events but rapidly self-organizing. Yet at the moment of the transition, there is high uncertainty, such that a sudden smile from mother could shift the microdevelopmental trajectory to alternative attractors of shared laughter or a comforting hug.

This picture of cognition–emotion interaction is consistent with Magai's claim that emotion traits select recurrent interpretations that are most compatible with them, while these interpretations contribute to ongoing emotional states (Magai & McFadden, 1995; Malatesta & Wilson, 1988). However, our global forms are attractors, not traits, thus highlighting the variable, stochastic nature of real-time processes. Moreover, the stability of emotional interpretations, and their recurrence over development, need not indicate "optimal" means of dealing with negative emotions (Thompson, 1993). Rather, stability results simply from the tendency for particular appraisals and particular emotions to enhance each other continuously and repeatedly. Contrary to conventional arguments, we suggest that cognitive strategies that smoothly and easily resolve distressing situations are not likely to be the building blocks of personality development. Rather, EIs that constitute flawed or incomplete resolutions are most likely to proliferate, because they keep the emotion system activated and supply the energy needed for continuing self-organization (Lewis & Junyk, 1997).

THE DEVELOPMENT OF EMOTIONAL LANDSCAPES

So far, we have looked at the self-organization of emotional interpretations in the moment, or microdevelopment. We have described this process as movement to attractors at which cognitive elements and emotions couple to form stable, coherent patterns. Self-organization at a (macro)developmental scale can be viewed as the emergence and crystallization of these attractors over months and years. For this crystallization to occur, recurrent emotional interpretations must alter the structure of their constituent elements, affecting their future activity.

When particular ways of seeing the world recur over occasions, attractors become deeper and more specific, constituting developmental change (Thelen & Smith, 1994). This occurs because coupling or cooperation on each occasion influences the way elements fit together on subsequent occasions. At the physiological level, coherent, recurring, neural firing patterns result from the simultaneous activation of neuronal groups within occasions (Edelman, 1987; Kelso, 1995). But what goes on at the psychological level? Particular concepts, micropropositions, images, and associations become more congruent with each other and fit more quickly and easily together (e.g., in scripts, plans, or propositions) as they become increasingly refined with use (e.g., Nelson, 1986). What develops, then, is complementarity. Of particular importance to social/personality development, complementarity arises between evaluations of the self and evaluations of the other (Sullivan, 1953). For example, a view of the self as needy emerges alongside a view of the other as unavailable, or of the self as "bad" and the other as rejecting. These concepts of self and other seem to be key semantic subsystems that become adjusted to each other over many occasions, resulting in appraisals or scripts that cohere rapidly in real time. Moreover, a considerable number of such scripts are available to each individual, giving the impression of a multiplicity of selves (Baldwin, 1992; Hermans, 1996).

In applying this principle to emotional development, we postulate emerging conceptual complementarities that select, and are selected by, particular emotions over repeated occasions. Thus, a likely interpretation of an emotional event grows out of the increasing compatibility of an ensemble of cognitive constituents with each other *and* with an emotion. At the same time, this emotion arises more rapidly and more predictably whenever this ensemble reconverges. Eventually, emotions may arise "automatically" from well practiced associations (Power & Dalgleish, 1997), but we suggest that the rest of the ensemble converges soon afterward. This view of recurrent coselection is consistent with evidence for enduring emotional biases and attributions resulting from repeated negative emotional experiences (Cicchetti et al., 1991; Dodge, 1991). But normative forms may arise through the same process. Most children begin to claim "It's not fair!" starting about the age of 5 or 6. This interpretation arises from components that are all compatible with anger (e.g., loss to self, violation of standards, inaccessibility of resources) and with each other. These components may not be able to coassemble before a certain stage of cognitive development (Case, 1985; Fischer, 1980). However, a corresponding emotion of anger may also be necessary to galvanize their links with each other. Thus, in both normative and idiosyncratic development, the honing of connections within the cognitive system, and between cognitive ensembles and emotions, may be responsible for a crystallizing repertoire of interpretations about the world.

In individual development, interpretations of emotional experiences converge to pervasive themes, sometimes called *emotion traits* (Malatesta & Wilson, 1988), and these themes can be seen as attractors on an emotional landscape. An emerging mosaic of attractors constitutes each child's developing landscape. As described earlier, these attractors include normative and idiosyncratic features. For example, the large-chinned individual in Proulx's (1993) novel exhibits "a smile, downcast gaze, the right hand darting up to cover the chin" (p. 2) whenever social anxiety arises. This attractor is idiosyncratic in its behavioral content, resilience, and accessibility from other states (its basin), but it includes the normative features of shame and hiding. Moreover, as these themes become more refined in macrodevelopment and quicker to emerge in microdevelopment, they also become enacted in increasingly diverse situations—and hence more "trait-like." This is because fewer contextual cues are required to trigger their assembly. However, in our view, context always plays a role, and the notion of traits needs to allow for indeterminacy and selection in real-time processes.

In summary, emotional interpretations of the social world self-organize on two time scales. They self-organize in microdevelopment with the convergence of an EI to an attractor. They self-organize in macrodevelopment as particular attractors become increasingly influential. To the extent that these attractors are idiosyncratic, they give rise to descriptions of personality development. To the extent that they are shared among members of a culture at a given age, they give rise to descriptions of normative cognitive and emotional development.

Yet the consolidation of cognition–emotion attractors does not proceed in a smooth, linear fashion with development. Development is marked by periods of rapid change and reorganization (Emde, Gaensbauer, & Harmon, 1976; Kagan, 1984; Spitz, 1965) and, as noted earlier, these reorganizations have been described as phase shifts by dynamic systems theorists (van der Maas & Molenaar, 1992; van Geert, 1991). Normative shifts in emotional development have long been related to parallel shifts in cognitive development. Examples include Spitz's (1965) 8-month anxiety, self-conscious emotions at 21 months (Lewis, Sullivan, Stanger, & Weiss, 1989), and the rapprochement crisis at 18–21 months (Mahler, Pine, & Bergman, 1975). However, personality changes also tend to be abrupt and dramatic (Magai & McFadden, 1995), and these transitions may coincide with normative changes when cognitive and emotional turbulence are at their height (Kegan, 1982; Magai & Hunziker, 1993; Mahler et al., 1975).

We view such developmental junctures as phase shifts at which novel cognition–emotion attractors emerge. At critical fluctuations in development, including maturational and environmental changes, coupling among cognitive and emotional constituents breaks down. The system has increased degrees of freedom, and novel patterns of coupling proliferate. These are chaotic junctures at which new interpretations, feeding back with emotions, can build on themselves over a small number of occasions. Coupling on each occasion increases the likelihood of their recurrence on subsequent occasions. Interpersonal factors are thus hugely important at these junctures and far less important between them. Some of these transformations are relatively common across children as a result of shared species-specific, maturational, or cultural constraints (Lewis, 1997). For example, the onset of defiance for many children just prior to 2 years of age may involve feedback between anger and self-assertion when the capacity for self-referencing matures (Lewis & Brooks-Gunn, 1979). However, there is also good opportunity for idiosyncratic interpretations to converge at these junctures. Some children become negativistic, others whiny and demanding, at this age. We are very much in agreement with Magai and McFadden (1995), who argue that a shake-up of expectancies and conceptualizations combined with strong emotions are at the root of abrupt changes in personality development.

Thus, at each developmental phase shift, some attractors on the emotional landscape shift and reform. New attractors may be globally consistent with those of other children, idiosyncratic variants of those forms, or highly individualistic. Yet the landscape as a whole becomes increasingly refined with development as new attractors reconfigure the orderliness already present in the system. As shown in Figure 3, this partial reshuffling of personality at developmental phase shifts results in a branching pathway of emotional diversification and specialization. New configurations are constrained by the "habits" acquired by cognitive and emotional elements from past constellations, tracing a history of increasingly specialized assemblies. In Figure 3, this specialization is denoted by finer branchings with age. The tendency for developmental progressions to fashion their own constraints, both resulting from and contributing to day-to-day experiences, is a chief implication of self-organization modeling (Smith, 1995). Thus, each newly achieved coherence affects the direction of further development in a progression of *cascading* constraints (Lewis, 1997). Yet each developmental juncture also provides opportunities to change directions (Kagan, 1984), including convergence toward the norm, because the system is highly sensitive to all kinds of influences—both universal and idiosyncratic—at phase shifts.

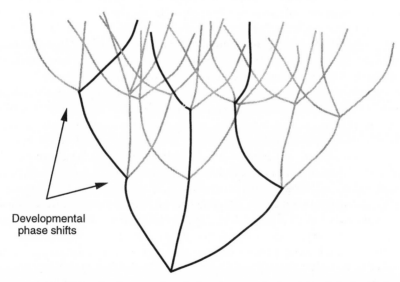

Developmental
phase shifts

Figure 3. A branching developmental path showing many potential trajectories. Trajectories represent emotional landscapes that become partially reconfigured and increasingly specialized with each phase shift.

EMOTION REGULATION AND SELF-ORGANIZING DEFENSES

Like other DS approaches, we have emphasized the bottom-up, non-directed features of development. But developmental outcomes reflect directed cognitive activities as well, including the intentions, goals, and plans that are crucial aspects of emotional behavior. A universal goal related to emotion is the reduction and avoidance of painful feelings, referred to as coping, defense, or emotion regulation. In this section, we ask how coping or defensive processes self-organize in development, and how they affect the development of emotional landscapes in general.

Emotion theorists view goals and plans as both antecedents and consequences of emotions. Emotions are elicited when goals or plans are implemented, achieved, or thwarted (Frijda, 1986; Oatley & Johnson-Laird, 1987), and emotions activate new goals and plans through their global effects on cognitive activity (Stein & Trabasso, 1992). If we consider goals and plans as ongoing concomitants of cognition–emotion feedback, then EIs become inherently dynamic. They not only change with the ebb and flow of new information, but they are also *about* change. They are about events over time, or changes in situations, through which goals are intentionally pursued.

Of all the goals we pursue through time, reducing or avoiding painful emotional states is among the most compelling. What sort of EIs could self-organize in the service of such "defensive" goals? Their cognitive constituents would have to include the registration or anticipation of painful emotions and a plan (conscious or not) to avoid or escape them. Their emotional constituents should then include fear or anxiety—emotions that activate plans to escape or withdraw from something aversive (Davidson, 1992) and prevent its recurrence (Stein & Trabasso, 1992). We know that anxiety motivates infants to look away from an aversive experience of mother in early coping behavior (Malatesta, Culver, Tesman, & Shepard, 1989). Later in development, anxiety may motivate *cognitive* disengagement by shifting attention to alternative interpretations of potentially painful events (Case, Hayward, Lewis, & Hurst, 1988; Lazarus & Folkman, 1984). If anxiety causes attention to move away from an anticipated painful EI, either through behavior or distraction, and if a new locus of attention stabilizes in its place, then a defensive *plan* has been served by self-organizing processes.

The self-organization of a defense can be traced through four phases: (1) the consolidation of a painful EI; (2) the elaboration of this EI to include anticipation, anxiety, and the intention to escape; (3) a phase shift to an alternative EI that accomplishes this escape; and (4) the stabilization of this defensive EI to an increasingly strong attractor. In the first phase, a painful EI of a familiar situation (e.g., being abandoned by mother at nap time + sadness) recurs over several occasions, coalescing to an attractor on the emotional landscape. In the second phase, this EI expands to include anticipation of this outcome and plans for escape (e.g., anticipation of a painful separation + anxiety + search for a stuffed animal to ease it). As argued by Thelen and Smith (1994), attractors *are* expectancies: Movement to an attractor is subjectively experienced as anticipation of a particular state. From the perspective of emotion theory, anticipation is a potent element of appraisal in its own right and has distinct emotional consequences, such as anxiety. Anxiety, in turn, induces goals and plans to avert the anticipated outcome. All these components become coupled with the original, painful EI. In the third phase, the coupling of these elements is critically perturbed by the amplification of anxiety, thus catapulting the system through another phase shift. At the same time, a new EI draws attention toward a more tolerable version of the present situation (e.g., "I don't need Mommie; my stuffed animals are much nicer"). Thus, anxiety disorganizes attention to the old EI and propels attention to a new EI that serves the venue of escape. Finally, in the fourth phase, the new EI consolidates sufficiently to capture and maintain attention. This results from feedback and coupling between a new emotional state (e.g., excitement, interest) and an altered cognitive appraisal (e.g., the attractiveness of the stuffed animal). Although residual negative emotion (e.g., residual or "signal" anxiety) may contribute to this new state, the meaningfulness of the situation has now been recreated.

Defensive self-organization may be aided by a specific effect of anxiety: cognitive disorganization. Anxiety is thought to hinder performance on various tasks by interfering with attention (Eysenck, 1979; Sarason, 1984). But anxiety also increases attention to threat-related stimuli (Mogg, Mathews, Eysenck, & May, 1991). Thus, cognitive disorganization may result from conflict between positive and negative feedback—a generic cause of fluctuations (Kelso, 1995). Anxiety may both draw attention to the original threat-related EI (positive feedback) and away from it, toward the sought-after distraction (negative feedback). These incompatible attentional targets are difficult to resolve and can perpetuate further anxiety. As a result of anxiety, then, attention may fluctuate chaotically, such that a practiced and familiar EI is unable to stabilize. According to DS theory, this may be exactly what is needed for the rapid assembly of novel (e.g., defensive) forms. For example, in neural networks, chaotic activation elicits autonomous search and the spontaneous formation of novel patterns (Happel & Murre, 1994).

What sort of state-space transformation might be expected in the microdevelopment of a defense? We propose that the original, painful EI changes from an attractor to a repellor, forcing trajectories outward, while other, less obvious interpretations become attractors that capture attention and emotion. These attractors are what serve as defenses. If this shift recurs over occasions, one or more defensive attractors become increasingly influential. Before long, the system gravitates directly to a defensive attractor, or moves from one defensive attractor to another, with the onset of anxiety in a certain region of

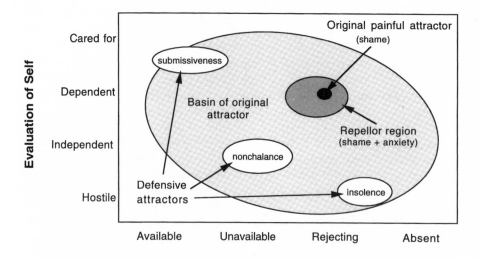

Figure 4. Defensive configuration containing shame/anxiety repellor surrounded by defensive attractors. These attractors (1) provide stable outcomes following chaotic fluctuations in microdevelopment, and (2) crystallize over repeated occasions in macrodevelopment.

the state space. The landscape portrait in Figure 1 represents this configuration. Several defensive attractors surround a predominant yet painful EI that has now become a repellor. The large basin represents all the states that initially gravitated to this EI. These states remain influenced by the *possibility* of returning to it, but gravitate instead to one of the defensive attractors that have sprung up in its basin. In Figure 4, we provide a concrete example of this defensive pattern, using the notion of self–other complementarity developed earlier. Anxious anticipation of shame has become a repellor surrounded by defensive attractors in which the self is construed as safe or invulnerable. Note that many states in the region *could* reflect complementarity between view of self and view of other, and thus be potentially stable. But the final outcome can only be specified through self-organizing processes. Moreover, the actual behavior of the other person is sure to be a strong influence, at least initially, among the forces driving the system toward one defensive attractor or another.

We also propose that defensive attractors are not particularly good solutions to emotionally challenging events. In fact, their inefficiency may be the very condition that favors their resilience. This follows from the postulate that ongoing emotion—in this case, negative emotion—is essential to maintain the coupling of conceptual elements in a coherent interpretation. Thus, we suspect that the best defense, if not a good offense, perpetuates some residual negative emotion, and most probably anxiety, in order to cohere, recur, and eventually crystallize (Lewis & Junyk, 1997).

If anxious EIs are indeed more chaotic than other EIs, they may provide a crucial inroad for intentionality. Chaos implies that the system has temporary access to a wide variety of potential states and can rapidly select any of them (Skarda & Freeman, 1987). This sensitivity may permit intentional mediation in the assembly of a defense, like jiggling a pinball machine while the path of the ball is still indeterminate. Children may learn to guide themselves toward defensive EIs as soon as they are aware of them. With development, this self-guidance grows from volitional motor behavior, to strategy rehearsal, and finally to verbal and subverbal self-cueing. In infancy, we see deliberate gaze aversion when mother returns from an absence, whereas preschoolers admonish themselves out loud, and later adopt an inner voice, to stave off helplessness and maintain a sense of control. Intention can be said to deepen attractors and guide trajectories toward them (Kelso, 1990). But its impact may be greatest when cognitive turbulence maximizes the potential for change.

Defensive phase shifts can be located on a macrodevelopmental scale as well. At developmental junctures, maturational changes and environmental perturbations set the occasion for new anxieties, and stable defensive EIs may become increasingly chaotic and repel trajectories toward new EIs. For example, the gaze aversion of the young infant becomes an inadequate means of emotion regulation when infants can no longer forget about hidden objects (Case, 1988), and the toddler's defiance becomes a source of anxiety when parents begin to punish disobedience (Dunn, 1988). The progression from defensive attractor to repellor to new defensive attractor may well be recursive at each developmental juncture, tracing a branching pathway of character defenses over a sequence of developmental phase shifts. As implied by Figure 3, branchings from one attractor to the next reflect cumulative individual constraints as well as novel influences (see Smith, 1995). To the extent that these attractors are defensive, each may resolve earlier conflicts while paving the way for new ones. These steps can lead to an enormous range of personality characteristics as habits of thinking and feeling become increasingly specialized.

Although defensive configurations are among the most important emotional interpretations, we believe that the role of anxiety and cognitive turbulence is more general still, influencing every aspect of emotional behavior and development. Whenever mental activity drifts toward painful interpretations in microdevelopment, anxiety concerning those interpretations can have a disorganizing effect on cognitive coherence. The vicinities of painful interpretations therefore provide less hospitable environs for the consolidation of new attractors in macrodevelopment. Regardless of the role of defenses, then, our capacity to form stable, coherent appraisals of life's painful junctures may be inevitably compromised.

DEVELOPING EMOTIONAL LANDSCAPES OF TWO INFANTS: AN EMPIRICAL ANALYSIS

The model presented in this chapter includes a number of propositions that have begun to be tested empirically, but this work is still at a preliminary stage. To give a flavor of where we are going, this section reports on part of a study conducted with Douglas (1996), following methods developed by Lewis, Zimmerman, Douglas, and Irving-Neto (1995) and Smith (1995). Our objective here is not so much to confirm the present model as to show how some of its terms and postulates can be demonstrated using a new type of dynamic systems methodology. We examined infants' emotional behavior following a brief separation from mother within and across three developmental periods. Infants are ideal subjects because they permit ready operationalization of cognitive and emotional constructs. Attention, a key feature of cognitive activity, was operationalized as gaze direction, whereas emotion was operationalized as intensity of facial distress. The principal goal of the methodology was to build state-space maps from the ordinal coding of videotape data. Here, we present maps for two infants at 2 and 6 months, and a descriptive follow-up at 10 months, to depict the development of individual emotional landscapes.

We videotaped the emotional behavior of 38 infants after a brief separation from mother, over three sessions (one per week) at each of the three waves (Lewis, Koroshegyi, Douglas, & Kampe, 1997). Separations were terminated when infants reached a predetermined criterion of 5 seconds of vocal distress, and reunions lasted 30 seconds (2 months), 45 seconds (6 months), and 90 seconds (10 months). The present analysis was conducted with a subsample of 4 infants, selected on the basis of diversity in reunion behavior at 10 months (Douglas, 1996). At 2 and 6 months, we coded gaze location and intensity of facial distress second-by-second on two 5-point ordinal scales (see Table 1). Distress intensity ranged from neutral to full distress. The categories of gaze direction represented gradations of engagement–disengagement, defined by the angle of the infant's gaze relative to the mother (Beebe & Stern, 1977). Interrater reliability kappas were .86 for distress and .91 for gaze (on 14% of all coded sessions). The corresponding values of the two variables were plotted as circles in the cells of a five-by-five grid, representing the state space for real-time self-organization. Event durations were denoted by the area of each circle. To show the sequence of activity in microdevelopment, we connected successive events (circles) with a line and included event numbers and arrows indicating the direction of time.

Attractors (outlined in grey) were provisionally demarcated as single cells, or clusters of *adjacent* cells, each containing behavior lasting at least 5 seconds in total duration. This arbitrary technique for defining attractors clearly needs formalizing, but it did an adequate job of discriminating dense clusters from relatively sparse regions of behavior.

Table 1.   Scales for Assessing Distress Intensity and Angle of Gaze

Intensity of distress
  (0) Contentment (happiness, interest or puzzlement)
  (1) Mild distress (troubled, uncomfortable or mildly anxious expression involving only one or two regions of the face, as defined by AFFEX)
  (2) Low-moderate distress (involving at least two regions of the face, i.e., eyebrows and eyes, or eyebrows and mouth)
  (3) Moderate distress (fully articulated negative expression, i.e., in all three regions)
  (4) Intense distress (cry-face)

Angle of gaze (Note: mother was positioned 45 degrees from infant's midline)
  (1) On-face (focal gaze at mother's face)
  (2) Peripheral engagement (within 15 degrees of on-face, including mother's hair, body or clothes)
  (3) Neutral (gaze at midline, plus or minus 30 degrees, playing with own hands, clothing, etc.)
  (4) Gaze aversion (gaze 30–60 degrees beyond midline)
  (5) Cut-off (gaze 60–90 degrees beyond midline)

At 10 months, gaze angle and facial distress could not be assessed due to infant locomotion, and we relied instead on verbal description. Here we present two infants only—those whose profiles changed the most from wave to wave. One session is omitted due to spoiled data.

A number of general predictions were made. Our first prediction was that cognitive–emotional activity would be concentrated in clusters defining attractors and return to these clusters regularly following perturbations or fluctuations. Second, these identified attractors were expected to be more consistent within waves than across waves, demonstrating stability of emotional landscapes within developmental periods and reorganization of landscapes across developmental periods. Third, identified attractors that were most consistent within waves were expected to demonstrate most continuity across waves, reflecting the crystallization of patterns involving frequently coupled elements. Fourth, however, qualifying this prediction, we expected high-distress attractors at one point in development to become repellors at some subsequent point, consistent with our model of defensive self-organization.

Jenny

2 Months

Globally speaking, at the age of 2 months, Jenny's attractive region varied across the engaged (right-hand) portion of the map (Figure 5), from mostly peripheral gazing at low distress to consistent, on-face gazing at high distress. In all sessions, behavior returned to identified attractors consistently following fluctuations. For example, in Session 2, the behavioral trajectory left

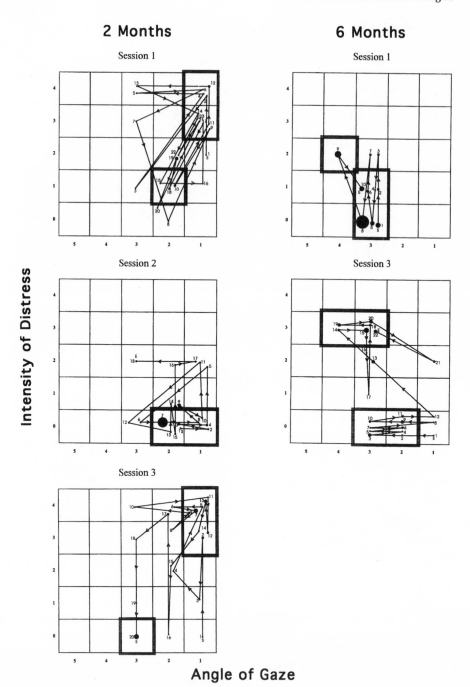

Figure 5. Emotion landscapes for Jenny at 2 and 6 months.

the attractor as distress rose, at Event 5, then shifted left to neutral gaze when distress dropped, and then "settled" once again. This cycle was repeated a second time. Thus, behavior was unstable outside a small, bounded zone, consistent with the definition of an attractor on a state space. The character of microdevelopment within sessions can easily be compared by glancing at the maps. For example, in both Sessions 1 and 3, behavior stabilized in the upper right corner (direct gaze) when distress was high. However, in Session 1, this organization competed with a second attractor in an ongoing oscillation, whereas in Session 3, the trajectory returned to the attractor following scattered fluctuations (until Event 15), became increasingly "wobbly" (at Events 16–17), and then left the attractor for good. Again, surrounding behavioral patterns were generally unstable. Overall, there was moderate consistency in the location of identified attractors across the three sessions.

6 Months

While trajectories generally remained in the engaged region at 2–3 months, behavior at 6 months shifted to the left, denoting a global tendency toward disengagement and gaze aversion. In both sessions, behavior tended toward neutral or peripheral engagement at low/absent distress—quite similar to 2 months. However, higher distress at 6 months moved behavior further left to moderate gaze aversion—a robust change from on-face engagement during distress at 2 months. Thus, a stable relation between distress and disengagement was a novel attractor, denoting a developmental reorganization. In session 3, for example, we see microdevelopment to this attractor with the onset of distress at Event 13. Subsequently, Event 21 provides a good example of a fluctuation, when a brief gaze at mother is insufficient to capture attention, indicating Jenny's refusal or inability to attune to mother even peripherally when distressed. Moreover, the absence of any activity in the upper right-hand region at 6 months suggests a repellor in a location of the state space that was previously a high-distress attractor. We therefore infer that the new disengagement attractor emerged as a joint product of normative change (Kaye & Fogel, 1980) and idiosyncratic, defensive reorganization.

10-Month Follow-Up

At 10 months, Jenny's style of engagement varied with distress once more. When distress was absent, she initiated affectionate behaviors (hugging, kissing). In two of the three sessions, however, mild distress emerged at the first physical contact following mother's absence, there was little successful modulation of this distress, and her behavior alternated between clinging and pushing away. She also initiated less face-to-face involvement, instead making self-soothing noises and facing away. This picture of variable, partially successful emotion regulation, somewhat suggestive of an ambivalent attachment style, provides an interesting sequel to the two phases of development preceding it. Most important, there was a clear shift from disengagement/avoidance to partial engagement during distress, indicating another reorganization. We speculate that this reorganization involved the breakdown of a defensive style, now ineffective due to normative developmental change (Case, 1988), replaced by a more specialized pattern drawing on tendencies from both prior waves. At the same time, developmental continuity was evident in the tendency *away* from full engagement when distressed, a pattern that was foreshadowed by the apparent emergence of an engagement-repellor at 6 months.

Scott

2 Months

In contrast to Jenny, Scott showed no consistency in behavior across the three sessions at 2 months (Figure 6). However, behavior regularly bounced back to transient attractors following fluctuations within each of the three sessions. Thus, our attractor construct remained useful for describing micro-developmental stability, but the prediction of within-wave consistency was not supported. The use of this methodology helped reveal an unexpected pattern: In each of the three sessions, angle of gaze remained constant despite fluctuations in distress, unlike the other three infants we analyzed. This may indicate less temperamental flexibility in attention allocation, hypothesized to impede the development of competent emotion regulation (Rothbart & Derryberry, 1981).

6 Months

At this age, however, the state space converged to what looked like the same attractor in all three sessions—peripheral engagement at moderate distress. The shift from transient attractors at 2 months to a single attractor at 6 months is an interesting example of developmental reorganization: Not only the content but also the "texture" of the state space changed. Also, the high degree of consistency across sessions at 6 months met and surpassed our predictions—a possible result of Scott's tendency toward attentional fixation. Yet the 6-month attractor was not a very effective resolution to negative emotion: Distress was much higher for Scott, on average, than for the other three infants at this age. This outcome is consistent with Rothbart and Derryberry's (1981) prediction, but it also indicates tight and recurrent coupling in the presence of ongoing negative emotion, consistent with our model. At 6 months, no other infant demonstrated this degree of consistency, and no other infant demonstrated this much negative emotion.

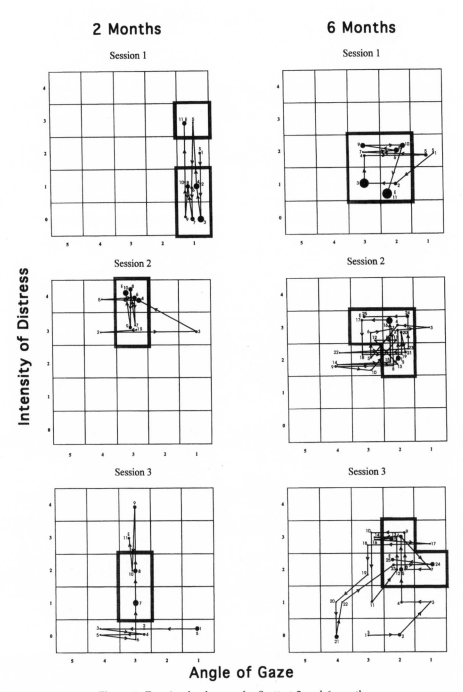

Figure 6. Emotion landscapes for Scott at 2 and 6 months.

10-Month Follow-Up

Scott's engagement with his mother was somewhat more variable at 10 months, but he generally showed little distress and no positive affect. In two sessions of very occasional distress, he began to approach mother immediately, but then directed his gaze at the door beyond her. In both sessions, this brief contact was followed by movement away from mother, increased independent activity, and sporadic eye contact from across the room. Although Scott usually tolerated contact initiated by mother, he did not reciprocate warmly. As with Jenny, both continuity and change were evident between 6 and 10 months. Scott continued to show disengagement from mother and absence of positive affect but changed from a stable, peripheral gaze fixation at 6 months to a more complex pattern of sporadic, distal contact at 10 months. Again, this reorganization may reflect a normative developmental advance, the wish to explore the world through locomotion, combined with an idiosyncratic defensive need to keep mother in sight.

These developmental portraits provide empirical demonstrations of some of the constructs and propositions we have presented. First, behavior was consistently found in a narrow range of values on both cognitive (attentional) and emotional variables, and returned to that range following fluctuations. This fit our prediction and provided a concrete instantiation of the idea of attractors on an emotional landscape. Also as predicted, these identified attractors were generally much more consistent within than across waves. More interestingly, reorganizations across waves lent themselves to reasonable interpretations based on our theoretical premises. Yet some behavioral characteristics remained similar across waves, hypothetically reflecting pervasive patterns of coupling among subsets of elements. Finally, in one instance, recurring high distress at one wave seemed to sew the seeds of a repellor at the next wave, consistent with our model. Overall, both infants showed branching pathways of increasingly specialized configurations, apparently integrating normative developmental influences with emergent tendencies from previous waves.

This analysis was intended to demonstrate how a nonmathematical, dynamic systems approach can capture the variability, diversity, and crystallization of emotional development in a coherent framework, and to show that the constructs we have presented theoretically can be translated into empirical measures. We see this as a step toward the development of a more precise, testable account.

ACKNOWLEDGMENTS.   Work on this chapter and the reported research were assisted by grants from the Hospital for Sick Children Foundation and the Social Sciences and Humanities Research Council of Canada. We are also grateful to Hal White for his valuable comments on an earlier draft of this chapter.

REFERENCES

Abraham, R. H., & Shaw, C. D. (1987). Dynamics: A visual introduction. In F. E. Yates (Eds.), *Self-organizing systems: The emergence of order* (pp. 543–597). New York: Plenum Press.

Baldwin, M. W. (1992). Relational schemas and the processing of social information. *Psychological Bulletin, 112,* 461–484.

Beebe, B., & Stern, D. N. (1977). Engagement–disengagement and early object experiences. In M. Freedman & S. Grand (Eds.), *Communicative structures and psychic structures* (pp. 35–55). New York: Plenum Press.

Camras, L. A. (1992). Expressive development and basic emotions. *Cognition and Emotion, 6,* 269–283.

Case, R. (1985). *Intellectual development: Birth to adulthood.* New York: Academic Press.

Case, R. (1988). The whole child: Toward an integrated view of young children's cognitive, social, and emotional development. In A. D. Pellegrini (Ed.), *Psychological bases for early education* (pp. 116–184). New York: Wiley.

Case, R. (1996). The role of psychological defenses in the representation and regulation of close personal relationships across the lifespan. In G. Noam & K. Fisher (Eds.), *Development and vulnerability in close relationships* (pp. 59–88). Mahwah, NJ: Erlbaum.

Case, R., Hayward, S., Lewis, M. D., & Hurst, P. (1988). Toward a neo-Piagetian theory of cognitive and emotional development. *Developmental Review, 8,* 1–51.

Cicchetti, D., Beeghly, M., Carlson, V., Coster, W., Gersten, M., Rieder, C., & Toth, S. (1991). Development and psychopathology: Lessons from the study of maltreated children. In D. P. Keating & H. Rosen (Eds.), *Constructivist perspectives on developmental psychopathology and atypical development* (pp. 69–102). Hillsdale, NJ: Erlbaum.

Davidson, R. J. (1992). Prolegomenon to the structure of emotion: Gleanings from neuropsychology. *Cognition and Emotion, 6,* 245–268.

Dodge, K. A. (1991). Emotion and social information processing. In J. Garber & K. A. Dodge (Eds.), *The development of emotion regulation and dysregulation* (pp. 159–181). Cambridge, UK: Cambridge University Press.

Douglas, L. (1996). *Emerging styles of emotion regulation in the first year of life.* Unpublished master's thesis, University of Toronto, Canada.

Dunn, J. (1988). *The beginnings of social understanding.* Cambridge, MA: Harvard University Press.

Edelman, G. M. (1987). *Neural Darwinism.* New York: Basic Books.

Ekman, P. (1984). Expression and the nature of emotion. In K. Scherer & P. Ekman (Eds.), *Approaches to emotion* (pp. 319–344). Hillsdale, NJ: Erlbaum.

Emde, R., Gaensbauer, T., & Harmon, R. (1976). *Psychological issues: Vol. 10. Emotional expression in infancy: A biobehavioral study.* New York: International Universities Press.

Eysenck, M. W. (1979). Anxiety, learning, and memory: A reconceptualization. *Journal of Research in Personality, 13,* 363–385.

Fischer, K. W. (1980). A theory of cognitive development: The control and construction of hierarchies of skills. *Psychological Review, 87,* 477–531.

Fischer, K. W., Shaver, P. R., & Carnochan, P. (1990). How emotions develop and how they organize development. *Cognition and Emotion, 4,* 81–127.

Fogel, A. (1993). *Developing through relationships: Origins of communication, self, and culture.* Chicago: University of Chicago Press.

Fogel, A., Nwokah, E., Dedo, J. Y., Messinger, D., Dickson, K. L., Matusov, E., & Holt, S. A. (1992). Social process theory of emotion: A dynamic systems approach. *Social Development, 1,* 122–142.

Freeman, W. J. (1995). *Societies of brains.* Hillsdale, NJ: Erlbaum.

Frijda, N. H. (1986). *The emotions.* Cambridge, UK: Cambridge University Press.

Frijda, N. H. (1993a). Moods, emotion episodes, and emotions. In M. Lewis & J. M. Haviland (Eds.), *Handbook of emotions* (pp. 381–403). New York: Guilford.

Frijda, N. H. (1993b). The place of appraisal in emotion. *Cognition and Emotion, 7,* 357–387.

Frijda, N. H., Mesquita, B., Sonnemans, J., & van Goozen, S. (1991). The duration of affective phenomena, or emotions, sentiments and passions. In K. T. Strongman (Ed.), *International review of studies on emotion* (pp. 187–225). New York: Wiley.

Haken, H. (1977). *Synergetics—An introduction: Nonequilibrium phase transitions and self-organization in physics, chemistry and biology.* Berlin: Springer-Verlag.

Haken, H. (1987). Synergetics: An approach to self-organization. In F. E. Yates (Ed.), *Self-organizing systems: The emergence of order* (pp. 417–434). New York: Plenum Press.

Happel, B. L. M., & Murre, J. M. J. (1994). Design and evolution of modular neural network architectures. *Neural Networks, 7,* 985–1004.

Hermans, H. J. M. (1996). Voicing the self: From information processing to dialogical interchange. *Psychological Bulletin, 119,* 31–50.

Higgins, E. T. (1987). Self-discrepancy: A theory relating self and affect. *Psychological Review, 94,* 319–340.

Isen, A. M. (1984). Toward understanding the role of affect in cognition. In R. S. Wyer & T. K. Srull (Eds.), *Handbook of social cognition* (pp. 179–236). Hillsdale, NJ: Erlbaum.

Izard, C. E. (1984). Emotion–cognition relationships and human development. In C. E. Izard, J. Kagan, & R. B. Zajonc (Eds.), *Emotions, cognition and behavior* (pp. 17–37). Cambridge, UK: Cambridge University Press.

Izard, C. E. (1993). Four systems for emotion activation: Cognitive and noncognitive processes. *Psychological Review, 100,* 68–90.

Izard, C. E., & Malatesta, C. (1987). Perspectives on emotional development I: Differential emotions theory of early emotional development. In J. D. Osofsky (Ed.), *Handbook of infant development* (pp. 494–554). New York: Wiley.

Jantsch, E. (1980). *The self-organizing universe.* Oxford, UK: Pergamon.

Kagan, J. (1978). On emotion and its development: A working paper. In M. Lewis & L. Rosenblum (Eds.), *The development of affect.* New York: Plenum Press.

Kagan, J. (1984). *The nature of the child.* New York: Basic Books.

Kaye, K., & Fogel, A. (1980). The temporal structure of face-to-face communication between mothers and infants. *Developmental Psychology, 16,* 454–464.

Kegan, R. (1982). *The evolving self.* Cambridge, MA: Harvard University Press.

Kelso, J. A. S. (1984). Phase transitions and critical behavior in human bimanual coordination. *American Journal of Physiology, 15,* A1000–A1004.

Kelso, J. A. S. (1990). Phase transitions: Foundations of behavior. In H. Haken & M. Stadler (Eds.), *Synergetics of cognition.* Berlin: Springer-Verlag.

Kelso, J. A. S. (1995). *Dynamic patterns: The self-organization of brain and behavior.* Cambridge, MA: Bradford/MIT Press.

Killeen, P. R. (1989). Behavior as a trajectory through a field of attractors. In J. R. Brink & C. R. Haden (Eds.), *The computer and the brain: Perspectives on human and artificial intelligence* (pp. 53–82). North-Holland: Elsevier.

Lazarus, R. S. (1966). *Psychological stress and the coping process.* New York: McGraw-Hill.

Lazarus, R. S. (1984). On the primacy of cognition. *American Psychologist, 39,* 124–129.

Lazarus, R. S., & Folkman, S. (1984). *Stress, appraisal, and coping.* New York: Academic Press.

Lewis, M. (1992). *Shame: The exposed self.* New York: Free press.

Lewis, M., & Brooks-Gunn, J. (1979). *Social cognition and the acquisition of self.* New York: Plenum Press.

Lewis, M., Sullivan, M. W., Stanger, C., & Weiss, M. (1989). Self-development and self-conscious emotions. *Child Development, 60,* 146–156.

Lewis, M. D. (1995). Cognition–emotion feedback and the self-organization of developmental paths. *Human Development, 38,* 71–102.

Lewis, M. D. (1996). Self-organising cognitive appraisals. *Cognition and Emotion, 10,* 1–25.

Lewis, M. D. (1997). Personality self-organization: Cascading constraints on cognition–emotion interaction. In A. Fogel, M. C. Lyra, & J. Valsiner (Eds.), *Dynamics and indeterminism in developmental and social processes* (pp. 193–216). Mahwah, NJ: Erlbaum.

Lewis, M. D., & Junyk, N. (1997). The self-organization of psychological defenses. In F. Masterpasqua & P. Perna (Eds.), *The psychological meaning of chaos: Translating theory into practice* (pp. 41–73). Washington, DC: American Psychological Association.

Lewis, M. D., Koroshegyi, C., Douglas, L., & Kampe, K. (1997). Age-specific associations between emotional responses to separation and cognitive performance in infancy. *Developmental Psychology, 33,* 32–42.

Lewis, M. D., Zimmerman, S., Douglas, L., & Irving-Neto, R. L. (1995, March). *Self-organization of infant distress: New methods for studying dynamic systems in development.* Poster presented at the meeting of the Society for Research in Child Development, Indianapolis, IN.

Magai, C., & Hunziker, J. (1993). Tolstoy and the riddle of developmental transformation: A lifespan analysis of the role of emotions in personality development. In M. Lewis & J. M. Haviland (Eds.), *Handbook of emotions* (pp. 247–259). New York: Guilford.

Magai, C., & McFadden, S. H. (1995). *The role of emotions in social and personality development: History, theory, and research.* New York: Plenum Press.

Mahler, M. S., Pine, F., & Bergman, A. (1975). *The psychological birth of the human infant.* New York: Basic Books.

Malatesta, C. Z., Culver, C., Tesman, J., & Shepard, B. (1989). The development of emotion expression during the first two years of life. *Monographs of the Society for Research in Child Development, 54*(1-2, Serial No. 219).

Malatesta, C. Z., & Wilson, A. (1988). Emotion/cognition interaction in personality development: A discrete emotions, functionalist analysis. *British Journal of Social Psychology, 27,* 91–112.

Maturana, H. R., & Varela, F. J. (1980). *Autopoiesis and cognition: The realization of the living.* Boston: Reidel.

Mogg, K., Mathews, A., Eysenck, M., & May, J. (1991). Biased cognitive operations in anxiety: Artifact, processing priorities or attentional search? *Behaviour Research and Therapy, 29,* 459–467.

Nelson, K. (1986). Event knowledge and cognitive development. In K. Nelson (Ed.), *Event knowledge: Structure and function in development* (pp. 231–247). Hillsdale, NJ: Erlbaum.

Oatley, K., & Johnson-Laird, P. N. (1987). Towards a cognitive theory of emotions. *Cognition and Emotion, 1,* 29–50.

Ortony, A., and Turner, T. J. (1990). What's basic about basic emotions? *Psychological Review, 97,* 315–331.

Power, M. J., & Dalgleish, T. (1997). *Cognition and emotion: From order to disorder.* Hove, UK: Psychology Press.

Prigogine, I., & Stengers, I. (1984). *Order out of chaos.* New York: Bantam.

Proulx, E. A. (1993). *The shipping news.* New York: Simon & Schuster.

Rothbart, M. K., & Derryberry, D. (1981). Development of individual differences in temperament. In M. E. Lamb & A. L. Brown (Eds.), *Advances in developmental psychology* (pp. 37–86). Hillsdale, NJ: Erlbaum.

Sarason, I. G. (1984). Stress, anxiety, and cognitive interference: Reactions to tests. *Journal of Personality and Social Psychology, 46,* 929–938.

Skarda, C. A., & Freeman, W. J. (1987). How brains make chaos in order to make sense of the world. *Behavioral and Brain Sciences, 10,* 161–195.

Smith, L. B. (1995). Self-organizing processes in learning to learn words: Development is not induction. In C. A. Nelson (Ed.), *New perspectives on learning and development: Minnesota Symposium for Child Development* (pp. 1–32). New York: Academic Press.

Spitz, R. (1965). *The first year of life.* New York: International Universities Press.

Stein, N. L., & Trabasso, T. (1992). The organisation of emotional experience: Creating links among emotion, thinking, language, and intentional action. *Cognition and Emotion, 6,* 225–244.

Sullivan, H. S. (1953). *The interpersonal theory of psychiatry.* New York: Norton.

Thelen, E. (1989). Self-organization in developmental processes: Can systems approaches work? In M. R. Gunnar & E. Thelen (Eds.), *Minnesota Symposia on Child Psychology: Vol. 22. Systems and development* (pp. 77–117). Hillsdale, NJ: Erlbaum.

Thelen, E., & Smith, L. B. (1994). *A dynamic systems approach to the development of cognition and action.* Cambridge, MA: Bradford/MIT Press.

Thelen, E., & Ulrich, B. D. (1991). Hidden skills: A dynamic systems analysis of treadmill stepping during the first year. *Monographs of the Society for Research in Child Development, 56*(1, Serial No. 223).

Thom, R. (1975). *Structural stability and morphogenesis.* Reading, MA: Benjamin.

Thompson, R. A. (1993). Socioemotional development: Enduring issues and new challenges. *Developmental Review, 13,* 372–402.

van der Maas, H. L. J., & Molenaar, P. C. M. (1992). Stagewise cognitive development: An application of catastrophe theory. *Psychological Review, 99,* 395–417.

van der Maas, H. (1995). Beyond the metaphor? *Cognitive Development, 10,* 621–642.

van Geert, P. (1991). A dynamic systems model of cognitive and language growth. *Psychological Review, 98,* 3–53.

van Geert, P. (1994). *Dynamic systems of development: Change between complexity and chaos.* New York: Prentice-Hall/Harvester Wheatsheaf.

Wright, J. C., & Mischel, W. (1987). A conditional approach to dispositional constructs: The local predictability of social behavior. *Journal of Personality and Social Psychology, 53,* 1159–1177.

8

Toward a Component Systems Approach to Emotional Development

Michael F. Mascolo and Debra Harkins

During the past decades, theorists and researchers have offered a wide range of perspectives on the nature and development of emotion. Toward one end of a continuum, theorists define emotions in terms of specific patterns of feeling and behavior organized by innate neurological pathways and biological substrates (Ackerman, Abe, & Izard, Chapter 4, this volume; Ekman, 1984; Izard & Malatesta, 1987; Panksepp, Knutson, & Pruitt, Chapter 3, this volume; Tomkins, 1962, 1984). At the other end, theorists suggest that emotions consist of socially constructed syndromes of cognition, feeling, and action (Averill, 1982; Mancuso & Sarbin, Chapter 12, this volume; Oatley, 1992; Shweder, 1994). A component systems approach to emotions (Scherer, 1984, 1994) holds out the possibility of integrating these two diverse traditions. From this view, emotional episodes consist of multiple component processes and systems that mutually regulate each other at the biological, psychological, and socio-cultural levels of functioning. In what follows, we elaborate on a component systems approach to emotional development, focusing specifically on the development of pride as a social, self-evaluative emotional experience. There-

Michael F. Mascolo • Department of Psychology, Merrimack College, North Andover, Massachusetts 01845.   **Debra Harkins** • Department of Psychology, Suffolk University, Boston, Massachusetts 02114.

What Develops in Emotional Development? edited by Michael F. Mascolo and Sharon Griffin. Plenum Press, New York, 1998.

after, we report the results of a preliminary study assessing developmental changes in pride-relevant behavior of infants and toddlers as they interact with their caregivers in achievement-related tasks.

A COMPONENT SYSTEMS APPROACH TO EMOTIONAL DEVELOPMENT

A component systems approach bears much in common with epigenetic systems (Bidell & Fischer, 1995; Gottleib, 1992; Mascolo, Pollack, & Fischer, 1997) and dynamic systems (Barton, 1994; Dickson, Fogel, & Messinger, Chapter 10, this volume; Fogel, 1993; Fogel & Thelen, 1987; Lewis, 1995, 1996; Lewis & Douglas, Chapter 7, this volume; Thelen, 1990; Thelen & Smith, 1994) approaches to emotion and psychological development. From these views, living processes consist of *integrative, self-organizing, multileveled* systems that coact with other such self-organizing systems throughout development. Systems are *integrative* in the sense that they are composed sets of interacting, interdependent elements that function together as an organized whole. The components of any system are dependent upon one another and cannot exist apart from one another. System elements are related such that a change in one part can create changes in other parts of the system.

A central component of systems is that they *self-organize* (Fischer & Bidell, in press; Lewis, 1996; Lewis & Douglas, Chapter 7, this volume). This concept of self-organization implies that no single element in the system is responsible for the functioning of that system. *Self-organization* refers to the process by which order arises from the interaction among system components. Elements within a system *mutually regulate* each other (Fischer & Bidell, 1996; Fogel, 1993). Mutual regulation involves the simultaneous adjustment of the activity of system elements to each other. For example, although the circulatory system is partially independent of the respiratory system, changes in respiration directly and simultaneously affect changes in heart rate and vice versa. Living systems are also *multileveled* in the sense that they are composed of hierarchies of multiply embedded component processes and subsystems (Bidell & Fischer, 1996; Mascolo et al., 1997). For example, the genome functions as the lowest level in the organism–environment system. Genes are located on chromosomes, which themselves are located within cell nuclei, which are located within cells, tissues, organs, organ systems, organisms, and a variety of embedded physical, dyadic, and sociocultural systems. As such, coactions among system components occur both *horizontally* within levels (e.g., cell–cell, organ–organ, organism–organism) and *vertically* between levels (e.g., gene–cell, organ–organ system, organ system–organism, organism–society) (Gottleib, 1991, 1992; Weiss, 1970).

The concept of mutual regulation directly implies that systems are open to outside influence and are thus *context-sensitive* (Bidell & Fischer, 1996). In this regard, the concept of *context* must be seen as a relative term. Context refers to that which lies outside of any given system or system component under analysis. The respiratory system may function as a context to the circulatory system; cellular activity can function as the context of gene action, and, of course, sociocultural systems function as contexts of organismic activity. Within development, transactions between a developing system and its context exert profound effects on the system in question (see Gottleib, 1992).

Thus, a component systems approach implies that behavior is neither a simple product of innate programs nor fixed stimuli from the outside environment. As stated by Thelen (1990), "Within a set of initial conditions and constraints, complexity arises that is nowhere contained in the initial elements alone" (p. 24). However, although systems are not fully determined by either their constituents or by their surrounds, systems are not infinitely flexible. As Fogel (1993) asserts, "Complex systems are more likely to be *ordered* than disordered, to settle into a small number of relatively stable modes of functioning, in which only particular degrees of freedom are permitted to the component parts" (p. 48, italics in original). Thus, systems theory provides a framework to conceptualize both stability and flux in living processes.

Emotional Episodes as Self-Organizing Component Systems

Traditional models of emotion proceed from the premise that emotions are discrete states defined by a central core. For example, Izard and Malatesta (1987) have suggested that "a *discrete emotion* can be defined as a particular set of neural processes that lead to a specific expression and a corresponding feeling tone" (p. 496, italics in original). Others have taken similar positions (Ackerman, et al., Chapter 4, this volume; Ekman, 1984; Tomkins, 1992; Panksepp, 1989, 1993; Panksepp et al., Chapter 3, this volume). Alternatively, a component systems approach proceeds from the premise that emotional episodes are composed of sets of interacting subsystems or component processes (Dickson, Fogel, & Messinger, Chapter 10, this volume; Fogel et al., 1992; Lewis, 1996; Chapter 2, this volume). From a component process view, emotion components mutually influence each other at all points throughout the emotion process. No single element in the system is primary in the organization of an emotional experience or episode. Rather, coherence in emotional functioning is achieved by the mutual interplay among elements in the emotion process as they function within social contexts. Thus, different patterns of emotional experience emerge through the self-organization of emotion components within a given context. Thus, emotional episodes function as sets of dynamic processes rather than as steady states, and are composed of multiple, interacting subsystems rather than fixed cores (Fogel, 1993; Fogel et al., 1992; Lewis, 1996).

Components of the Emotion Process

Emotional experiences and episodes consist of systematic changes in a variety of component processes or organismic subsystems (e.g., appraisal/ cognition/motivation systems, central nervous system (CNS), autonomic nervous system (ANS), actions, experiential/feeling, etc.). They involve the detection of notable changes in events, which then undergo meaning analysis. Meaning analysis occurs at various levels of complexity, from low-level, nonconscious information processing to complex and conscious representational activity. We use the term *appraisal* to refer to assessments of the relations between perceived events and one's goals, motives, or concerns (Frijda, 1986; Lazarus, 1991; Lazarus & Smith, 1988; Smith & Ellsworth, 1985, 1987). Note that appraisals are not primarily cognitive affairs; appraisals reflect evaluations of the *significance* of events for individuals (Lazarus, 1991) and thus are more about the fate of one's motives (Roseman, 1984) than they are defined by cognitive activity per se. Appraisal processes are involved in the orchestration of patterns of *bodily change*, including CNS (Ledoux, 1994; Panksepp et al., Chapter 3, this volume) and ANS activity (Ekman, Levenson, & Friesen, 1983; Levenson, 1994). Feedback from such physiological processes contributes to the *feeling tone* of any given emotional experience. Physiological activity accompanies and supports emotion-typical *motive-action-tendencies*. Motive-action-tendencies refer to the propensity of an individual to want to do something, and to do something within a given appraised context. Motive-action-tendencies include instrumental actions as well as facial and vocalic activity. The awareness of feedback from all ongoing emotion components provides the feeling tone of a given experience.

Mutual Regulation and Self-Organization of System Components

There is no prescribed sequence of emotion processes. From a component systems perspective, there are many routes to the formation of any given emotional experience or episode, and emotional components interact in many ways. For example, consider the interaction between appraisal and affective (feeling) tone in emotional processes. As indicated earlier, appraisal refers to the interpretation of the significance of events to organisms, and thus implies information processing and cognitive activity. Prior to any particular emotional experience, appraisal processes functions to monitor *all* incoming patterns of sensory data *in parallel*. Appraisal processes function by comparing such sensory data to complex hierarchies of goals, motives, and concerns. Much of this appraisal activity is nonconscious. Event appraisals implicating important motives and concerns generate physiological (CNS and ANS) reactions and concomitant feeling tone. The feeling tone provides feedback, which *selects* the initial feeling-generating appraisals from among all other competing appraisals for conscious attention (Brown, 1994; Brown & Kozak, Chapter 4, this volume; Lewis, 1995, 1996; Lewis & Douglas, Chapter 7, this volume). Thus, even though event-appraisals participate in generating physiological changes and corresponding feeling tone, feeling tone functions to bring these appraisals into the psychological foreground, and the emotion process continues. Of course, the route to this effect is not unidirectional. One's existing feeling state or mood strongly influences cognition and appraisal (Isen, 1990). Temperament, mood, and ongoing emotional episodes predispose an individual to appraise situations in diverse and complex ways. In this way, appraisal, CNS, ANS, and experiential systems coact and mutually regulate each other in the formation and evolution of an emotional episode.

To help clarify the concept of mutual regulation, the top panel of Figure 1 provides a sample illustration of one of the many ways that mutual regulation might take place. It depicts a simple example of mutual regulation as positive feedback between two simple component processes. Units A and B can represent any two specific emotion components (e.g., particular appraisal, arousal, or action elements). We assume that each unit both sends output to and receives input from other units (or from sensory changes from the social environment). Each unit functions according to its own operating principles, represented in Figure 1 by mathematical functions mapping patterns of input to patterns of output. Despite their independence as separate units, system elements mutually regulate each other and self-organize into fairly ordered patterns. For example, Unit A produces output based upon a simple linear function of the inputs it receives from the environment and from Unit B ($O_a = e_i + O_b$), leveling out at some maximum value. Unit B becomes activated as a function of the output from Unit A ($O_b = O_a$), also leveling out at some maximum value. In this simple network, in the context of patterned sensory input from the environment (e_i), Unit A would send output to Unit B, which would thereupon send output back to Unit A, amplifying Unit A's output. The process would continue until maximum output values for Units A and B are reached. In this model, because of their interconnections and output functions, Units A and B mutually regulate each other by sustaining and amplifying each other's activity in the presence of some pattern of sensory input.

Thus, if Unit A represented a particular appraisal that an event matched or violated a goal or standard, and Unit B represented a particular arousal component, the top panel of Figure 1 would provide a simple model of how appraisal and affect mutually amplify each other within a given context. For example, if a child were to run in front of one's moving car, an incipient appraisal similar to "a child is in danger" (Unit A) would excite experience-

Mutual Regulation between Two Units

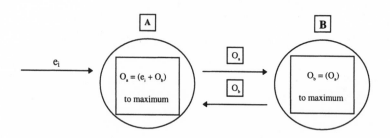

Mutual Regulation among Multiple Units

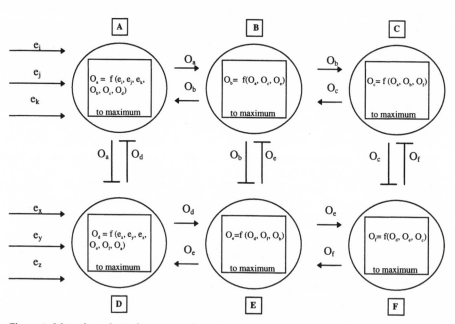

Figure 1. Mutual regulation between and among component processes. Letters indicate separate units that produce outputs according to output functions represented within each unit. Single arrows depict excitatory connections, whereas blunted lines depict inhibitory connections among units. Inputs e_i through e_z represent sensory inputs to the system.

related bodily changes (Unit B). As a result of the output functions and interconnection between Units A and B, bodily experience further excites the initial appraisal, which thereupon amplifies the bodily experience, and the reverberation continues to some maximum value. In this example, Units A and B have different functions in the creation of an emotional experience. Whereas Unit A processes motive-relevant events, affective reactions produced by Unit B function to amplify and *select* the appraisal "a child is in danger" (Unit A) from among all competing appraisals and inputs for conscious attention. In this way, neither the appraisal nor the bodily experience is primary; both organize each other in the production of an emotional episode.

Of course, the upper panel of Figure 1 depicts an extraordinarily simple case based on but one way in which system elements can coregulate each other, namely positive feedback. A somewhat more illustrative representation of the interplay among component systems could look more like the bottom panel of Figure 1, in which multiple units send both excitatory and inhibitory output to other such units on the basis of output functions that can be nonlinear as well as linear. Units A, B, and C might represent particular positive appraisal, affect and action components, whereas Units D, E, and F might represent parallel negative emotion components. Thus, any particular emotional episode is the product of mutual regulations among many emotion components, including appraisal, motivational, physiological, experiential, action, and other components. Indeed, each of these processes consists of systems composed of multiple component processes. As such, in a fully developed model of emotion, units such as those represented in Figure 1 would represent specific system elements (e.g., particular appraisal, arousal, or action components), rather than general categories of processes such as "appraisal" or "arousal."

Because there is a large number of component processes that are relevant to the construction of any given emotional experience, and because these component processes can combine in many different ways, it follows that the number of possible emotional episodes that can be constructed is extremely large. However, systems theory would predict that emotional processes have a tendency to settle into a smaller number of recurrent patterns, sometimes called *attractors* (Fogel, 1993; Lewis, 1995, 1996). Within each attractor pattern, system elements can assume an extremely large number of minor variations (Camras, 1992). This possibility is represented in the lower panel of Figure 1. As a result of the particular patterns of connections among units and their individual output functions, system units would self-organize into quasi-stable attractor patterns through mutual regulation. For example, activation of Unit A by environmental inputs e_i, e_j, and e_k would serve to mutually activate and amplify Units B and C, while inhibiting the activation of Units D, E, and F. Activation of Unit D by inputs e_x, e_y, and e_z would have the opposite effect. However, attractor patterns can assume a variety of minor fluctuations

depending upon many different factors, including the intensity and patterning of various inputs, the output functions of individual units, and the initial
states of activation of any given unit. For example, although environmental
inputs e_i, e_j, and e_k would mutually activate Units A, B, and C, the simultaneous activation of input e_x would modify the patterned activity across
Units A, B, and C through inhibition, while partially activating of Units D, E,
and F. In presenting Figure 1, we do not mean to propose any specific model of
emotion or mutual regulation. Figure 1 simply provides a general sense of
how mutual regulation might take place in a more specific component systems model of emotion.

Context as a Component of Self-Organizing Emotional Activity

According to the foregoing model, emotional episodes, like all psychological activity, are emergent phenomena that result from coordination and
mutual regulation of component subsystems. However, as discussed earlier,
living systems are highly context-sensitive. Organismic functioning is embedded in larger systems of social interaction and sociocultural activity. To the
extent that sociocultural and organismic systems mutually regulate each
other, social context must be seen as an actual *part* of the emotion process
(Fogel et al., 1992).

As an illustration of this notion, consider some observations that we have
made in a study on the development of emotional reactions that are generally
called pride. Parents were asked to play with their children and to prompt
them to perform a series of goal-directed tasks. Parent and children's behaviors
before and after success were recorded. Consider the following observation:

> A 19-month-old boy was being coaxed onto his fire truck by his father. The boy put
> one leg on the truck with an expressionless face. The father looked at the child, and,
> while smiling, said in an exaggerated high voice, "Can you get on? Can you do it?"
> The boy looked at the father, smiled, and sat on the fire truck. As the boy sat, the
> father said in a higher tone, "Yea! You did it! Yea! You did it!" After the first time the
> father said "yea," the child's smile widened, and the child clapped his hands. After
> the child had begun to clap, the father began clapping as well. The child then
> stopped smiling and looked down to the fire truck. The father indicated that in the
> past, he had often praised the child by saying "yea!" and applauding.

To the extent that pride experiences involve appraisals that the self is responsible for a socially valued outcome (Mascolo & Fischer, 1995), simultaneous
display of positive affect (i.e., smiling), social orientation (i.e., looking at the
father), and self-evaluation (i.e., clapping) in this situation suggest a pride-
like episode. We would argue that in this situation, the production of the
child's pride-relevant display was not simply a product of the processes that
occurred *within* the child. Rather, it required the mutual regulation of appraisal, affect, and action *between* the child and adult. The child's goal-directed

activity was directed and scaffolded by the parent's encouragement and directives. The child's smile and gaze at the parent was supported throughout task activity by the father's gaze, smile, and voice. The child's applause was prompted by the father's verbal praise ("yea!"). Because the history of similar interactions involving verbal praise ("yea!") and clapping by the parent, the child's applause can be seen as the result of the child's anticipation and adjustment of his behavior to familiar routines between the parent and child.

We would suggest that the pride-relevant behaviors displayed by the child in this example cannot be understood as a simple reaction to the child's success. Neither can they be understood as the simple expression of a discrete emotion encased within the child. In this situation, it is often difficult to determine where the father's emotional support ends and the child's emotional behavior begins, and vice versa. The emotional communication between the parent and child is continuous throughout dyadic interaction (Fogel, 1993). *The parent and child are simultaneously adjusting their behaviors to each other as they anticipate each other's ongoing behaviors.* Thus, the emotional behaviors observed were not simply products of activity within each partner; rather, they were *socially created* by processes that occurred *between* the child and the parent. In this way, emotional processes within both the child and the adult are context-sensitive. To the extent that the dynamic social context helps regulate and coordinate an individual's emotion components, context must be seen as an actual part of the emotion process.

The Functions of Emotional Processes

Emotional processes serve a variety of *functions* for individuals and their surrounding community, of which we will mention but three. A most important function of emotional processes, and particularly of emotional *feelings* is the *selection of perception* (Brown, 1994; see also Lewis, 1996; Mandler, 1984; Tomkins, 1984). If adaptation to one's environs were simply a "cognitive" or "rational" affair, a person would be required to constantly calculate the adaptive value of his or her actions. However, feelings that participate in emotional experiences serve the function of selecting from the vast number of perceived events that compete for attention those that have most significance for us. Within a systems perspective, because emotion components mutually regulate each other in the production of an emotional episode, appraisals both influence and are influenced by the very reactions they generate (Fogel et al., 1992; Lewis, 1996).

Emotional processes also function to *support and organize adaptive action* in the service of one's broad goals, motives, and concerns. Emotional action-tendencies function to maintain or advance the motives and concerns implicated in event appraisals as well as a person's broader concerns. Furthermore, changes in physiological arousal (CNS and ANS) that accompany emotional experiences support and facilitate adaptive action. The autonomic processes that underlie the supposed "fight or flight" reactions are a case in point. A third function of emotional processes is the *coregulation of social activity*. A large and still growing literature attests to the ways in which an individual's emotional facial, vocalic, and instrumental activity regulates social activity between them (Fogel, 1993; Trevarthen, 1984). Emotional behavior provides information to interactants that function to bring them closer together, create distance between them, or otherwise modulate social interactions relative to personal and socially created goals and concerns.

Defining Emotion from a Component Systems View

Based on all of the foregoing, we are now in a position to offer a definition of the events to which we refer when we speak of "emotion." In so doing, we differentiate between *emotional episodes* and *emotional experiences* (see Lewis, 1989, Chapter 2, this volume; Lewis & Brooks, 1978; Frijda & Mesquita, Chapter 11, this volume, for similar distinctions between emotional experience and other aspects of emotion). From a component systems perspective, an *emotional episode* refers to the patterning of all component systems (i.e., cognitive/information processing; appraisal/motivational; ANS/CNS; facial, vocalic, and instrumental action, etc.) in the context of notable changes in input from one's environment (Scherer, 1994). An *emotional experience* consists of the subjective awareness of feedback from the activity of the various component systems implicated in an emotional episode. In speaking of emotional episodes and experiences, we have refrained from offering a definition of "emotions" per se. This follows from the proposition that emotional episodes are the constructed products of ongoing organismic activity rather than independent entities or steady states encased within the individual.

If emotional episodes and experiences are defined in terms of patterned configurations of multiple organismic subsystems, what is it that makes a given episode or experience *emotional*? One important aspect that makes an experience emotional is the presence of affect or feeling. At least in the West, people tend to use the term *emotion* to refer to feeling tone (Lutz, 1988). As such, emotional experiences are felt experiences. However, there are several problems in defining emotion primarily in terms of feeling. First, although emotional episodes often involve feeling, they cannot be reduced to feeling tone alone; emotional feelings cannot be defined in isolation from other psychological processes. For example, there are many experiences that we call feelings that we do not call emotions (e.g., coldness, pain, the feel of one's hand on a table). One attribute that differentiates emotional feelings from other feelings is that emotional feelings most often have objects—they are *about* something (Campos, 1994; Solomon, 1976, 1980). I do not simply feel proud, I feel proud *of* myself *for* being a good provider or for getting an A on my physics test. This suggests that emotional experiences are like judgments or involve judgment processes. Although possible, it would be odd to say, "I feel proud, but I don't believe that I am responsible for performing a valued act." As such, emotional experiences go beyond mere feeling and include the functioning of appraisal and other organismic processes. To define emotional episodes as mere feelings would be tantamount to defining the whole in terms of a single part.

From a component systems view, in a given context, emotion components self-organize into quasi-stable patterns with many possible minor variations. As such, a component systems approach is compatible with prototype models of the structure and content of emotion categories (Lakoff, 1987; Russell, 1991; Shaver, Schwartz, Kirson, & O'Connor, 1987). Prototype models proceed from the view that emotion categories are not defined by sets of essential, necessary, or sufficient conditions, but rather are represented in terms of idealizations (Lakoff, 1987), prototypes (Rosch, 1978), or family resemblances (Wittgenstein, 1953). As such, any particular category of emotional states (e.g., joy, anger, pride) would be defined in terms of an idealized emotional theme or configuration of component processes, even though particular instances of any category of emotional episodes would vary widely.

Although a component systems approach provides a framework for representing the meaning of everyday emotion categories in terms of idealized or prototypical patterns of emotional elements, important issues arise in the use of everyday emotion terms to define the basic categories of emotional life. On the one hand, emotion words are an important way to communicate our subjective life to others. Everyday emotion terms represent emotional meanings that are salient to individuals within a given culture, and are thus worthy of study. As such, it would be a mistake to ignore everyday emotion categories in the study of emotional life. However, it would also be a mistake to assume that emotion words reflect fixed or final categories of extant emotional states. Everyday emotion words only make a series of more or less general distinctions that are salient to a given individual, linguistic community, or culture. Although emotion-related systems organize into ordered patterns, the number of possible emotional experiences is quite large. To the extent that there are more emotional patterns than there are words to describe them, thinking about emotion processes in terms of conventional emotion words may blind us to important distinctions.

Based on this sort of thinking, Kagan (1994) suggests that the study of emotion proceed from a Baconian inductivist strategy. Within this mode, instead of setting out to investigate affective states labeled by ordinary emotion words, psychologists would begin their research with detailed observation of emotional phenomena within specified or controlled contexts. The naming of emotional states would begin only after fine-grained observation produced evidence of the clustering of emotional components within and across contexts. Using such an approach, investigators might observe emotional patterns that would otherwise be obscured by everyday emotion words. However, although an inductivist approach offers the promise of precision, it brings its own problems. There is nothing in an individual's observable behavior that marks it as "emotional"; the characterization of another's behavior as "emotional" necessarily involves attributions that are founded upon subjective and intersubjective experience. As such, even the most careful observations of emotional behavior are ultimately informed by subjective and intersubjective meanings reflected by everyday emotion concepts.

Individual emotional episodes consist of both private and public elements. As such, it is unlikely that we can offer a precise model of the nature of individual emotional episodes based exclusively on the meaning of everyday emotion words or careful observations of emotional behavior in others. One strategy must inform the other. Our present work on the development of self-evaluative emotion is informed by the everyday concept of *pride*. In so doing, we use the everyday notion of pride to build an initial model of the development of children's positive, self-evaluative emotional reactions. Observations of children's behaviors in situations that may be regarded as "pride-relevant" can help us ultimately to extend or refine the concept of pride, or perhaps discard it as a more precise model of self-evaluative emotional development begins to take form.

THE DEVELOPMENT OF SELF-EVALUATIVE EMOTIONAL EXPERIENCES AND EPISODES

To the extent that emotional experiences and episodes involve the patterned activity of multiple component systems, it follows that emotional episodes would undergo developmental transformation as their components and relations among components change (Sroufe, 1979, 1996). To illustrate this process, we examine developmental changes in the self-evaluative emotional episodes that we call *pride*. Pride experiences involve complex social, self-evaluative processes. They not only require some awareness of self, but also that one adopt an evaluative stance toward the self with reference to social standards. The component systems that compose pride episodes and experiences involve *appraisals* that one is responsible for a socially valued activity or for being a socially valued person, *internal bodily reactions* including increased heart rate, changes in skin conductance and respiration, along with *motive-action-tendencies* to present one's worthy self or act to others. In pride, one *experiences* one's bodily state as bigger, stronger, taller, expanding, or "on top of the world" (see Barrett, 1995, Chapter 5, this volume; Davitz, 1969; Heckhausen, 1984; Lewis, Alessandri, & Sullivan, 1992; Mascolo & Fischer, 1995; Stipek, Recchia, & McClintic, 1992). Table 1 displays a model of develop-

Table 1. Developmental Changes in Pride-Relevant Appraisal, Action, and Social Systems

Step	Appraisal components	Action components	Social scaffolding
1	*Action-effect contingency.* Child connects sensorimotor action with its effect.	*Positive affect.* Single positive affective behaviors (e.g., smile, laugh).	*Emotional scaffolding.* Within coregulated parent–child interactions, parents not only scaffold the child's task activity by giving directives and by performing part of the task for the child, but they also "scaffold" and help regulate the child's emotional reaction itself. This is accomplished *throughout the entire course of goal-directed activity* through the parent's *gaze* (looking at the child), *tone of voice* (high affective content, heightened pitch), *facial behavior* (smiles), use of *encouragement, praise, frustration moderation*, and *direction of the child's attention* to positive aspects of her or his performance.
2	*Awareness of self as an agent of an outcome.* Child completes goal-directed action and is aware of the self as the cause of the outcome. Child is aware of meeting simple outcome standards (e.g., getting a ball in a container; knocking over a bowling pin). Child makes an appraisal like "I threw it!"	*Emergence of outcome, social, and evaluative orientation.* At least two of the following: (a) *positive affect*; (b) *outcome reaction* (i.e. behavior resulting from an outcome per se rather than an evaluation of an outcome, e.g., pausing to "regard the outcome" or excited exclamations or movements); (c) *social referencing* (e.g., looking at other); (d) *postural changes* (e.g., chin up, chest out); or (e) *self-evaluations* (e.g., clapping hands, hands in air, positive verbal comments).	
3	*Awareness of self as a competent agent.* Child completes out a goal-directed action evaluated as special, is aware that the outcome was caused by the self, and attributes the outcome to the self's competence. Child makes an appraisal such as "I can throw the ball far!" or "I'm good at throwing!"	*Affective self-evaluation.* Three or more pride-relevant components that reflect affective self-evaluation using social standards, for example, (a) *positive affect*, (b) *social referencing*, and (c) *self-evaluation.* Other combinations are also possible.	*Increasingly individuated emotional activity.* With development, the child's emotional behaviors become increasingly coordinated, internalized and produced by the child him- or herself. The child exhibits emotional behaviors that are less tied to direct parental input. In social interaction, coregulation may become more symmetrical as the child's emotional behaviors become increasingly coordinated and internalized.
4	*Comparative assessments of self's competence.* The child compares concrete competence in two situations ("I'm good at running and jumping!"), or engages in social comparisons of competence ("I can throw far, just like Mom!" or "I can throw farther than Dad!")	*Affective self-evaluation.* Child exhibits affective self-evaluation as in Step 3, but tied to social comparison. Self-evaluation is more complex (e.g., "I won"). Child may show more complex coordinations of multiple pride behaviors.	

mental changes within three pride-related subsystems, including appraisal, action, and social systems. Although each system is somewhat distinct from the others, they nevertheless coregulate each other and cannot function independently of one another. We first examine developmental changes in each subsystem separately and then discuss ways in which these systems interact in the development and production of pride experiences and episodes.

Developmental Changes in Pride-Relevant Appraisals

Table 1 proposes four steps in the development of pride-relevant appraisal processes. As indicated earlier, in general, pride episodes involve appraisals that the self is responsible for performing a socially valued action or for being a socially valued person. As such, each step in the proposed sequence represents an increasingly differentiated and coordinated form of making this appraisal from early infancy through the preschool years. These steps are only four in a series of steps that can be proposed between birth and adulthood (Mascolo & Fischer, 1995).

We suggest that the first step in the development of pride-relevant appraisals consists of the capacity to become aware of *action-effect contingencies*. This is a very early developing skill, which itself undergoes a series of transformations throughout infancy (Mascolo & Fischer, 1995). For example, Watson and Ramey (1972) demonstrated that within days of exposure to mobiles that responded to subtle head movements, 8-week-olds infants smiled as their actions resulted in movements of the mobiles. Piaget's (1952) descriptions of infant smiles during secondary circular reactions are also illustrative of such reactions. Although these data suggest that very young infants are capable of reacting emotionally to self-caused effects, children's awareness of self at these early ages is still quite undeveloped. At Step 2, beginning around 20 months of age, the child develops a more sophisticated *awareness of the self as an agent of outcomes*. This step corresponds with the development of the onset of self-recognition and the ability to represent simple outcome standards. At this step, the child can represent him- or herself as an agent who caused an outcome and is thus capable of making appraisals such as "I did it!" or a nonverbal equivalent. Children's emotional reactions to self-caused actions change around this age. Heckhausen (1987; J. Heckhausen, 1988) has reported that beginning around 14–20 months, children stop and notice results of their acts. Bullock and Lutkenhaus (1988) suggest that this occurs when children can focus on outcomes per se rather than on the flow of activity. Kagan (1981) reported that smiles on completion of goal-directed acts increased between 20 and 24 months, around the same time children show self-recognition (Bertenthal & Fischer, 1978; Lewis & Brooks-Gunn, 1978) and distress after inability to imitate modeled acts.

At Step 3, *awareness of self as a competent agent*, beginning around 2½ years of age, the child is not only able to construct an awareness that he or she performed an outcome, but also that the outcome is *valued* and/or that the self is *competent* (e.g., "I'm good at it!"). Several studies suggest that between about 2½ and 3 years of age, children begin to evaluate themselves positively in the context of achievement. Lewis et al. (1992) reported such reaction in 3-year-olds in basketball toss and drawing tasks. Halisch and Halisch (1980, cited in Heckhausen, 1984) reported pride-like reactions in 2½-year-olds in a ring-stacking task. Only indirect evidence suggests that such reactions are mediated by a sense of competence. Geppert and Kuster (1983) reported that although 18- 30-month-olds used their name, "I," or "me" to indicate that they wanted to complete interrupted tasks, only children older than 30 months made statements such as "I can do it alone" and tried to stop adults from completing the last step of tasks. This suggests that 30-month-olds were concerned with demonstrating their competence, whereas younger children simply wanted to continue to participate in interrupted activities.

At Step 4, *comparative assessments of the self's actions*, beginning around 3 or 3½ years of age, the child is able to compare his or her performance with that of others within a given context. Such comparisons can take place in a variety of contexts, including competition (winning or losing in a competitive task or game) or identification (comparing one's performance with that of a valued other). In studies employing competitive ring stacking, Stipek, Reccia, and McClintic (1992) reported that although children older than 32 months smiled more after winning than losing at competitive ball stacking, only 3½-year-olds appreciated competition as shown by pausing, slowing down, or stopping after losing. Of course, social comparisons are simply one step along the path in the development of pride-relevant appraisals; multiple additional forms of appraisal occur beyond this point (see Mascolo and Fischer, 1995, for further details).

Developmental Changes in Pride-Related Action-Tendencies

In the preceding section, we cited evidence from studies on the development of pride behaviors to make inferences about children's capacities to construct pride-relevant appraisals at various points in development. On the one hand, we believe that appraisal processes are powerful determinants of emotion action-tendencies and that much is to be gained by specifying the types of specific appraisals that can lead to specific emotional action-tendencies. On the other hand, we maintain that appraisal processes are not the only determinants of emotional action-tendencies. There is no reason to assume that there is a one-to-one correspondence with pride appraisals and pride behaviors. Appraisal and action components are partially independent systems that mutually regulate each other and coact with other systems in the production of any pride-relevant episode.

Different researchers have used different criteria to define and identify pride episodes in children and have thus reported the emergence of pride episodes at different ages (Heckhausen, 1988; Lewis et al., 1992; Stipek et al., 1992). For example, defining pride as the production of three or more pride-relevant behaviors, Lewis et al. (1992) reported the emergence of pride episodes around age 3. Using more permissive criteria, other researchers have reported the emergence of pride episodes (Heckhausen, 1988) and individual pride behaviors (e.g., smiles, clapping, positive exclamations, calling attention; Stipek et al., 1992) in 1- and 2-year-olds. Our interpretation of this conflict is that pride episodes do not emerge fully formed in the child but emerge in simpler forms prior to more complex forms (see Fischer & Bidell, 1991; Mascolo & Fischer, 1995).

Based upon our own research (which follows) and our review of the relevant literature, we have focused on five categories of behaviors that we consider pride-relevant in the context of success. They include (1) *positive affect* (e.g., smiling, laughter); (2) *outcome and excited reactions*, reactions to causing an outcome per se and which are not necessarily evaluative (e.g., pausing to "regard an outcome," excited movements, exclamations (e.g., "eek!")); (3) *social referencing* (e.g., looking to others); (4) *postural changes* (e.g., head up, shoulders back); (5) *self-evaluation* (e.g., clapping, raising hands in air, positive verbal comments). Although many of these behaviors emerge relatively early in development, Table 1 proposes developmental changes in pride-relevant behavior. At Step 1, emerging in early infancy, we postulate that children will exhibit single pride-behaviors, and particularly simple *positive affect*, in the context of success. At Step 2, during the second year of life, children's pride-relevant behaviors become more complex. Children begin to exhibit multiple pride-relevant behaviors, for example, smiles accompanied by outcome reactions or social referencing. We suggest that such behaviors show evidence that children are beginning to anticipate social approval for their successful outcomes but have not yet internalized such evaluations and directed them toward the self. At Step 3, beginning around age 3, children begin to exhibit three or more pride behaviors following a successful outcome and particularly coordinations of behavior that indicate *affective self-evaluation using social standards* (e.g., positive affect, social referencing, and self-evaluation). Thereafter, one would predict further development of pride-relevant behaviors. For example, self-evaluations may embody social comparisons or more elaborate evaluate categories.

Developmental Changes in Pride-Relevant Social Systems

As discussed earlier, from a component systems framework, the child's processes are part of a larger system of social interaction. Within that system, the psychological processes of the child and other persons mutually regulate each other. As such, it is difficult (and perhaps meaningless) to attempt to delimit where one person's influence over the other begins and the other's ends. As a result, social context must be regarded as an actual part of the emotion process.

Although child and adult mutually regulate each other in social interaction, their interactions are not necessarily symmetrical. Initially, adults take the lead, guiding children's participation in interaction. Bruner and his colleagues have invoked the metaphor of *scaffolding* to refer to the processes by which adults assist children in their learning in a way that is contingent upon the child's own actions (Wood, Bruner, & Ross, 1976). According to Wood et al., scaffolding proceeds as an interactive process whereby an expert recruits the child's interest in a task, reduces the number of steps required to perform the task, directs the child's attention in a way that maintains the goal of the task, highlights distinctions between the child's level of functioning and the adult's ideals, controls frustration, and may actually perform part of the task for the child. Scaffolding functions to increase the child's level of functioning at a task beyond that which the child could attain if working alone. It is assumed that over time, children will come to appropriate and internalize the skills that they are developing within scaffolded interactions with others (see Mascolo & Fischer, 1995; Rogoff, 1990; Wood, 1988).

We suggest that adults support children's emotional processes in similar ways. We refer to the process by which socialization agents support emotional activity within the child as *emotional scaffolding*. Throughout a child's task-relevant activity, adults engage in a variety of behaviors that direct, influence, or otherwise support the production of emotion in children. In such contexts, parents not only scaffold their young children's task activity, but also they provide emotional scaffolding. Parental gaze, tone of voice (e.g., affective quality, pitch), facial behavior (e.g., smiles), frustration modulation, and use of encouragement and praise throughout the entire task provide direct support for the production of pride-relevant behavior in children.

This process is illustrated by the example of the 19-month-old, described earlier, who evinced pride-like behavior upon sitting on his fire engine. The upper panel of Figure 2 provides a visual representation of the production of the child's pride-relevant behavior as a result of interactions between the child and father throughout the child's task activity. In the first segments of the interaction, the father entices the child onto the fire engine by making a request in an affectively positive way. In the context of the father's ongoing positive affective display, the child looks at the father and smiles. The mutual positive affect between the child and father begins prior to the child's goal-directed activity and is sustained even after the child's success. This coregulated affect is indicated by the double arrows between the child and father. The child's success prompts parental praise, which is followed by a self-evaluative display in the child (clapping the hands). It is only at this point that the child's behavior reflects three central pride-relevant behaviors: smiling,

Nineteen-month-old Boy with Father

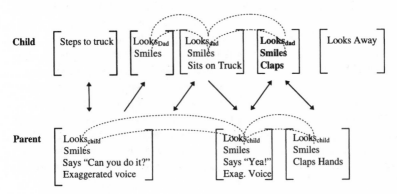

Thirty-six-month-old Boy with Mother

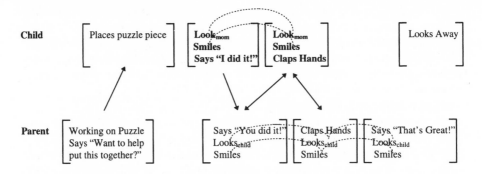

Time ──────▶

Figure 2. Structure of dyadic interactions contributing to the pride behavior in two children. Brackets indicate a single episode of activity coordinated over time. Curved dotted lines indicate that particular behaviors are sustained over time. Single arrows indicate inferred unilateral influence of one person on another. Double arrows indicate mutual influence (coregulation) of behavior. Note that both the 19-month-old's task behavior and pride reaction are supported by specific actions on the part of the parent. In contrast, the 3-year-old not only completes his task on his own, but it is his independently produced pride reaction that initiates affectively charged, coregulated interactions between the child and his mother.

looking at the father, and self-evaluation. Following this reaction, the father also applauds. In this example, the child's pride-relevant behaviors, marked in boldface, are the product of coregulated activity between the child and father. The father's emotional scaffolding is an actual part of the child's pride-like reaction, and the child may not have been able to produce pride reaction at this level of complexity without the parent's emotional support throughout the course of the event.

We suggest that such rich, social interactions provide the social matrix from which pride experiences and episodes are constructed in development. With continued immersion in social interaction, children appropriate and internalize emotional skills that allow them to construct pride episodes that are less directly tied to direct social interaction. To illustrate, consider the following observation of a precocious 36-month-old boy who exhibits pride-like behavior after putting puzzle pieces together:

> Mother and child are seated on the floor with puzzle pieces before them. Barely looking up from the puzzle, the mother says to child: "Wanna help me put these leaves together [motioning to two puzzle pieces]? I don't know. That might go there. Wanna try that one?" Mother and child look down at their respective pieces. Child puts two pieces together, looks up, smiles, and says, "Oh! I did it!" The mother then looks up and says in an affectively positive tone, "You did it!" The child begins to clap his hands, and then the mother claps her hands and says, "That's great!"

This interaction is represented in the bottom panel of Figure 2. Although the 36-month-old exhibited the same classes of pride-relevant behavior as did the 19-month-old (positive affect, social referencing, and self-evaluation), the 36-month-old's reaction requires little or no emotional scaffolding from the mother. In fact, the mother did not even notice the child's success until the child's pride reaction called her attention to it. Thereafter, the mother praised the child, which appeared to enhance the child's pride-like behavior. In turn, the child's pride reaction appeared to sustain the mother's positive affect in coregulated interaction. Thus, whereas the 19-month-old's pride behavior followed as a joint product of the activity of parent and child, the 36-month-old's behavior follows as a product of appropriated and internalized social evaluations.

These examples help illustrate the ways in which pride episodes and experiences are founded upon social relationships and are constructed in development through social interaction. They change gradually over time and take increasingly complex and internalized forms throughout development. As such, pride reactions are neither the result of the internalization of fixed cultural rules nor are they a result of the unfolding of a maturational plan. Pride episodes emerge from the coordination and mutual regulation of multiple emotion components as they function both within and between individuals.

AN EMPIRICAL ANALYSIS OF THE DEVELOPMENT OF PRIDE

This section describes a preliminary study examining the development of pride-relevant behavior in children between the ages of 1 and 3. In this study, we examined the types of pride-relevant behavior that children exhibit before and after success in achievement tasks, developmental changes in those behaviors, and the ways in which parents interact with children throughout children's goal-directed activity.

Twenty-eight children participated, 8 one-year-olds (4 boys and 4 girls, M age = 16 months), 12 two-year-olds (5 boys and 7 girls, M age = 26 months), and 8 three-year-olds (5 boys and 3 girls, M age = 36 months). Each child and a parent (all but one were mothers) were seen in their home. Children performed five tasks: bowling (five large plastic pins and a ball), ring toss (a plastic pole and three large rings for tossing), ring stacking (a sturdy wooden pole with five snugly fit wooden rings), basketball toss (small ball and a short, wide wastepaper basket accessible to young children), and jack-in-the-box. Parents demonstrated the use of the toy and then invited children to play. No additional instructions were given. Children played with the toys until distracted, began a new task, or were directed to a new task. Children's and parent's pride-relevant emotional behaviors before and after both success and failure were coded. Children's reactions were coded into the five categories described in Table 1. Parental behaviors included *positive affect* (e.g., smiling, laughter), *encouragement* (e.g., "You can do it," head nodding during goal-directed activity, etc.), and *praise* of child or outcome (e.g., "Good job!", "What a good bowler!").

Three sets of analyses were performed. The first concerned the development of children's pride-relevant behaviors. Children's pride-behaviors were aggregated across success in each of the five tasks. Table 2 displays the proportion of all success trials on which children exhibited each pride-relevant behavior. The main effects of age, individual pride behavior, and pride behavior produced before versus after success were significant ($F(2, 25) = 5.53$, $p < .01$; $F(4, 100) = 30.02$, $p < .0001$; and $F(1,25) = 54.30$, $p < .0001$, respectively) and indicated that the frequency with which children exhibited individual pride-behaviors after success increased with age. The most fre-

Table 2. Developmental Changes in Pride Components

Age	Smile	Excited reactions	Erect posture	Social orientation	Self-evaluation
1	.21	.37	.02	.27	.01
2	.38	.54	.06	.23	.07
3	.57	.52	.09	.37	.11

quent behaviors included smiles, excited reactions, and social referencing; note that self-evaluation and erect posture did not begin to increase in frequency until age 3. These results concur with Stipek et al. (1992), who reported developmental changes in positive affect (smiles) and social referencing after success in 1- to 3-year-olds, but extend her findings to include self-evaluations, excited movements, and erect posture as well.

The finding that individual, pride-relevant behaviors develop between the ages of 1 and 3 tells us nothing about changes in the complexity or patterns of pride-behavior. Stipek et al. (1992) reported that children exhibit individual pride behaviors upon success even at 1 year of age. Are these children proud of their accomplishments? Lewis et al. (1992) defined pride as the presence of three or more pride-relevant behaviors and reported the presence of such behaviors in 3-year-olds. To assess developmental changes in the complexity of children's pride behavior, we tabulated the mean number of different categories of pride-relevant behaviors (a number that ranges from 0 to 5) exhibited by each child before and after success and failure. The results indicate that across age, pride-relevant behaviors were more complex after than before success (Ms = 1.27 pride behaviors after success, .46 before success, $F(1,25) = 54.37, p < .001$). Most important, as indicated in Table 3, there was a trend toward greater complexity in children's pride-relevant behaviors with age, both before success and after success ($F(2,25) = 5.61, p < .01$). These results help resolve ambiguities in the field concerning the age of emergence of pride-like behavior in children. Like any psychological activity, pride does not emerge at any single point in development. Children begin to respond to success in affectively positive ways even at age 1. In so doing, they exhibit one or two pride behaviors, including smiling, social referencing, and outcome reactions (exciting reactions directed toward outcomes, enjoying the outcome). However, with age, children coordinate multiple pride behaviors upon success, such that the coordination of smile, social referencing, and self-evaluations begins to appear between 2½ and 3 years of age.

The second set of findings concerns the behaviors of parents to their children's task-related behaviors. Table 4 displays the proportion of trials on which parents smile at, praise, and encourage their children before versus after

Table 3. Complexity of
Children's Pride-Relevant
Displays by Age

Age	Before	After
1	.30	.88
2	.42	1.29
3	.68	1.65

Table 4. Maternal Behavior before and after Success

	Smile		Praise		Encouragement	
Age	Before	After	Before	After	Before	After
1	.42	.48	.17	.64	.41	.25
2	.18	.43	.06	.64	.22	.27
3	.33	.55	.07	.56	.17	.20

success. A significant age by pre–post success interaction, $F(2, 25) = 3.49$, $p < .05$, indicates that *after* success, parents smile at, praise, and encourage their younger and older children similarly. Interestingly, parents tend to smile at, praise, and encourage their 1-year-olds *before a success* more often than they do for their 2- and 3-year-olds. Parents tended to encourage 1-year-olds *more* often before than after success. The picture that emerges is one in which parents of young children lavish their young children in positive emotional support both before and after success, perhaps in an attempt to promote success and positive feelings. As children become older and more competent, parents become more discriminating in their positive reactions to children's behavior.

These conclusions are consistent with an analysis of the complexity of parental praise and encouragement. The complexity of parent's praise and/or encouragement was calculated both before and after success. This number was 0 if neither praise nor encouragement was present, 1 if either praise or encouragement was present, and 2 if both were present. As indicated in Table 5, parents exhibited more complex praise/encouragement after than before success at any age ($F(1,25), = 82.83, p < .001$). Furthermore, the complexity of parental praise/encouragement *declined* with age before success ($F(2, 25) = 3.64, p < .05$) but not after success, $F(2, 25) = .27$. This suggests that as

Table 5. Complexity of
Maternal Reaction before
and after Success

	Complexity	
Age	Before	After
1	.61	.88
2	.32	.81
3	.20	.77

children become older, parents become more discriminating by allocating less praise and encouragement to older children before a success.

A final set of analyses concerns the relations between parental pride-influencing behavior and pride-relevant behavior in children. Controlling for children's age, partial correlations were calculated between the complexity of parent praise and encouragement and various aspects of children's pride-relevant behavior. Significant relationships were observed between parental complexity and the complexity of children's pride behaviors ($r = .42, p < .05$), as well as the proportion of success trials on which children smiled ($r = .47$, $p < .01$), exhibited erect posture ($r = .33, p < .05$) and self-evaluation ($r = .44$, $p < .01$).

These results illustrate several aspects of a component systems approach to emotional development. First, from a component systems view, although emotional episodes are composed of relatively stable organizations of multiple components, such components can assume a wide variety of minor variations. Results indicate that children exhibit many types of pride-relevant behaviors following task success. With development, these pride components become combined in a variety of ways organized around the theme of affective self-evaluation using social standards. As such, pride episodes emerge as the product of the coordination of multiple component processes in both real time and in ontogenesis.

Second, results suggest that the formation of pride-relevant behaviors is not simply a product of processes that occur within children. Pride behaviors are affected by processes that occur between the child and others. Parents are not passive in the context of children's achievement behavior. Parents provide emotional scaffolding both before and after children's success, and parents who respond with complex positive reactions to children's success have children who themselves exhibit more complex pride-like behavior. Although care must be taken when making claims about the direction of causality in parent–child interaction, we suggest that parent–child interaction forms a dyadic system (Fogel, 1993) in which behaviors and characteristics of parents and children mutually regulate each other in achievement contexts.

Third, results suggest ways in which social interaction promotes the development of pride-relevant experiences. Although parents of 1-year-olds provided rich positive emotional support both before and after their children's success, as children became older, parents provided less emotional support prior to task success. This result bears similarity to the ways in which parental scaffolding of children's cognitive performance changes in development. As children become more competent with a given task, parents in Western European culture tend to "up the ante" and provide less scaffolding for their children's cognitive performance (Rogoff, 1990, 1992). Similarly, we suggest that emotional scaffolding of achievement behavior early in development helps to organize children's self-evaluations and pride-relevant behaviors. With development, children gain the capacity to produce for themselves the self-evaluations that were previously produced in joint interactions with others. As such, pride experiences emerge as children appropriate and coordinate self-evaluations and action patterns founded upon relationships with others.

Pride experiences arise at the intersection of emotion, self, and social relations. Each of these processes alone acts as an important organizer of human behavior. Emotion organizes behavior in contexts that have implications for the fate of one's motives; self-awareness organizes behavior as children attempt to make their actions conform to desired self-images; beyond its direct effect on behavior, social interaction provides the matrix from which individuals appropriate the standards they use to evaluate the self. Because pride experiences involve the coordination of these three spheres of activity, they function to organize the behavior and experience of the individual in social contexts that have implications for a sense of self-worth. Pride experiences make children feel good about their capacity to meet social standards of worth, which thereby organizes future standard-related behavior. Pride increases the child's sense of agency in a given task domain, which helps the child to approach related tasks with greater confidence in the future. Thus, pride experiences organize and are organized by children's evaluations of the self-position relative to the social order of which they are a part.

CONCLUSION

A component systems approach provides powerful metaphors for resolving many apparent contradictions in current discussions about the production of emotion. First, from a component systems perspective, different classes of emotional episodes are defined in terms of the patterned coordination of multiple component systems and processes. Even though emotional activity tends to become organized into stable general patterns, specific instances of an emotion category can exhibit an almost unlimited number of minor variations depending upon context and other local conditions. In this way, a component systems approach depicts emotional states as exhibiting both stability and plasticity. As such, a systems view (see also Lewis & Douglas, Chapter 7, this volume; Dickson et al., Chapter 10, this volume) can help resolve contradictions between models that portray emotions as tightly organized responses (Ackerman et al., Chapter 4, this volume; Izard & Malatesta, 1987; Ekman, 1984) and those that depict emotion as more dispersive syndromes (Averill, 1982; Harre, 1986; Mancuso & Sarbin, Chapter 12, this volume).

Second, from a component systems perspective, emotion-relevant component systems mutually regulate each other in the production of any given state or experience. As a result, no single emotional component is a primary determinant of an emotional experience. As such, a component systems view recasts the debate about the sequence or primacy of cognitive, affective, or behavioral components of emotion (Lazarus, 1984; Zajonc, 1984; Laird, 1984; Roseman, 1984). From a component systems approach, rather than working to determine any necessary sequence of events that occurs in the production of a discrete emotion, one would attempt to determine the ways in which emotional components mutually and continuously modulate each other throughout the course of an entire emotional episode.

Third, a component systems view embraces the notion that the affective activity of individuals is a product of coactions among multiple levels of the organism–environment system, including biogenetic, organismic, dyadic, and sociocultural levels of functioning. Functioning at any given level is never totally independent of the functioning of other levels. Emotional activity is thus the product of intersystemic functioning rather than functioning of any particular system or subsystem. Such a framework holds out the promise of integrating views of emotion that implicate genetic (Tomkins, 1962), psychological (Arnold, 1960) or sociocultural (Harre, 1986) determinants of emotion. Rather than reducing emotion to any single level of systemic functioning, a component systems view would attempt to specify the ways in which systems at various levels interpenetrate each other in the production of any given emotional episode.

A component systems approach provides powerful metaphors for conceptualizing emotion processes. Nevertheless, there is a need to move beyond metaphorical descriptions of emotion processes toward more specific models of emotion that build on ideas similar to those described in Figures 1 and 2. Researchers have enjoyed some success in proposing specific systems models of cognitive, social, and motor development (Fischer & Bidell, in press; Fogel & Thelen, 1987; Thelen & Smith, 1994; Van Geert, 1994), and such work is beginning in the domain of emotional development (Dickson et al., Chapter 10, this volume; Lewis, 1995, Chapter 2, this volume). Thus, to actualize the promise of a component systems approach, we need to particularize our metaphors into models that describe how specific emotion components coregulate each other to produce specific emotional episodes.

ACKNOWLEDGMENTS.   We wish to thank J. Nicholas Buehler, Kurt Fischer, Marc Lewis, and Raymond Shaw for their contributions to the arguments made in this chapter. We also thank Mark Morency and Mark Saviano for their assistance in data collection and analysis. This work was supported by a grant from Merrimack College to the first author.

REFERENCES

Arnold, M. B. (1960). *Emotion and personality*. New York: Columbia Press.
Averill, J. R. (1982). *Anger and aggression: An essay on emotion*. New York: Springer-Verlag.

Barrett, K. C. (1995). A functionalist approach to shame and guilt. In J. Tangney & K. W. Fischer (Eds.), *Self-conscious emotions: The psychology of shame, guilt, embarrassment and pride* (pp. 25–63). New York: Guilford.

Barton, S. (1994). Chaos, self-organization, and psychology. *American Psychologist, 49,* 5–14.

Bertenthal, B. L., & Fischer, K. W. (1978). Development of self-recognition in the infant. *Developmental Psychology, 14,* 44–50.

Bidell, T., & Fischer, K. W. (1996). Between nature and nurture: The role of human agency in the epigenesis of intelligence. In R. Sternberg & E. Grigorenko (Eds.), *Intelligence: Heredity and environment* (pp. 193–242). New York: Cambridge University Press.

Brown, T. (1994). Affective dimensions of meaning. In W. T. Overton & D. S. Palermo (Eds.), *The nature and ontogenesis of meaning* (pp. 167–190). Hillsdale, NJ: Erlbaum.

Bullock, M., & Lutkenhaus, P. (1988). The development of volitional behavior in the toddler years. *Child Development, 59,* 664–674.

Campos, J. J. (1994, Spring). The new functionalism in emotion. *SRCD Newsletter.*

Camras, L. A. (1992). Expressive development and basic emotions. *Cognition and Emotion, 6,* 269–283.

Davitz, J. R. (1969). *The language of emotions.* New York: McGraw-Hill.

Ekman, P. (1984). Expression and the nature of emotion. In P. Ekman & K. Scherer (Eds.), *Approaches to emotion* (pp. 319–344). Hillsdale, NJ: Erlbaum.

Ekman, P. (1992). Are there basic emotions? A reply to Ortony and Turner. *Psychological Review, 99,* 550–553.

Ekman, P., Levenson, R. W., & Friesen, W. V. (1983). Autonomic nervous system activity distinguishes between emotions. *Science, 221,* 1208–1210.

Ellsworth, P. E. (1994). Levels of thought and levels of emotion. In P. Ekman & R. J. Davidson (Eds.), *The nature of emotion: Fundamental questions* (pp. 192–196). New York: Oxford University Press.

Fischer, K. W., & Bidell, T. (1991). Constraining nativist inferences about cognitive capacities. In S. Carey & R. Gelman (Eds.), *The epigenesis of mind: Essays on biology and knowledge* (pp. 199–235). Hillsdale, NJ: Erlbaum.

Fischer, K. W., & Bidell, T. (in press). Dynamic development of psychological structures in action and thought. In W. Damon (Ed.), *Handbook of Child Psychology, Vol. I: Theory* (R. Lerner, Vol. Ed.). New York: Wiley.

Fogel, A. (1993). *Development through relationships: Origins of communication, self and culture.* Chicago: University of Chicago Press.

Fogel, A., Nwokah, E., Dedo, J. Y., Messinger, D., Dickson, K. L., Matusov, E., & Holt, S. A. (1992). Social process theory of emotion: A dynamic systems approach. *Social Development, 1,* 122–142.

Fogel, A., & Thelen, E. (1987). Development of early expressive and communicative action: Reinterpreting the evidence from a dynamic systems perspective. *Developmental Psychology, 23,* 747–761.

Frijda, N. (1986). *The emotions.* New York: Cambridge University Press.

Geppert, U., & Kuster, U. (1983). The emergence of "Wanting to do it oneself": A precursor to achievement motivation. *International Journal of Behavioral Development, 3,* 355–369.

Gottlieb, G. (1991). Experiential canalization of behavioral development: Theory. *Developmental Psychology, 27,* 4–13.

Gottlieb, G. (1992). *Individual development and evolution: The genesis of novel behavior.* New York: Oxford University Press.

Harré, R. (Ed.). (1986). *The social construction of emotions.* New York: Basil Blackwell.

Heckhausen, H. (1984). Emergent achievement behavior: Some early developments. In J. Nicholls (Ed.), *Advances in motivation and achievement, Vol 3: The development of achievement motivation* (pp. 1–32). Greenwich, CT: JAI Press.

Heckhausen, H. (1987). Emotional components of action: Their ontogeny as reflected in achievement behavior. In D. Gorlitz & J. F. Wohlwill (Eds.), *Curiosity, imagination and play: On the development of spontaneous cognitive and motivational processes* (pp. 326–348). Hillsdale, NJ: Erlbaum.

Heckhausen, J. (1988). Becoming aware of one's competence in the second year: Developmental progression within the mother-child dyad. *International Journal of Behavioral Development, 3,* 305–326.

Isen, A. (1990). The influence of positive and negative affect on cognitive organization: Some implications for development. In N. L. Stein, B. Leventhal & T. Trabasso (Eds.), *Psychological and biological approaches to emotion* (pp. 75–94). Hillsdale, NJ: Erlbaum.

Izard, C., & Malatesta, C. (1987). Perspective on emotional development I: Differential emotions theory of early emotional development. In J. Osofsky (Ed.), *Handbook of infant development* (2nd ed., pp. 494–554). New York: Wiley.

Kagan, J. (1981). *The second year: The emergence of self-awareness.* Cambridge, MA: Harvard University Press.

Kagan, J. (1994). On the nature of emotion. In N. Fox (Ed.), The development of emotion regulation: Biological and behavioral considerations. *Monographs of the Society for Research in Child Development, 59,* (2-3, Serial No. 240), 7–24.

Laird, J. (1984). The real role of facial response in the experience of emotion: A reply to Tourangeau and Ellsworth, and others. *Journal of Personality and Social Psychology, 47,* 909–917.

Lakoff, G. (1987). *Women, fire and dangerous things. What categories reveal about the mind.* Chicago: University of Chicago Press.

Lazarus, R. S. (1991). *Emotion and adaptation.* New York: Oxford University Press.

Lazarus, R. S. (1984). Thoughts on the relations between emotion and cognition. In P. Ekman & K. Scherer (Eds.), *Approaches to emotion* (pp. 247–258). Hillsdale, NJ: Erlbaum.

Lazarus, R. S., & Smith, C. A. (1988). Knowledge and appraisal in the cognition-emotion relationship. *Cognition and Emotion, 2,* 281–300.

Le Doux, J. E. (1994). Emotion-specific physiological activity: Don't forget about CNS physiology. In P. Ekman & R. J. Davidson (Eds.), *The nature of emotion* (pp. 248–251). New York: Oxford University Press.

Levenson, R. W. (1994). The search for autonomic specificity. In P. Ekman & R. J. Davidson (Eds.), *The nature of emotion* (pp. 252–257). New York: Oxford University Press.

Lewis, M. D. (1995). Cognition–emotion feedback and the self-organization of developmental paths. *Human Development, 38,* 71–102.

Lewis, M. (1989). Thinking and feeling—the elephant's tail. In C. A. Maher, M. Schwebel, & N. S. Fagley (Eds.), *Thinking and problem solving in the developmental process: International perspectives* (pp. 89–110). Hillsdale, NJ: Erlbaum.

Lewis, M., Alessandri, S., & Sullivan, M. W. (1990). Expectancy, loss of control and anger in young infants. *Developmental Psychology, 26,* 745–751.

Lewis, M., Alessandri, S., & Sullivan, M. W. (1992). Differences in shame and pride as a function of children's gender and task difficulty. *Child Development, 63,* 630–638.

Lewis, M., & Brooks, J. (1978). Self-knowledge and emotional development. In M. Lewis & L. Rosenblum (Eds.), *The development of affect* (pp. 205–226). New York: Plenum Press.

Lewis, M., & Brooks-Gunn, J. (1979). *Social cognition and the acquisition of self.* New York: Plenum Press.

Lutz, C. (1988). *Unnatural emotions.* Chicago: University of Chicago Press.

Mandler, G. (1984). *Mind and body.* New York: Norton.

Mascolo, M. F., & Fischer, K. W. (1995). Developmental transformations in appraisals for pride, shame and guilt. In J. Tangney & K. W. Fischer (Eds.), *Self-conscious emotions: The psychology of shame, guilt, embarrassment and pride* (pp. 64–113). New York: Guilford.

Mascolo, M. F., Pollack, R., & Fischer, K. W. (1997). Keeping the constructor in development: An epigenetic systems approach. *Journal of Constructivist Psychology, 10,* 25–49.

Oatley, K. (1992). Social construction in emotions. In M. Lewis & J. M. Haviland (Eds.), *Handbook of emotions* (pp. 341–352). New York: Guilford.

Panksepp, J. (1989). The neurobiology of emotions: Of animal brains and human feelings. In H. Wagner & A. Manstead (Eds.), *Handbook of social psychophysiology* (pp. 5–26). New York: Wiley.

Panksepp, J. (1993). Neurochemical control of moods and emotions: Amino acids to neuropeptides. In M. Lewis & J. Haviland (Eds.), *Handbook of emotions* (pp. 87–107). New York: Guilford.

Piaget, J. (1952). *The origins of intelligence in children.* New York: Norton.

Rogoff, B. (1990). *Apprenticeship in thinking.* New York: Oxford University Press.

Rogoff, B. (1992). Children's guided participation and participatory appropriation in sociocultural activity. In R. H. Wozniak & K. W. Fischer (Eds.), *Development in context: Acting and thinking in specific environments* (pp. 121–153). Hillsdale, NJ: Erlbaum.

Rosch, E. (1978). Principles of categorization. In E. Rosch (Ed.), *Cognition and categorization* (pp. 28–49). Hillsdale, NJ: Erlbaum.

Roseman, I. J. (1984). Cognitive determinants of emotions: A structural theory. In P. Shaver (Ed.), *Review of personality and social psychology* (vol. 5, pp. 11–36). Beverly Hills, CA: Sage.

Russell, J. A. (1991). In defense of a prototype approach to emotion concepts. *Journal of Personality and Social Psychology, 60,* 37–47.

Scherer, K. (1984). On the nature and function of emotion: A component process approach. In K. R. Scherer & P. Ekman (Eds.), *Approaches to emotion* (pp. 293–317). Hillsdale, NJ: Erlbaum.

Scherer, K. (1994). Toward a concept of "modal emotions." In P. Ekman & R. J. Davidson (Eds.), *The nature of emotion* (pp. 25–31). New York: Oxford University Press.

Shaver, P., Schwartz, J., Kirson, D., & O'Connor, C. (1987). Emotion knowledge: Further exploration of a prototype approach. *Journal of Personality and Social Psychology, 52,* 1061–1086.

Shweder, R. A. (1994). "You're not sick, you're just in love": Emotion as an interpretive system. In P. Ekman & R. J. Davidson (Eds.), *The nature of emotion: Fundamental questions* (pp. 32–44). New York: Oxford University Press.

Smith, C. A., & Ellsworth, P. C. (1985). Patterns of cognitive appraisal in emotion. *Journal of Personality and Social Psychology, 48,* 813–838.

Smith, C. A., & Ellsworth, P. C. (1987). Patterns of appraisal and emotion related to taking an exam. *Journal of Personality and Social Psychology, 52,* 475–488.

Solomon, R. C. (1976). *The passions.* Garden City, NJ: Doubleday.

Solomon, R. C. (1980). Emotions and choice. In A. O. Rorty (Ed.), *Explaining emotions* (pp. 251–279). Berkeley: University of California Press.

Sroufe, L. A. (1979). Socioemotional development. In J. Osofsky (Ed.), *Handbook of infant development* (Vol. 1) (pp. 462–516). New York: Wiley.

Sroufe, L. A. (1996). *Emotional development: The organization of emotional life in the early years.* New York: Cambridge University Press.

Stipek, D. J., Recchia, S., & McClintic, S. (1992). Self-evaluation in young children. *Monograph of the Society for Research in Child Development, 57* (1, Serial No. 226).

Thelen, E. (1990). Dynamic systems and the generation of individual differences. In J. Colombo & J. Fagen (Eds.), *Individual differences in infancy: Reliability, stability, prediction* (pp. 19–43). Hillsdale, NJ: Erlbaum.

Thelen, E., & Smith, L. B. (1994). *A dynamic systems approach to the development of cognition and action.* Cambridge, MA: MIT Press.

Tomkins, S. S. (1962). *Affect, imagery, consciousness: Vol. 1. The positive affects.* New York: Springer.

Tomkins, S. S. (1984). Affect theory. In K. S. Scherer & P. Ekman (Eds.), *Approaches to emotion* (pp. 163–197). Hillsdale, NJ: Erlbaum.

Trevarthen, C. (1984). Emotions as regulators of contact and relationships with persons. In P. Ekman & K. Scherer (Eds.), *Approaches to emotion* (pp. 129–162). Hillsdale, NJ: Erlbaum.

Watson, J. S., & Ramey, C. T. (1972). Reactions to response-contingent stimulation in early infancy. *Merrill–Palmer Quarterly, 18,* 219–227.

Weiss, P. (1970). The living system: Determinism stratified. In A. Koesler & J. Smythies (Eds.), *Beyond reductionism: New perspectives in the live sciences* (pp. 3–55). New York: Macmillan.

Wittgenstein, L. (1953). *Philosophical investigations*. New York: Macmillan.

Wood, D. J. (1988). *How children think and learn*. New York: Basil Blackwell.

Wood, D. J., Bruner, J., & Ross, G. (1976). The role of tutoring in problem solving. *Journal of Child Psychology and Psychiatry, 17*(2), 89–100.

van Geert, P. (1991). A dynamic systems model of cognitive and language growth. *Psychological Review, 98,* 3–53.

Zajonc, R. B. (1984). On the primacy of affect. In P. Ekman & K. Scherer (Eds.), *Approaches to emotion* (pp. 259–270). Hillsdale, NJ: Erlbaum.

9

Alternative Trajectories in the Development of Anger-Related Appraisals

Michael F. Mascolo and Sharon Griffin

Looking at her mother with her eyebrows drawn, an 8-month-old protests loudly after being held tightly by an unfamiliar friend of the family. After being pushed by his sibling, a 7-year-old boy yells, "You can't do that! I'm telling!" After a close friend reveals a secret to a disliked other, a 14-year-old boy confronts his friend, saying, "You broke your promise. I can't trust you anymore!" After witnessing a televised report of a brutal beating of an illegal Mexican immigrant by American officers of the law, a woman writes a letter to the editor to declare her moral outrage. Each of these hypothetical incidents portrays an individual who can be considered angry. However, although one might apply a common label in each case, the episodes differ markedly in the angry behaviors displayed, the situations in which the behaviors occurred, and the ways in which the situations were interpreted. Whereas the infant's angry display may have been precipitated by an impediment to her action, the anger of the older individuals involves appraisals that embody increasingly complex violations of beliefs about the ways events ought to be. In this

Michael F. Mascolo • Department of Psychology, Merrimack College, North Andover, Massachusetts 01845.   **Sharon Griffin** • Frances L. Hiatt School of Education, Clark University, Worcester, Massachusetts 01610.

What Develops in Emotional Development? edited by Michael F. Mascolo and Sharon Griffin. Plenum Press, New York, 1998.

chapter, we examine alternative trajectories in the development of appraisals involved in the experience of anger.

APPRAISAL AS A COMPONENT OF EMOTIONAL EPISODES

Our thinking about the production of emotional processes proceeds from a component systems approach, which is elaborated in more detail elsewhere (Mascolo & Harkins, Chapter 8, this volume; Mascolo, Pollack, & Fischer, 1997). Briefly, emotional episodes and experiences consist of coordinations of multiple component processes that mutually regulate each other in any given social context (Camras, 1992; Dickson, Fogel, & Messinger, Chapter 10, this volume; Fogel et al., 1992; Lewis, 1995, 1996, Chapter 2, this volume; Scherer, 1984, 1994). Emotional episodes involve the detection of *notable changes* in events that then undergo appraisal (Fischer, Shaver, & Carnochan, 1990). The concept of *appraisal* refers to the evaluation of the relation between perceived events and one's goals, motives, standards, and concerns (Frijda, 1986, 1988; Lazarus, 1991a; Roseman, 1984). Appraisal processes, which may be nonconscious, operate to determine the significance of events to an organism (Smith & Lazarus, 1990). Appraisals influence patterns of *bodily change*, which involve patterned *central* and *autonomic* nervous system activity (Ekman, Levenson, & Friesen, 1983; LeDoux, 1994; Levenson, 1994). Such physiological changes support the production of *motive action-tendencies* (Frijda, 1986), which consist of the organism's disposition to perform certain classes of actions within a given appraised context. These include instrumental actions as well as patterns of facial activity and vocal quality. Feedback from the various emotion components contributes to the *feeling tone* of any given emotional experience (Kagan, 1978). Considering all the foregoing, we define an *emotional episode* as that patterning of all component systems in the context of notable changes in one's environs. An *emotional experience* refers to the subjective aspects of feedback from the activity of the various systems that compose an emotional episode (e.g., awareness of appraisal, feeling tone, action-tendencies, etc.).

For example, emotional episodes that we call anger often involve *appraisals* that events are unwanted or perceived as blocking one's goals or actions; however, they can also involve appraisals that events are illegitimate or otherwise contrary to the way they "ought" to be. Anger episodes also involve *felt bodily reactions* that are experienced as "heat," "pressure," "tension," as well as a characteristic feeling tone. Anger involves *motive action-tendencies* to remove the unwanted or illegitimate event (de Rivera, 1981). This can be done in a variety of ways, including physical aggression, verbal aggression, angry looks and gestures, verbal discussion, as well as a variety of indirect angry communications (e.g., door slamming, silence, etc.) (Shaver, Schwartz, Kirson, & O'Conner, 1987). Angry episodes may be accompanied by prototypical *facial* (Russell, 1991, 1994) and *vocalic* patterns (Scherer, 1979).

From a component systems viewpoint, although each component system functions somewhat independently from the others, emotional episodes *self-organize* through the *mutual regulation* of emotion components within a given context (Dickson et al., Chapter 10, this volume; Fogel et al., 1992; Lewis, 1995, 1996; Lewis & Douglas, Chapter 7, this volume). From this view, no single component system is primary in creating any given pattern of emotional activity within a given context. Furthermore, there is no necessary or fixed sequence of events that produces any given emotional experience. Because emotion components can combine in many ways, the number of possible patterns of emotional episodes is very large (Mascolo & Harkins, Chapter 8, this volume; Scherer, 1984). However, component systems mutually regulate each other by placing constraints on each other's activity. Because of these mutual constraints, emotional episodes have a tendency to settle into stable patterns (Fogel, 1993; Lewis, 1995). Still, such patterns can assume a virtually infinite number of minor variations (Camras, 1992).

Appraisals play an important role in the emotion process. Appraisals continuously monitor the significance of event-related input for one's goals, motives, and concerns (Frijda, 1988), and prompt patterned changes in other emotional components (e.g., bodily transformation, motive action-tendency, feeling tone, etc.). As such, appraisals and emotional episodes function in the service of one's central goals, motives, and concerns (Lazarus & Smith, 1988; Roseman, 1984). We assume that appraisals themselves consist of multiple component processes. For example, anger often involves the appraisal that an individual who is capable of behaving otherwise has acted illegitimately. This appraisal consists of multiple component subappraisals. These include component appraisals that the event in question is unwanted, that it violates certain standards of appropriate conduct, and that the other could have and should have controlled his or her behavior relative to those standards. Such component appraisals, either independently or in coaction with each other, influence the activity of other emotional components (Ortony & Turner, 1990). Beyond primary appraisals of the relations between events and one's goals, motives, and concerns, emotional episodes also involve secondary appraisals of one's capacity to cope with events in question (Folkman & Lazarus, 1990). Thus, appraisals act as important organizers of emotional episodes and experiences.

Despite their importance, appraisals consist of but one component in the emotion process. Because emotion components mutually regulate each other, appraisal processes both organize and are organized by the activity of other components throughout the course of the emotion process (Lewis, 1995, 1996; Lewis & Douglas, Chapter 7, this volume). For example, imagine that, in a hurry to leave the supermarket, one encounters a long line at the checkout counter. The appraisal of this event as motive-inconsistent may give rise to internal changes, bodily tensions, and concomitant feeling tone. Feedback from such reactions may influence appraisal processes in such a way as to

prompt greater attention to the circumstances causing one's wait. Such affectively charged attention may prompt one to attribute blame to the clerk,
perhaps for working too slowly. This could generate still further affective and
bodily activity, and the process would continue. Thus, appraisal processes
both influence and are influenced by multiple emotion-relevant component
systems throughout the course of an emotional episode (Lewis, 1996; Lewis &
Douglas, Chapter 7, this volume).

Thus, emotional episodes and experiences consist of the coordination of
multiple component systems within a given context (Dickson et al., Chapter
10, this volume; Fogel et al., 1992). We suggest that in ontogenesis, emotional
episodes undergo developmental transformation (Sroufe, 1979, 1996) as their
elements change and reorganize in relation to each other. Transformations in
emotion-relevant appraisals are among the factors that lead to developmental
changes in emotional experiences and episodes. Keeping in mind that appraisals function as but one element in the emotion process, in what follows,
we examine developmental changes in appraisals that participate in the
emotional episodes we call anger.

THE DEVELOPMENT OF APPRAISALS IN ANGER

An analysis of the literature on the determinants of anger in infancy and
adulthood reveals some striking differences. Theoretical approaches to anger
in infants generally characterize the antecedents of anger in terms of obstacles
and blocked goals (Barrett & Campos, 1987; Lewis, 1993; Lewis, Alessandri, &
Sullivan, 1990; Stenberg & Campos, 1990). Such a view of the determinants of
anger is often shared by those who offer theories of emotion drawn from
Darwinian or ethological theory (Izard, 1991; Plutchik, 1984; Tomkins, 1984).
However, theorists who analyze anger in adults often offer different views.
From these views, anger is generated by event-appraisals that have a significant moral dimension, including ought violations (de Rivera, 1981), attributions of blame or accountability to others (Smith & Ellsworth, 1985; Weiner,
1985), or slights to the ego (Lazarus, 1991a). The idea that anger among adults
involves a moral dimension suggests that anger processes undergo developmental changes in ontogenesis.

Anger in Infancy

Theorists and researchers who examine the determinants of anger in
infancy often define anger and its determinants in terms of obstacles or
blocked goals. For example, according to Barrett and Campos (1987), anger
involves the appreciation that "there is an obstacle to my obtaining my goal"
(p. 564) where the goal involves any significant end state. Such appreciations
give rise to forward movements directed at eliminating obstacles. According

to Izard (1991), causes of anger include restraint, blocking, or interrupting goal-oriented behavior, and aversive stimulation. Although aversive stimulation (e.g., pain) is sufficient to evoke anger, higher-order cognition can act as a secondary stimulus that can strengthen or weaken angry states. Tomkins (1984) links different "basic emotions" to variations in the intensity of stimulus gradients. Within this framework, anger involves intense stimulation sustained over a period of time, rather than increasing or decreasing stimulus intensity. Pain, frustration, or distress, which involve lower levels of stimulation, can lead to anger if stimulation is sustained or augmented. Lewis (1993, Lewis et al., 1990) explicitly differentiates between the concepts of frustration and anger. Lewis suggests that frustration is a motivational concept that refers to the increase in general behavior that occurs when goal-directed behavior is blocked. Anger is the emotional response to frustration that functions to overcome the source of the frustration: "The anger response consists of a particular neuromusculature facial expression and bodily activity designed to overcome the source of frustration" (Lewis, 1993, p. 159). As such, Lewis views anger in infancy as a response to goal frustration.

Research on the development of anger suggests that goal blockage evokes anger-relevant reactions in infants as young as 2 months of age. Lewis et al. (1990) studied the development of angry facial expressions in two groups of 2-, 4-, 6-, and 8-month-olds. During an initial learning period, for one group of infants, the production of an audiovisual stimulus was made contingent upon infant arm movement; control groups experienced the stimulus display in the absence of this contingency. After the learning period, both groups of infants experienced a period of nonstimulation during which the audiovisual display did not occur. During the period of nonstimulation, infants who formerly controlled the stimulus display exhibited heightened levels of angry facial behavior, whereas control infants did not. The pattern of findings was the same for all age groups, suggesting that even 2-month-olds exhibit angry facial behavior in the context of goal frustration.

In an elegant follow-up study, Sullivan and Lewis (1993) demonstrated that anger reactions in 4- to 6-month-olds were not attributable to the withdrawal of the contingent event itself, but rather to "the disruption of the infant's perceived control of an outcome" (p. 3). After contingency learning, infants were exposed to one of three types of frustrating conditions: extinction (cessation of stimulation), partial reinforcement (outcome occurs on every third pull), and noncontingency (stimulation levels maintained independent of the child's activity). Results indicated that infants displayed the highest levels of angry facial behavior in response to noncontingent stimulation, followed by extinction and partial reinforcement. These results clearly link angry faces most strongly to frustration that involves *loss of perceived control* rather than simply to loss of stimulation or general frustration (i.e., violations of any expectancy or goal).

Other studies have produced similar results. Stenberg and Campos

(1990) sought to determine the most suitable stimulus conditions to evoke angry reactions in infants, which were defined in terms of facial, vocalic, and instrumental activity. After investigating a series of anger-eliciting tasks, they reported that arm restraint proved to be the most effective elicitor. The investigators found that after arm restraint, 4- and 7-month-olds, but not 1-month-olds, exhibited angry facial patterns. One-month-olds exhibited angry facial components, but these components could not be differentiated from facial components associated with other emotional episodes, particularly discomfort–pain. In addition, after arm restraint, 4-month-olds tended to look at their arms, whereas 7-month-olds tended to look at their mothers or the experimenter. These data suggest that angry reactions to frustrating events emerge by 4 months. The finding that 7-month-olds look to their mothers upon arm restraint may suggest that these infants may begin to see others as objects of their anger, or at least as persons who can help alleviate negative events.

Appraisal Theory and Anger in Adults

In the past decade, theorists and researchers have proposed appraisal theories of emotion. Appraisal theories generally assume that emotional experiences are generated by assessments of the relations between perceived events and an individual's goals, motives, and concerns (Frijda, 1986, 1988; Lazarus, 1991a; Roseman, 1984; Scherer, 1988; Smith & Ellsworth, 1985; Smith & Lazarus, 1988). Such theorists have attempted to map out the appraisal dimensions that differentiate experiences of different emotions. Almost without exception (see Berkowitz, 1990, for an opposing view), appraisal theorists have proposed models that link anger to appraisals that embody morally relevant content. Smith and Lazarus (1990) hold that the "core emotional theme" of anger consists of "other-blame," which is a necessary component of anger. de Rivera (1981) suggests that anger involves a psychological situation in which there is a challenge to what one asserts ought to exist. Such challenges strengthen an individual's will to remove the challenge to what ought to be. In his dimensional theory of emotions, Roseman (1984) differentiates between frustration and anger as discrete emotional responses. According to Roseman, frustration involves appraisals that circumstances have resulted in motive-inconsistent events, whereas anger involves judgments that motive-inconsistent events are illegitimate and precipitated by responsible others. Weiner (1985) also differentiates between frustration and anger. To Weiner, frustration is an outcome-related emotion, linked only to the appraisal of motive-inconsistency. However, anger is a dimension-related emotion, and thus requires appraisals of the justifiability of the other's behavior (see Scherer, 1988, and Frijda, 1986, for similar discussions).

Using self-report and emotion-rating techniques, appraisal researchers have amassed a large body of empirical research supporting these assertions. For example, Smith and Ellsworth (1985) factor-analyzed participant ratings of self-reported emotional experiences using 15 different ratings dimensions. Of interest here, anger was associated with high ratings on *human rather than situational control*, and *other-rather than self-responsibility/control*. Although frustration was judged as similar to anger, frustration was less associated with *human control* than was anger. Similar findings were reported in a series of follow-up studies (Smith & Ellsworth, 1987; Ellsworth & Smith, 1988). In a similar study, Roseman, Spindel, and Jose (1990, see also Roseman, 1991) participants recalled and rated actual experiences of emotions on a series of judgment dimensions. Results indicated that whereas both anger and frustration were seen as evoked by illegitimate events, other persons were seen as causes of anger to a greater degree than for frustration. Shaver et al. (1987) reported that 95% of participant-generated descriptions of anger included references to events that were judged as unfair, illegitimate, wrong, or contrary to the way they were "supposed" to be. In a series of studies involving ratings of protagonists in vignettes, Weiner and his colleagues have reported that participants claim higher levels of anger when the actions of individuals were judged to result from internal and controllable causes (Weiner, 1985; Weiner, Amirkhan, Folkes, & Verette, 1987; Weiner, Graham, Stern, & Lawson, 1982; Weiner & Handel, 1985; Weiner, Russell, & Lerman, 1979).

Are Infants Capable of Making Adult-Like Appraisals?

Lazarus (1991b) has considered the question of whether infants are capable of making adult-like appraisals in anger. According to Lazarus, studies that link angry facial expressions in infants to the loss of control over contingent events (Lewis et al., 1990) suggest that infants have a primitive sense of ego-identity and are capable of appraising goal-relevance and goal-incongruence. The Stenberg and Campos (1990) finding that upon arm restraint, 4-month-olds look at their hands and 7-month-olds look at others suggests that infants are capable of viewing the cause of motive-inconsistent events as external to them. Lazarus suggests that it is unclear whether infants are able to attribute control to human agents for negative events, and thus concludes that other-blame may be necessary for adult but not infant anger.

We suggest that the appraisals involved in anger undergo developmental change. In infancy, anger-relevant behavior is evoked primarily by blocked goals and actions, conditions that we will call *want violations*. With development, anger experiences increasingly involve judgments that events violate conditions that ought to be, appraisals that we will call *ought violations*. To say that anger appraisals develop in the direction of increasingly sophisticated ought violations is not to say that older children and adults never experience anger in reaction to want violation. Rather, with development, ought violations become increasingly salient components of anger appraisals and experiences. Ought violations embody at least two related components that are absent in simple want violations. First, ought violations involve appraisals that events are inconsistent with morally relevant *standards* of value, worth, or legitimacy. Second, ought violations generally involve the ascription of *blame* to agents that can be held accountable for violating such standards.

We define moral standards in anger broadly to include not only one's sense of right or wrong, but also one's sense of what is valuable, worthy, honorable, socially appropriate, or legitimate. Moral judgments not only involve standards for what is considered right but also standards for what is regarded as good or valued (McIntyre, 1984; Taylor, 1989). Defined in this way, we suggest that the appraisals we call *ought violations* begin to develop around 18–24 months of age with the emergence of semiotic function and the capacity to form representations of one's world (Case, 1991; Fischer, 1980; Fischer & Hogan, 1989; Piaget, 1951). This follows for several reasons. An ought violation implies that an event *should not* have occurred. As such, it requires the articulation of a *negative*. However, there are no negatives in nature (Burke, 1952). The articulation of the negative is made possible by the ability to represent not only the way the world is, but also alternative ways the world *could* be. As such, a person who appraises an event as an ought violation must compare the perceived event to standards that define a possible, normative, valued, or ideal state of the world. Furthermore, such normative representations of the world are not simple products of the child's individual experience. Rather, they reflect the appropriation of rules, norms, standards, or ideals from interaction with others within sociocultural contexts. Thus, the participation of moral standards in anger not only requires an ability to go beyond the present to represent possible states of the world, but also the capacity to evaluate existing conditions against socially relevant standards for how the world should be. These skills only begin to develop with the onset of representations between 18 and 24 months of age and then undergo massive transformation throughout development.

Similarly, ought violations involve the attribution of *blame* to others for the violation of standards of value or legitimacy. The allocation of blame to others goes beyond the capacity to attribute simple causality for an event to some external source. In blame, we make judgments that an other who can control his or her actions has violated a moral standard. This not only requires a rudimentary understanding that others are intentional agents—that they have mental states that guide and control their behavior—but also an understanding that others should control their behavior in line with acceptable standards of conduct, however rudimentary.[1] When are children able to perform the requisite judgments?

[1]One might object that anger need not be preceded by sophisticated assessments of the extent to which others could have controlled the actions that precipitated a negative event. Some might object that such an conception of blame makes the appraisal processes in anger appear too

Research on "intentional communication" in infancy suggests that by 9 months of age, infants alternate their gaze between a desired object and the adult's eyes or gesture in order to make a request (Bates, Camaioni, & Volterra, 1975; Bretherton, Fritz, Zahn-Waxler, & Ridgeway, 1986; Bruner, 1975; Rogoff, 1990). Although such research suggests that infants in the last quarter of the first year can regard others as agents (persons who produce their own behavior), we agree with Poulin-Dubois and Shultz (1988), who suggest that it is not until later that infants are aware that the behavior of others is under the control of inner intentions. Research on children's internal-state language suggests that by 24 months of age (Bretherton & Beeghly, 1982; Bretherton et al., 1986; Huttenlocher & Smiley, 1990), children use words for themselves (e.g., *me*) as well as words for intentional actions (e.g., *get*, *give*) and inner states (e.g., *want*), but only in reference to the self. It is not until about 30 months of age that children begin to use such words in reference to others. We suggest that children begin to ascribe intentions to others at around 2½ years of age.

If 2½-year-olds are capable of understanding that others have intentions that control their behavior, when are children able to understand that others can and should regulate their behavior in accordance with rudimentary social standards? That is, when are children able to make judgments about the legitimate ways in which one ought to control one's behavior? Several studies have suggested that 3-year-olds are capable of differentiating intentional actions from accidents in allocating blame to others for negative events (Nelson, 1980; Yuill, 1984; Yuill & Perner, 1988). Using stories in which negative outcomes are explicitly described as either intended acts or accidents, 3-year-olds indicated that intended negative outcomes were more blameworthy than accidental outcomes. Dunn and Munn (1987) reported that 2- and 3-year-old children sometimes justify their positions in disputes with siblings and parents in terms of simple social rules (e.g., protesting "That doesn't belong to you" when a sibling takes a toy, or "No, it was Mummy's go again!" in a

---

deliberative or cognitive. We would address this issue in two ways. First, the emergence of the capacity to blame others in anger does not mean that individuals lose the capacity to become angry in the context of want violations. Persons can still become angry when events prevent them from fulfilling their local or long-term goals. We sometimes call such experiences *frustration*. Second, it is interesting to note that in anger, we often turn "want violations" into "ought violations." Even if an affective experience is initially precipitated by a want violation, we often look for others to blame for the violation. For example, we might become frustrated when, in a hurry, we encounter a long line at the checkout counter at the local supermarket. We may, in anger, blame the cashier for working too slowly, even though the wait is beyond anyone's control. As such, the attribution of blame in anger need not precede the onset of an anger episode; it can arise during the course of an angry episode. Furthermore, the attribution of blame need not be deliberate, well reasoned, or even appropriate to the situation from the perspective of onlookers. These arguments do not undercut the role of ought violations and attributions of blame in the experience of anger. Rather, they accentuate the difficulty of experiencing anger in the absence of appraisals involving ought violations.

dispute about turn taking). After 3 years of age, there is considerable development in children's ability to use a variety of dimensions to mediate judgments
of blame, including causality (Fincham, 1981), controllability (Mant & Perner,
1988), foreseeability (Yuill & Perner, 1988), negligence (Shultz, Wright, &
Schleifer, 1986), mitigating circumstances (Darley, Klosson, & Zanna, 1978),
and avoidability and motive acceptability (Olthof, Ferguson, & Luiten, 1989).
Thus, we suggest that the development of the capacity to attribute blame in
anger begins to develop between the ages of 2 and 3 years of age and
undergoes massive development thereafter.

Why Do Anger Appraisals Shift from Want to Ought Violations?

If anger-related appraisals develop from want violations toward ought
violations, what accounts for this transition? Why would standards of value
or legitimacy become so important to the experience of anger, but less salient
in the development of other emotional reactions, such as sadness or joy? There
are at least three responses to this question. The first two are variants of the
thesis that anger appraisals do not actually undergo developmental transformation at all. The first would suggest that anger episodes are always defined
primarily by obstacles and blocked goals, and that ought violations are of
secondary concern. From this view, the moral aspects of anger would serve
mainly to regulate angry interactions between individuals. Because we become angry when our goals are violated, society needs a mechanism to ensure
that individuals do not move against others in anger upon just any goal
frustration. The prescription that anger may only be experienced or enacted
when others can be held responsible for ought violations would thus serve to
keep anger and conflict in check. A second explanation would stipulate that
anger appraisals always consist of ought violations and thus never undergo
developmental change. One might argue that infants who encounter violations of their expectations experience something like "This shouldn't be
happening!" From this view, goal violations in infancy would be seen as a
rudimentary form of ought violation.

Our position is that there is both continuity and transformation in the
development of anger-relevant appraisals. The social circumstances under
which infants and children experience anger contain the seeds for the subsequent development of ought violations in the child. Infants become angry
when they fail to control wanted or anticipated outcomes (Lewis et al., 1990).
Many instances of a child's failure to control outcomes occur in social interaction, including occasions on which parents do not respond to children when
wanted, when parents remove prohibited objects, and in the context of
conflicts among toddlers. Contexts involving interpersonal conflict naturally
raise the question of how best to deal with such conflict. As such, dealing with
conflict raises issues at the intersection of morality and identity: What can I

claim as legitimately mine? What can you claim as legitimately yours? Where does what is considered "mine" end and what is considered "yours" or "ours" begin? What are the appropriate ways in which I should relate to you? How should you relate to me? Answers to these questions are elaborated in social interactions between children and agents of culture. Subsequent to the onset of representational intelligence, children develop the capacity to use social representations of worth, value, or legitimacy to make judgments of how events should be in various contexts, including situations that involved interpersonal conflict. With development, children not only gain the capacity to represent such standards, but they also *appropriate* such standards *as their own*. As such, social standards of value, worth, and legitimacy become part and parcel of the goals, motives, and concerns that define the child's developing sense of self. Thus, in the development of anger, want violations can become ought violations as children appropriate social standards to define the self and to evaluate the legitimacy of the behaviors of self and others in social interaction. Of course, the assertion that ought violations increasingly participate in anger with development does not imply that older children and adults cannot experience anger in the context of want violations; the capacity to experience anger in the context of want violations is not lost with development.

DIVERGENT AND CONVERGENT ENDPOINTS IN THE DEVELOPMENT OF EMOTION: ANGER AND GENDER

Traditionally, theorists have assumed that development follows a single, linear trajectory. The staircase provides a convenient metaphor for conceptualizing linear development (Freud, 1940; Inhelder & Piaget, 1955-1958; Kohlberg, 1969). From this view, development begins at a single, common point and proceeds in a step-by-step fashion toward a singular endpoint. Within recent decades, however, it has become clear that development proceeds as a multidirectional, dynamic process (Valsiner, 1987; Bidell & Fischer, 1996; Mascolo & Fischer, in press). Not only do persons begin development from a variety of different starting points, but behavior both within and between individuals develops toward a variety of different endpoints. Developmental pathways can diverge or converge as a result of a multiplicity of factors that affect development.

Toward the end of mapping out alternative pathways in emotional development, one might begin by specifying convergent and divergent endpoints of development in adulthood. The analysis of gender differences in anger may provide a window into alternative pathways and endpoints. Theorists and researchers have examined gender-related differences that bear on the issue of the development of anger. For example, theorists have suggested that men and women in Western culture often differ in their ways of approaching issues of morality and value (Brown, Tappan, & Gilligan, 1995; Gilligan, 1982; Gilligan & Attanucci, 1988). Others have noted differences in the extent to which men and women are able to command power in a male-dominated society (Miller, 1988). To the extent that anger involves moral violations within social contexts involving power as a salient component, there are likely to be differences in the appraisals that mediate experiences of anger among men and women. Such differences would mark alternative endpoints in the development of anger-related appraisals.

Gilligan and her colleagues (Brown et al., 1995; Gilligan, 1982; Gilligan & Attanucci, 1988) have postulated that both women and men use two orientations in approaching moral issues. These include an ethos of *care* and an ethos of *justice*. The justice orientation is structured around the conceptions of equality, fairness, and reciprocity among persons. The care orientation is founded upon ideals of connection, attachment, loving and being loved, listening and being listened to. As such, moral violations within a justice orientation would embody instances of domination, oppression, unfairness, or inequality; moral violations emanating from a care perspective would involve detachment, abandonment, inattentiveness, or lack of responsiveness. If adult anger involves appraisals that involve standards of legitimacy and value, and if men and women often differ in their moral orientations, then one might predict that the appraisals that mediate anger among men and women would tend to differ.

To investigate this possibility, sixty-seven (31 men and 36 women) undergraduates attending a small liberal arts college in Massachusetts provided written narratives about their actual experiences of anger. Participants were asked to recall an actual recent occasion on which they felt angry and to describe in as much detail as possible the circumstances that caused them to become angry, and their reasons for becoming angry. Resulting anger narratives were parsed into a series of segments. *Context* included any background material that set up or supported the narrative. *Precipitating events* included descriptions of the actual events or actions that caused the person to become angry. *Action sequences* included particular actions that were taken as a result of one's anger. *Interpretations* included the participants' statements describing why they felt angry, and constituted the primary focus on the present study. Interpretations included all statements that completed phrases such as "I was angry because ..." or otherwise provided reasons for feeling angry. Interpretive statements were further parsed into a series of *interpretive chunks*, which consisted of a single, distinct reason for why the individual felt angry. A single reason corresponded to any single criterion falling under the three general categories of ought violations described later (e.g., the reason "unfair" under the sociomoral category). (A complete description of the coding categories and subcategories are provided in Mascolo & Griffin, 1994). If multiple adjacent sentences elaborated upon a single reason for feeling angry, they were considered part of the same chunk. Parsing the text sequentially, a new chunk began when the individual focused on a different reason explaining why she or he felt angry, even if the person shifted to a reason that had been involved at an earlier point in the narrative.

Using existing theory and an analysis of a subset of the data, we identified three types of ought violations into which the responses could be classified. *Relational violations* were defined in terms of failures of others to extend appropriate care, nurturance, or sensitivity to the self or to others (e.g., being uncaring, insensitive, selfish, hurtful), and/or violations of the basis of an existing interpersonal relationship (e.g., violation of a traust, betrayal). Examples of relational violations included "He had me trusting him and even loving him as a friend, and he turned around and proved to me that trust and love could never be felt," "I became angry at my roommate's selfishness," "I was angry because my Grandmother let this girl come between my family, and my Grandmother was letting her ruin a special bond between my brother and my Grandmother," "I felt that he did not care about my son and myself." *Personal violations* included obstructions of personal motives or autonomy (e.g., blocked goals or desires; infringement upon one's independence, efficacy, or freedom), intrusions of the physical or psychological self (e.g., violations of the body, or what is considered me or mine), or assaults on one's self-esteem (e.g., insults, criticism). Examples include "I felt that he was useless to me," "I was angry because my privacy was totally violated," "[My parents] try to invoke the 'if you live under my house you live by my rules' approach. I am not asking to leave my house and be totally on my own, just a little freedom," "When he comes home and cracks on me or my other roommate on a grade or other important matter, its as if he's invading our personal life." *Sociomoral violations* included transgressions of moral principles (e.g., inequality, injustice, dishonesty, etc.), social conventions (i.e., violation of rules for socially appropriate behavior, e.g., lack of courtesy, bad manners), accepted standards of personal conduct (e.g., lacking integrity, being irresponsible or negligent). Examples of sociomoral violations included "I became angry because I perceived that I was being treated unfairly ...," "I love him, but he had no right to overstep his bounds and get fired again ...," "I knew the real reason [for not getting promoted] was because he was a guy and my bosses are very chauvinistic, and all the men that started made more than the women no matter who had more experience or who was better," "What really pissed me off was the fact that he kept denying to my face that he took the mug." Thus, personal, relational, and sociomoral violations reflect three ways in which individuals can interpret social situations. These include intrusions to the self, violations of connections between persons, and violations of generally accepted conventions and moral standards that regulate the behavior and relations within a community.

Men and women differed in the interpretations they offered for the range of anger-eliciting events they provided. Two analyses were performed. Table 1 depicts the proportion of men and women who exhibited at least one instance of each ought violation (i.e., at least one interpretive chunk) in their narratives about anger. Women's anger narratives were more likely to contain at least one relational violation ($\chi^2(1) = 10.43, p < .01$), whereas men's narratives were more likely to contain at least one personal violation ($\chi^2(1) = 3.99, p < .05$). In addition, a higher proportion of women's narratives contained at least one sociomoral violation, but this difference was only marginally significant ($\chi^2(1) = 3.13, p < .10$). It is important to note that whereas women reported relational violations more often than men, almost one-fourth of men reported such violations. Similarly, although men reported personal violations more often than women, well over half of all women reported personal violations.

We also analyzed the predominance of personal, relational, and socio-moral violations within the anger narratives of men and women. In so doing, we calculated the proportion of interpretive chunks that were categorized in terms of each type of ought violation. The results are depicted in Table 2. Relational violations occupied a larger proportion of women's rather than men's narratives ($t(62) = 2.07, p < .05$), and personal violations consisted of a larger proportion of men's narratives ($t(56) = 3.63, p < .01$). In addition, sociomoral violations occupied a larger proportion of women's narratives ($t(65) = 2.18, p < .05$). Taken together, these results suggest that relational violations are more salient for women than for men, whereas personal violations are more dominant for men than for women. Results also suggest that women may be more likely than men to view anger-related violations in terms of sociomoral violations. The dominance of personal violations in men's narratives may help explain why sociomoral violations were not more prominent in men's anger narratives.

Despite these patterns, it is important to note that neither men's nor women's anger narratives were exclusively defined by any single class of

Table 1. Proportion of Men and Women Reporting Moral Violations

Violation type	Women	Men
Personal	.66	.87
Relational	.61	.23
Sociomoral	.83	.64

Note. Entries denote the proportion of men and women who reported each moral violation across anger narratives.

Table 2. Dominance of
Anger Narratives by Type
of Moral Violation

Violation type	Women	Men
Personal	.26	.54
Relational	.25	.11
Sociomoral	.49	.31

Note. Entries denote the mean proportion of chunks across anger narratives categorized in terms of each violation type.

ought violations. Although relational violations were more dominant in women's than men's narratives, only .25 of the content of women's narratives were categorized as relational. Conversely, although over .50 of men's narratives involved personal violations, personal violations accounted for .25 of the content of women's narratives. In addition, both men and women's narratives contained sizable proportions of sociomoral violations. Although there were differences in the extent to which the different ought violations were represented in women's and men's anger narratives, *each* type of ought violation could be found in *both* men's and women's anger. As such, individual anger narratives were characterized by what Gilligan calls a "polyphony" of different voices (Brown et al., 1995). Thus, although the participation of specific moral violations is clearly not *gender-specific*, the engagement of relational and personal (and perhaps sociomoral) violations in anger is nevertheless *gender-related*[2] (see Brown et al., 1995). As a result, personal, relational, and sociomoral violations provide examples of both converging and diverging endpoints toward which anger-relevant appraisals develop.

ALTERNATIVE TRAJECTORIES IN THE DEVELOPMENT OF APPRAISALS IN ANGER

Based on these three types of violations, we suggest three alternative trajectories in the development of anger-related appraisals, one for personal,

[2]We regard the results of this study as initial and tentative. We caution against drawing general conclusions that link men's anger to personal violations and women's anger to relational violations. Although consistent with sex differences reported by others, the results are based on data culled from college students from a primarily white, middle-class, and Catholic background. It is plausible that the moral violations involved in men's and women's anger will vary as a function of a variety of factors, including age, social context (e.g., workplace vs. the home), socioeconomic status, and cultural, ethnic, and religious background.

one for relational, and one for sociomoral violations. Within each trajectory, appraisals develop in a series of steps that reflect different and increasingly complex forms of the appraisals in question. In proposing these trajectories, we first considered specific types of personal, relational, and sociomoral violations that can occur within Western European culture. We then used neo-Piagetian models of development (Biggs & Collins, 1982; Case, 1991; Halford, 1982) and in particular dynamic skills theory (Fisher, 1980; Fischer, et al., 1990) to chart developmental changes in the appraisals that can participate in anger episodes.

Neo-Piagetian models of development share with Piaget a concern for the ways in which children's cognitive and affective processes undergo qualitative transformations in development. In general, like Piaget, such models suggest a series of major transformations in children's cognitive development at 24 months of age with the transition from sensorimotor to representational activity, at 5–7 years with the transition to more complex systems of representational thought, and again at around 10–12 years with the transition from systems of representations to abstract thinking. Despite this similarity, neo-Piagetian approaches differ from Piagetian theory in several ways. First, they offer much more sensitive tools for predicting fine-grained changes in children's activities and representational structures as a function of age, psychological domain, and context. For example, in dynamic skills theory, Fischer (Fischer et al., 1990) postulates four major tiers of development (reflexes, sensorimotor acts, representations, and abstractions), each of which is further specified into four levels (sets; mappings; systems; and systems of systems, which produce the next major tier of development). This produces a series of 13 levels of skills development, which can be further specified into a series of substeps. Using the steps specified by skills theory, it is not useful to ask at what *point* a behavior or psychological structure emerges in development. All behavior develops gradually and assumes a series of increasingly complex *forms* in ontogenesis.

Neo-Piagetian approaches generally grant a more important role for social context in children's psychological functioning than did Piaget. For example, in dynamic skills theory (Fischer, 1980; Fischer, Bullock, Rotenberg, & Raza, 1983), the basic unit of analysis in the study of psychological development is the skill, which refers to the capacity to organize or control one's actions and meaning structures within a given psychological *domain*, and within a given social or physical *context*. Because skills are inherently tied to contexts and particular domains, they represent a property of the child-in-a-context rather than an abstract competence located within the child. Thus, a change in context or content domain will result in a change in skill. An important aspect of dynamic skills theory is that children will display a skill within a context that offers assistance, aid, or support of the behavior in question before they will display the skill on their own. As such, the age of emergence of any given step in a developmental sequence will depend upon the specific form of the skill in question as well as the level of support and assistance provided in the context.

In what follows, we propose three trajectories in the development of appraisals in anger. In so doing, we use dynamic skills theory to specify the components necessary to make the appraisal in question within a given context. The appraisals were then ordered in terms of developmental complexity. Within each trajectory, anger appraisals develop from simple want violations toward increasingly sophisticated ought violations. We suggest that ought violations can only begin to appear after 24 months of age, with the emergence of representational intelligence and the capacity to represent valued ways in which events can and should be. At the very least, an ought violation requires the participation of some value or standard beyond a simple violated goal, however rudimentary, concrete, implicit, or incomplete. We suggest that such standards begin to appear around the second birthday and become more complex, elaborated, and explicit with subsequent development. Of course, the fact that such standards are available to children does not mean that children or even adults do not continue to become angry in the context of simple want violations. Want violations are necessary components of anger appraisals and continue to organize anger reactions throughout development.

Because the developmental levels and steps proposed by skills theory have been articulated elsewhere (Fischer, 1980; Fischer & Hogan, 1989; Fischer et al., 1990), they will not be elaborated upon here. Rather, we discuss relevant terms and concepts as we elaborate the proposed sequences. Because we explicitly assume that developmental changes in cognitive and emotional processes are strongly tied to context and task domain, the developmental sequences proposed here are not meant to reflect general stages or structured wholes such as those proposed by Erikson (1963), Inhelder and Piaget (1955/1958), or Kohlberg (1969). Rather, each step is defined by the coordination of select appraisal components within a given psychological domain and within a particular context. Thus, even though there are parallels in the steps proposed for personal, relational and sociomoral violations, one would not predict that parallel steps would necessarily emerge at the same time.

Steps in the Development of Personal Violations

Table 3 contains a proposed developmental sequence of appraisals involving personal violations in anger. Personal violations entail any intrusion on the self's personal motives, goals, or actions, as well as violations of the self, or what is considered me or mine. Step P1, distress over failure to control outcomes, occurs with the development of reflex mappings that begin to emerge around 8 weeks of age. With reflex mappings, the infant can coordi-

Table 3. Steps in the Development of Personal Violations

Step	Form of appraisal	Age of onset	Example of step
P1: Reflex mappings	Distress over failure to control simple contingency or effect	3–4 weeks	Swiping of the arm that formerly led to pleasurable outcome is disrupted
P2: Sensorimotor actions	Frustration over failure to achieve controlled outcome	4 months	Controlled movement to obtain seen ball is thwarted
P3: Sensorimotor mappings	Frustration over failure to obtain covered wanted object; anger over negative outcome seen as caused by other	7–8 months	Barrier is placed between child and wanted ball. Infant sees other as cause of negative event, looks at other and becomes angry
P4: Single representations	Anger over intrusion on objects considered "mine"	18–24 months	Other takes toy that child considers "mine"; child becomes angry and says "mine" or "my ball", etc.
P6: Representational mappings	Anger over violation of one's concrete sense of competence by agentive other. Child holds agentive other responsible for criticizing self's ability to perform concrete action	3½–4 years	Other laughs at child for spilling milk, not being able to climb tree, etcc.; child explicitly links violation to the agentive acts of other (e.g., "You laughed at me because I spilled my milk! You shouldn't laugh!")
P7: Representational systems	Anger over criticism of self's sense of competence in a concrete trait domain. Violation of concrete trait-like sense of self, which is coordinated from multiple concrete actions in a given behavioral domain.	5–7 years	Child becomes angry when playmate demeans child's concrete trait-like skills (e.g, math class, soccer); other attempts to give child guidance and child sees other as criticizing a concrete trait or ability.
P8: Single abstractions and beyond	Anger over violation of self's abstract personal boundaries; anger over impediments to child's attempt to define identity as free, autonomous, or independent from others.	10–11 years and beyond	Child's room is "private"; others enter and child feels violated; child wants to see self as "independent"; parental restriction of activity seen as impediment to freedom or autonomy.

nate two simple reflex acts, which consist of innate voluntary action patterns such as looking or swiping the arm (Fischer & Hogan, 1989). Using reflex mappings, an infant can detect contingencies between simple actions and their effects (e.g., performing an uncontrolled arm swipe and looking at its effect). Evidence for this step comes in the form of Lewis et al.'s (1990) finding (described earlier) that loss of control over contingent feedback is associated with the production of angry faces in 2-, 4- and 8-month-old children. Because several researchers have reported relative lack of differentiation between angry and distress faces in the first half-year of life (Camras, 1992; Camras, Malatesta, & Izard, 1991; Stenberg & Campos, 1990), we refer to this step as distress rather than anger.

Step P2 begins with the onset of a sensorimotor tier of development at around 4 months of age. At about this time, infants can begin to use sensori-motor acts, which consist of single, controlled actions on objects involving the coordination of multiple reflex acts (e.g., controlled reaching for a seen ball) (Fischer & Hogan, 1989). At this step, infants may experience frustration over failure to achieve controlled outcome. Attempts to thwart the child's con-trolled movements directed toward objects may produce angry displays (Case, Hayward, Lewis, & Hurst, 1988). Angry facial behavior is also more pronounced at this age (Stenberg & Campos, 1990). Step P3 emerges with the onset of sensorimotor mappings, which begin to emerge around 8 months of age. At this step, the child can coordinate two sensorimotor actions toward a single goal (e.g., lift a cover in order to obtain an object). Thus, a barrier between a wanted object and the child may prompt angry behavior (Case et al., 1988). Stenberg and Campos's (1990) finding that upon arm restraint, 7-month-olds directed their gaze toward other people suggests that infants may be able to connect the negative input to seen others.

With the onset of the representational tier of development at around 18–24 months of age, children become capable of representing the properties of simple objects, events, or people independent of their own actions. The onset of representation sparks important changes in self- and other-awareness (Bertenthal & Fischer, 1978; Kagan, 1981; Lewis & Brooks-Gunn, 1979; Lewis et al., 1990; Mascolo & Fischer, in press). At this step, the child becomes capable of representing simple standards that define the boundaries of what is legit-imately considered "me" or "mine." Children also are able to construct representations of other people as intentional agents of action. Thus, at this step, anger may become mediated appraisals that others have removed objects that are conceived of as possessions, or as "mine." Although children may use statements that an object is "mine" as a simple attempt to maintain possession of a wanted object, the categorization of a toy as "mine" neverthe-less involves the use of a socially negotiated standard that defines the "appro-priate" boundaries between self and other. As such, the violation of what is considered "mine" can be seen as a rudimentary form of ought violation.

Indirect evidence for the participation of appraisals involving personal violations in young children's anger comes from a longitudinal study on children's justifications in child–sibling and child–mother disputes in children between 18 and 36 months of age (Dunn & Munn, 1987). The researchers reported that 36-month-olds offered justifications for their positions in disputes about .30 of the time, whereas 24-month-olds offered justifications between .11 and .18 of the time. Most of these justifications involved reference to children's own feelings and concerns (e.g., a child whose sibling took a spoon with which the child was previously playing said, "I need that!"). Beyond justifications based on simple wants and needs, children also offered justifications based on simple social rules, such as possession (e.g., saying "That doesn't belong to you!" after a sibling removed a child's toy). At all ages, anger accompanied approximately .05 of the child–mother disputes and about .10 of the child–sibling disputes. These data are consistent with the notion that anger in 2- and 3-year-olds not only involves violations of wants but also self-relevant standards.

Subsequent steps in the proposed sequence involve increasingly sophisticated ways in which other people can be seen as intruding upon standards that define a child or adolescent's self- or personal boundaries. At Step P5, with the onset of the ability to construct representational mappings, children between the ages of 3½ to 4 years of age become capable of understanding relationships between at least two representations. At this step, for example, a child can form a mapping that links the intentional behavior of another child to violations of one's perceived competence to perform a given concrete action. Such a violation might occur, for example, in the context of teasing. After being teased for causing a mishap, the offended child might construct a representational mapping such as "You laughed at me because I spilled my milk!" Such an appraisal consists of a mapping in which a threat to one's concrete sense of competence to perform a specific, concrete action is explicitly linked to the agentive actions of the other. At Step P6, with the onset of representational systems at around 6–7 years of age, children can coordinate two representational mappings into a representational system. At this step, children are able to coordinate representations of multiple, concrete actions in several contexts into a single, concrete trait representation (e.g., the child might coordinate representations for success on several math tests with representations of success in several reading tests into the general concrete trait "I'm smart at school"). At this step, children can place value on self-relevant traits and are often sensitive to intrusions on such concrete self-assessments. Thus, a child may become angry when judging that classmates have insulted his or her valued concrete traits. Similarly, children may begin to see reprimands, criticisms, and offers of guidance from adults as attacks on their valued, concrete self-representations. Although evidence is sparse, Gessell and Ilg (1946) report that children around the age of 7 often respond with anger to punishment or attempts to offer the self-guidance. Such children might view offers of guidance as violations of their concrete trait-like sense of self-as-competent in a given behavioral domain.

With the onset of single abstractions and abstract mappings in early and middle adolescence, individuals become capable of coordinating multiple trait and action representations into valued, identity-related abstractions. Such abstractions may support the adolescent's activity toward abstract, identity-related goals such as "seeking freedom from parents" or "becoming independent." Furthermore, the onset of abstractions may support the adolescent's attempt to define certain areas of his or her world (e.g., room, possessions, inner thoughts and desires) as "private." Actions by others that intrude upon these self-related goals may elicit angry reactions. Although evidence supporting these speculations is sparse, many theorists have suggested that adolescents become increasingly concerned with values related to identity, privacy, and individuation in Western cultures (Damon & Hart, 1988; Erikson, 1963).

Steps in the Development of Relational Violations

Relational violations include breaches of the basis of interpersonal relationships, or failures by others to extend the appropriate levels of care or nurturance to the self. Table 4 depicts a developmental trajectory for appraisals involving relational violations. Although it is unlikely that infants are able to psychologically differentiate between appraisals involving personal and relational violations, Case et al. (1988) proposes a series of developmental changes in infant anger reactions that can be considered instances of relational violations. At Step R1, with the onset of single, sensorimotor actions at around 4 months, infants may experience frustration over the failures of a seen caregiver to respond when wanted. At Step R2, with the onset of sensorimotor mappings at around 7–8 months, infants can keep in mind the goal of seeing their mothers, even when the mother is out of sight. As such, infants can exhibit angry reactions upon separation from their mother. In a variety of cultures, separation protest, which may include anger, begins to emerge between 6 and 12 months and declines in the latter part of the second year of life (Kagan, 1976).

Step R3 emerges with the onset of representational thought, around 18 to 24 months of age. With advances in self-awareness, children come to solicit their parent's attention and expect it to be directed toward them, perhaps exclusively toward them. As a result, young children may begin to exhibit angry reactions when parents begin to attend to other children. Haywood (reported in Case et al., 1988) reported a spurt in negative mood when children between 16 and 20 months witnessed mothers attending to another child, peaking at around 20 months (about the age that most children exhibit

Table 4. Steps in the Development of Relational Violations

Step	Form of appraisal	Age of onset	Example of step
R1: Sensorimotor actions	Frustration over failure of caregiver to respond to child when wanted	4 months	Seen caregiver who previously responded to child's cries fails to respond
R2: Sensorimotor mappings	Frustration/anger over separation between caregiver and self	7–8 months	Caregiver separates from child by leaving room to an unseen location
R3: Single representations	Anger over parent's attending to other child; anger when caregiver violates child's concrete standards and expectations that caregiver should be "generally available."	18–24 months	Parent holds and talks to a neighbor's child and child wants parent to attend to self; child is angry when attachment figure violates child's expectation that she should be available to self.
R4: Representational systems	Anger/hurt over parental reprimand or criticism seen as indicative of lack of love or caring. Child sees others as violating concrete expectations for "appropriate" amount of care other should provide.	5–7 years	Parent reprimands child; child says angrily, "When you yell at me, I think you don't love me! If I got hurt you wouldn't even help me!" or something similar.
P8: Single abstractions and beyond	Anger over violations of basis of close friendship/interpersonal relationship; involves violation of abstract standards and expectations that define interpersonal relationship.	10–11 years and beyond	Adolescent becomes angry when close friend reveals shared secret or becomes friends with a disliked third person; with development, relationship violations seen in terms of violation of trust or betrayal.

self-recognition in mirror tasks; Bertenthal & Fischer, 1978). It is possible that with the onset and further development of representational intelligence after 24 months, children may begin to construct standards and expectations for "appropriate" types of attention or care that parents should extend to them (Bretherton, Ridgeway, & Cassidy, 1990).

With further development along the representational tier, children come to elaborate increasingly clear representations of appropriate types of nurturance and care they expect from others. At Step R4, with the development of representational systems beginning around 6–7 years, children develop increasingly textured representations of the way in which caregivers should extend care to them. As a result, children may begin to become angry or justify their anger when they feel that their parents do not extend the appropriate degree of care toward them. Bretherton et al. (1986) reported examples of 6- to 7-year-olds who express concerns about their parent's care for them in reprimand contexts. For example, following a maternal reprimand, one female child said, "You don't care for me. If I were sick, you wouldn't give me medicine … and if I got really sick, you wouldn't even call the doctor to see what to do, because you don't care" (p. 541). Although these words were not necessarily stated in anger, they suggest the possibility that children may interpret other's actions to imply lack of care. Furthermore, they suggest that 6- and 7-year-olds can construct clear, concrete standards for the appropriate ways in which caregivers should care for them, and that children may invoke such considerations of care in reprimand-related exchanges with caregivers.

Step R5 marks the onset of abstractions during adolescence. At this step, teenagers become capable of representing relationships more explicitly and defining them in terms of mutual interpersonal expectations (Selman, 1980). As such, relational violations may involve violations of mutually agreed-upon standards and expectations about the nature of interpersonal relationships, especially with peers. At this age, for example, anger may result when close friends reveal shared secrets, or when close friends "betray" a relationship by making friends with a disliked other. Such transgressions may be understood in terms of increasingly abstract, value-laden notions such as "betrayal" or the violation of an explicit "trust." This proposal is supported by Gesell, Ilg, and Ames (1956), who report that beginning around 10 years, many children place great importance on trust among friends and become angry if friends associate with disliked others.

Steps in the Development of Sociomoral Violations

Sociomoral violations consist of transgressions of social and moral standards or rules. Table 5 displays a proposed developmental trajectory for the participation of sociomoral violations in anger. Because sociomoral violations involve violations of social rules, standards, or norms, we propose no steps in

Table 5. Steps in the Development of Sociomoral Violations

Step	Form of appraisal	Age of onset	Example of step
SM1: Single representations and compounded representations	Anger involving appraisals that intentional agents who can control their actions have violated rudimentary social rules or standards.	2–3 years	Sibling takes child's toy; child responds angrily, "That's not yours!"; child wants other to yield toy and says angrily, "My turn!"
SM2: Representational mappings	Anger mediated by simple social comparisons	3.5–4.5 years	Parent gives a larger piece of cake to sibling than to self; child becomes angry over difference; does not necessarily categorize difference as "unfair"
SM3: Representational systems	Anger over events categorized as unfair or in violation of clearly understood concrete rules based on reciprocity or fairness.	5–7 years	Child becomes angry at sibling who takes toy and says angrily, "No fair. I didn't take your ball when you were playing with it so don't you take my doll when I'm playing" or something similar.
SM4: Single abstractions and beyond	Anger/moral outrage over abstract sociomoral rules. Adolescent's anger is increasingly mediated by abstract moral rules, ideologies, or generalized values or beliefs about proper social behavior.	10–11 years and beyond	Adolescent can become angry at violations of increasingly abstract rule systems and idealizations (e.g., oppression, social injustice, hypocrisy, discrimination, violation of generalized social rules, etc.).

the development of sociomoral violations prior to 24 months of age. The first step in the development of sociomoral violations, SM1, occurs around 2 to 3 years of age, soon after the emergence of the representational tier of development. At this step, the child can begin to see others as intentional agents who can control their behavior relative to rudimentary sociomoral or rule-relevant standards, at least in contexts that support these judgments. As reported earlier, in their naturalistic analysis of children's disputes with siblings and parents, Dunn and Munn (1987) found that 2- and 3-year-olds sometimes justified their positions in disputes using simple social rules (e.g., "No! It's mommy's go again!" or "Get down. You don't walk on tables"). The capacity of these young children to offer socially appropriate justifications or reasons why others should forestall their behavior suggests a rudimentary capacity to represent concrete, rule-related, sociomoral violations.

Later on, with the onset of representational mappings at 3½ to 4½ years, the child is able to keep in mind the relationship between two or more representations. At such, rudimentary social comparisons occur. Thus, at Step SM2, the child's anger may be accompanied by appraisals involving social comparisons. For example, a child may become angry when a sibling is given a bigger piece of cake, or a toy that is perceived as nicer than his or her own. With the development of representational systems at step SM3, the child may begin to connect multiple representations of an event into more stable and generalized concrete social or moral rules. As such, children's anger may be mediated by more coordinated appraisals that events are "unfair" or in violation of more clearly articulated but concrete family rules, rules about lying and truth telling (Strichartz & Burton, 1990), or other sociomoral concerns (Jose, 1990). Finally, with the onset of abstractions at Step SM4, adolescents begin to experience anger or moral outrage mediated by rule systems that embody principles alluding to abstract "rights," "responsibilities," "social injustice," or other principles that define morally appropriate social relations.

CONCLUSION

From a component systems approach, emotional experiences and episodes are composed of multiple component systems and processes, including appraisal, affective, motive–action, and other systems. Although each component system is partially independent of others, they nevertheless fully interpenetrate each other in the production of emotional experiences. Emotional episodes self-organize into relatively stable patterns through the mutual regulation of component systems within a given sociocultural context. In this chapter, we examined the nature and development of appraisal processes as one component of anger episodes and experiences. We argued that whereas anger in infancy is precipitated by obstacles to action and blocked goals, adult anger often involves appraisals defined by ought violations—judgments that events challenge conditions that one asserts ought to exist. We presented evidence suggesting that ought violations in adulthood occur in a variety of forms, including personal, relational, and sociomoral violations, and argued that these appraisal patterns may be gender-related, but not gender-specific. Finally, we proposed alternative pathways in the development of these ought violations in anger. Of course, any single, angry episode may involve appraisals that embody aspects of different types of ought violations.

Anger is an adaptive reaction. Anger functions to remove conditions that violate an individual's goals, motives, or concerns. However, as anger-related appraisals develop from "want violations" to "ought violations," the functions of anger become elevated to a higher plane. With this transition, anger episodes no longer function simply to remove obstacles to what an individual wants or desires; they function to remove challenges to what an individual asserts *ought* to exist (de Rivera, 1981). The development of "ought violations" reflects important transformations in the evolution of the child's sense of self. A significant aspect of the self consists of the awareness of one's "moral position" in relation to others within a given context (Damon, 1988; Taylor, 1989). According to Harre and Gillett (1994), "[p]ersonal identity is one's sense of being located in space and having a position in the moral order of the little group with which one is conversing" (p. 107). As standards of value, worth, and moral standing become fundamental aspects of one's developing identity, anger episodes that result from violations of such standards support the assertion of one's moral position in the face of challenges to it by others.

ACKNOWLEDGMENTS.   We thank Kurt Fischer and Marc Lewis for their contributions to the arguments advanced in this chapter. We wish to acknowledge the assistance of Erik Riera and Lisa Kulpinski for their assistance in data collection. This work was supported by a grant from Merrimack College to the first author.

REFERENCES

Barrett, K. C., & Campos, J. J. (1987). Perspectives on emotional development II: A functional approach to emotions. In J. D. Osofsky (Ed.), *Handbook of infant development* (2nd ed., pp. 555–578). New York: Wiley.

Bates, E., Camaioni, L., & Volterra, V. (1975). The acquisition of performance prior to speech. *Merrill–Palmer Quarterly, 21*, 205–226.

Berkowitz, L. (1990). On the formation and regulation of anger and aggression: A cognitive-neoassociationistic analysis. *American Psychologist, 45*, 494–503.

Bertenthal, B. L., & Fischer, K. W. (1978). Development of self-recognition in the infant. *Developmental Psychology, 14*, 44–50.

Bidell, T., & Fischer, K. W. (1996). Between nature and nurture: The role of human agency in the epigenesis of intelligence. In R. Sternberg & E. Grigorenko (Eds.), *Intelligence: Heredity and environment* (pp. 193–242). New York: Cambridge University Press.

Biggs, J., & Collis, K. (1982). *Evaluating the quality of learning: The SOLO taxonomy (structure of the observed learning outcome)*. New York: Academic Press.

Bretherton, I., & Beeghly, M. (1982). Talking about internal states: The acquisition of an explicit theory of mind. *Developmental Psychology, 18*, 906–921.

Bretherton, I., Fritz, J., Zahn-Waxler, C., & Ridgeway, D. (1986). Learning to talk about emotions: A functionalist perspective. *Child Development, 57*, 529–548.

Bretherton, I., Ridge way, D., & Cassidy, J. (1990). The role of internal working models in the attachment relationship: Can it be assessed in 3-year-olds? In M. Greenberg, D. Cicchetti, & E. M. Cummings (Eds.), *Attachment during the preschool years: Theory, research, and intervention* (pp. 273–308). Chicago: University of Chicago Press.

Brown, L. M., Tappan, M. B., & Gilligan, C. (1995). Listening to different voices. In W. M. Kurtines & J. L. Gewirtz (Eds.), *Moral development: An introduction* (pp. 311–336). Boston: Allyn & Bacon.

Bruner, J. (1975). The ontogenesis of speech acts. *Journal of Child Language, 2*, 1–19.

Burke, K. (1952). A dramatistic view of the origins of language. *Quarterly Journal of Speech, 38*, 251–264.

Camras, L. A. (1992). Expressive development and basic emotions. *Cognition and Emotion, 6*, 269–283.

Camras, L. A., Malatesta, C., & Izard, C. E. (1991). The development of facial expressions in infancy. In R. S. Feldman & B. Rime (Eds.), *Fundamentals of nonverbal behavior* (pp. 73–105). New York; Cambridge University Press.

Case, R. (Ed.). (1991). *The mind's staircase*. Hillsdale, NJ: Erlbaum.

Case, R., Hayward, S., Lewis, M., & Hurst, P. (1988). Toward a neo-Piagetian theory of cognitive and emotional development. *Developmental Review, 8*, 1–51.

Damon, W. (1988). *The moral child*. New York: Free Press.

Damon, W., & Hart, D. (1988). *Self-understanding in childhood and adolescence*. New York: Cambridge University Press.

Darley, J. M., Klosson, E. C., & Zanna, M. P. (1978). Intentions and their contexts in moral judgments of children and adults. *Child Development, 49*, 66–74.

de Rivera, J. (1981). The structure of anger. In J. H. de Rivera (Ed.), *Conceptual encounter* (pp. 35–82). Washington, DC: University Press of America.

Dunn, J., & Munn, P. (1987). Development of justification in disputes with mother and siblings. *Developmental Psychology, 23*, 791–798.

Ekman, P., Levenson, R. W., & Friesen, W. V. (1983). Autonomic nervous system activity distinguishes between emotions. *Science, 221*, 1208–1210.

Ellsworth, P. C., & Smith, C. A. (1988). From appraisal to emotion: Differences among unpleasant feelings. *Motivation and Emotion, 12*, 271–302.

Erikson, E. (1963). *Childhood and society* (2nd ed.). New York: Norton.

Fincham, F. D. (1981). Perception and moral evaluation in young children. *British Journal of Social Psychology, 20*, 265–270.

Fischer, K. W. (1980). A theory of cognitive development: The control and construction of hierarchies of skills. *Psychological Review, 87*, 447–531.

Fischer, K. W., Bullock, D. H., Rotenberg, E. J., & Raya, P. (1993). The dynamics of competence: How context contributes directly to skill. In R. Wozniak & K. W. Fischer (Eds.), *Development in context: Acting and thinking in specific environments* (pp. 93–117). JPS Series on Knowledge and Development. Hillsdale, NJ: Erlbaum.

Fischer, K. W., & Hogan, A. E. (1989). The big picture in infant development: Levels and variations. In J. Lockman & N. Hazan (Eds.), *Action in social context: Perspectives on early development* (pp. 275–305). New York: Plenum Press.

Fischer, K. W., Shaver, P. R., & Carnochan, P. (1990). How emotions develop and how they organize development. *Cognition and Emotion, 4*, 81–128.

Fogel, A. (1993). *Development through relationships: Origins of communication, self and culture.* Chicago: University of Chicago Press.

Fogel, A., & Thelen, E. (1987). Development of early expressive and communicative action: Reinterpreting the evidence from a dynamic systems perspective. *Developmental Psychology, 23*, 747–761.

Folkman, S., & Lazarus, R. S. (1990). Coping and emotion. In N. L. Stein, B. Leventhal, & T. Trabasso (Eds.), *Psychological and biological approaches to emotion* (pp. 313–332). Hillsdale, NJ: Erlbaum.

Fogel, A., Nwokah, E., Dedo, J. Y., Messinger, D., Dickson, K. L., Matusov, E., & Holt, S. A. (1992). Social process theory of emotion: A dynamic systems perspective. *Social Development, 1*, 122–142.

Freud, S. (1940). *At outline of psychoanalysis* (J. Strachey, trans.). New York: Norton.

Frijda, N. H. (1986). *The emotions.* New York: Cambridge University Press.

Frijda, N. H. (1988). The laws of emotion. *American Psychologist, 43*, 349–358.

Gessell, A., & Ilg, F. L. (1946). *The child from five to ten.* New York: Harper & Brothers.

Gessell, A., Ilg, F. L., & Ames, L. B. (1956). *Youth: The years from ten to sixteen.* New York: Harper & Row.

Gilligan, C. (1982). *In a different voice.* Cambridge, MA: Harvard University Press.

Gilligan, C., & Attanucci, J. (1988). Two moral orientations: Gender differences and similarities. *Merrill–Palmer Quarterly, 34*, 223–237.

Halford, G. S. (1982). *The development of thought.* Hillsdale, NJ: Erlbaum.

Harre, R., & Gillett, G.(1994). *The discursive mind.* Thousand Oaks, CA: Sage.

Huttenlocher, J., & Smiley, P. (1990). Emerging notions of persons. In N. L. Stein, B. Leventhal, & T. Trabasso (Eds.), *Psychological and biological approaches to emotions* (pp. 283–296). Hillsdale, NJ: Erlbaum.

Inhelder, B., & Piaget, J. (1958). The growth of logical thinking from childhood to adolescence (A. Parsons & S. Milgram, trans.). New York: Basic Books. (Original published 1955.)

Izard, C. (1977). *Human emotions.* New York: Plenum Press.

Izard, C. (1991). *The psychology of emotions.* New York: Plenum Press.

Kagan, J. (1976). Emergent themes in human development. *American Scientist, 64*, 186–196.

Kagan, J. (1978). On emotion and its development: A working paper. In M. Lewis & L. A. Rosenblum (Eds.), *The development of affect* (pp. 11–42). New York: Plenum Press.

Kagan, J. (1981). *The second year: The emergence of self-awareness.* Cambridge, MA: Harvard University Press.

Kohlberg, L. (1969). Stage and sequence. A cognitive developmental approach to socialization. In D. A. Goslin (Ed.), *Handbook of socialization theory and research* (pp. 347–480). Chicago: Rand McNally.

Jose, P. E. (1990). Just-world reasoning in children's immanent justice judgments. *Child Development, 61*, 1024–1033.

Lazarus, R. S. (1991a). *Emotion and adaptation.* New York: Oxford University Press.

Lazarus, R. S. (1991b). Progress on a cognitive–motivational–relational theory of emotion. *American Psychologist, 46*, 819–834.

Lazarus, R. S., & Smith, C. A. (1988). Knowledge and appraisal in the cognition–emotion relationship. *Cognition and Emotion, 2*, 281–300.

Le Doux, J. E. (1994). Emotion-specific physiological activity: Don't forget about CNS physiology. In P. Ekman & R. J. Davidson (Eds.), *The nature of emotion* (pp. 248–251). New York: Oxford University Press.

Lewis, M. (1993). The development of anger and rage. In R. A. Glick & S. P. Roose (Eds.). *Rage, power and aggression* (pp. 148–172). New Haven, CT: Yale University Press.

Lewis, M., Allessandri, S., & Sullivan, M. W. (1990). Expectancy, loss of control and anger in young infants. *Developmental Psychology, 26,* 745–751.

Lewis, M., & Brooks-Gunn, J. (1979). *Social cognition and the acquisition of self.* New York: Plenum Press.

Lewis, M. D. (1995). Cognition–emotion feedback and the self-organization of developmental paths. *Human Development, 38,* 71–102.

Levenson, R. W. (1994). The search for autonomic specificity. In P. Ekman & R. J. Davison (Eds.), *The nature of emotion* (pp. 252–257). New York: Oxford University Press.

Mant, C. M., & Perner, J. (1988). The child's understanding of commitment. *Developmental Psychology, 24,* 343–351.

Mascolo, M. F., & Fischer, K. W. (1995). Developmental transformations in appraisals for pride, shame and guilt. In J. Tangney & K. W. Fischer (Eds.), *Self-conscious emotions: The psychology of shame, guilt, embarrassment and pride* (pp. 64–113). New York: Guilford.

Mascolo, M. F., & Fischer, K. W. (in press). The development of self as the coordination of component systems. In M. Ferrari & R. Sternberg (Eds.), *Self-awareness: Its nature and development.* New York: Guilford.

Mascolo, M. F., & Griffin, S. (1994). *Sex differences in anger coding manual.* North Andover, MA: Merrimack College Human Development Laboratory.

Mascolo, M. F., & Mancuso, J. C. (1990). The functioning of epigenetically evolved emotion systems: A constructive analysis. *International Journal of Personal Construct Theory, 3,* 205–222.

Mascolo, M. F., Pollack, R., & Fischer, K. W. (1997). Keeping the constructor in development: An epigenetic systems approach. *Journal of Constructivist Psychology, 10,* 25–49.

McIntyre, A. (1984). *After virtue: A study in moral theory.* Notre Dame: IN: University of Notre Dame Press.

Miller, J. B. (1991). The construction of anger in women and men. In J. V. Jordan, A. G. Kaplan, J. B. Miller, I. P. Stiver, & J. L. Surrey (Eds.), *Women's growth in connection* (pp. 181–196). New York: Guilford.

Nelson, S. A. (1980). Factors influencing young children's use of motives and outcomes as moral criteria. *Child Development, 51,* 823–829.

Olthof, R., Ferguson, T. J., & Luiten, A. (1989). Personal responsibility antecedents of anger and blame reactions in children. *Child Development, 60,* 1328–1336.

Ortony, A., & Turner, T. J. (1990). What's basic about basic emotions? *Psychological Review, 97,* 315–331.

Piaget, J. (1951). *Play dreams and imitation.* Melbourne: William Heineman Ltd.

Piaget, J. (1983). Piaget's theory. In Mussen, P. H. (Ed.), *Handbook of child psychology, Vol. 1, History, theory and methods* (pp. 103–128). (W. Kessen, Vol. Ed.). New York: Wiley.

Plutchik, R. (1984). Emotions: A general psychoevolutionary theory. In K. S. Scherer & P. Ekman (Eds.), *Approaches to emotion* (pp. 197–219). Hillsdale, NJ: Erlbaum.

Poulin-Dubois, D., & Schultz, T. R. (1988). The development of the understanding of human behavior: From agency to intentionality. In J. W. Astington, P. L. Harris, & D. Olson (Eds.), *Developing theories of mind* (pp. 109–127). New York: Cambridge University Press.

Radke-Yarrow, M., & Kochanska, G. (1990). Anger in young children. In N. L. Stein, B. Leventhal, & T. Trabasso (Eds.), *Psychological and biological approaches to emotions* (pp. 297–310). Hillsdale, NJ: Erlbaum.

Rogoff, B. (1990). *Apprenticeship in thinking.* New York: Oxford University Press.

Roseman, I. J. (1984). Cognitive determinants of emotions: A structural theory. In P. Shaver (Ed.), *Review of personality and social psychology* (vol. 5, pp. 11–36). Beverly Hills, CA: Sage.

Roseman, I. J. (1991). Appraisal determinants of discrete emotions. *Cognition and Emotion, 5,* 161–200.

Roseman, I. J., Spindel, M. S., & Jose, P. E. (1990). Appraisals of emotion-eliciting events: Testing a theory of discrete emotions. *Journal of Personality and Social Psychology, 59,* 899–915.

Russell, J. A. (1991). Culture and the categorization of emotions. *Psychological Bulletin, 110,* 426–450.

Russell, J. A. (1994). Is there universal recognition of emotion from facial expressions? A review of the cross-cultural studies. *Psychological Bulletin, 115,* 102–141.

Scherer, K. (1979). Nonlinguistic vocal indicators of emotion in psychopathology. In C. E. Izard (Ed.), *Emotions in personality and psychopathology.* New York: Plenum Press.

Scherer, K. (1984). On the nature and function of emotion: A component process approach. In K. R. Scherer & P. Ekman (Eds.), *Approaches to emotion* (pp. 293–317). Hillsdale, NJ: Erlbaum.

Scherer, K. (1988). Criteria for emotion-antecedent appraisal: A review. In V. Hamilton, G. H. Bower, & N. H. Frijda (Eds.), *Cognitive perspectives on emotion and motivation* (pp. 89–126). Norwell, MA: Kluwer Academic.

Scherer, K. (1994). Toward a concept of "modal emotions." In P. Ekman & R. J. Davidson (Eds.), *The nature of emotion* (pp. 25–31). New York: Oxford University Press.

Schultz, T., Wright, K., & Schleifer, M. (1986). Assignment of moral responsibility and punishment. *Child Development, 57,* 177–184.

Selman, R. (1980). *The growth of interpersonal understanding.* New York: Academic Press.

Shaver, P., Schwartz, J., Kirson, D., & O'Connor, C. (1987). Emotion knowledge: Further exploration of a prototype approach. *Journal of Personality and Social Psychology, 52,* 1061–1086.

Smetana, J. G., Killen, M. & Turiel, E. (1991). Children's reasoning about interpersonal and moral conflicts. *Child Development, 62,* 629–644.

Smith, C. A., & Ellsworth, P. C. (1985). Patterns of cognitive appraisal in emotion. *Journal of Personality and Social Psychology, 48,* 813–838.

Smith, C. A., & Ellsworth, P. C. (1987). Patterns of appraisal and emotion related to taking an exam. *Journal of Personality and Social Psychology, 52,* 475–488.

Smith, C. A., & Lazarus, R. S. (1990). Emotion and adaptation. In L. A. Pervin (Ed.), *Handbook of personality: Theory and research* (pp. 609–637). New York: Guilford.

Sroufe, L. A. (1979). Socioemotional development. In J. Osofsky (Ed.), *Handbook of infant development* (Vol. 1, pp. 462–516). New York: Wiley.

Sroufe, L. A. (1996). *Emotional development: The organization of emotional life in the early years.* New York: Cambridge University Press.

Stenberg, C. R., & Campos, J. J. (1990). The development of anger expressions in infancy. In N. L. Stein, B. Leventhal, & T. Trabasso (Eds.), *Psychological and biological approaches to emotions* (pp. 247–282). Hillsdale, NJ: Erlbaum.

Strichartz, A. F., & Burton, R. V. (1990). Lies and truth: A study of the development of the concept. *Child Development, 61,* 211–220.

Stipek, D. J., Recchia, S., & McClintic, S. (1992). Self-evaluation in young children. *Monographs of the Society for Research on Child Development, 57*(1, Serial No. 226).

Sullivan, M. W., & Lewis, M. (1993, March). *Determinants of anger in young infants: The effect of loss of control.* Poster presented at the 30th meeting of the Society for Research in Child Development, New Orleans, LA.

Taylor, C. (1989). *Sources of the self.* Cambridge, MA: Harvard University Press.

Thelen, E., & Smith, L. B. (1994). *A dynamic systems approach to the development of cognition and action.* Cambridge, MA: MIT Press.

Tomkins, S. S. (1984). Affect theory. In K. S. Scherer & P. Ekman (Eds.), *Approaches to emotion* (pp. 163–197). Hillsdale, NJ: Erlbaum.

Valsiner, J. (1987). *Human development and culture.* Lexington, MA: Lexington Books.

Van Geert, P. (1994). *Dynamic systems of development: Change between complexity and chaos.* London: Harvester Wheatsheaf.

Weiner, B. (1985). An attributional theory of achievement motivation and emotion. *Psychological Review, 92,* 548–573.

Weiner, B., Amirkhan, J., Folkes, V. S., & Verette, J. A. (1987). An attributional analysis of excuse giving: Studies of a naive theory of emotion. *Journal of Personality and Social Psychology, 52,* 316–324.

Weiner, B., Graham, S., Stern, P., & Lawson, M. (1982). Using affective cures to infer causal thoughts. *Developmental Psychology, 18,* 278–286.

Weiner, B., & Handel, S. J. (1985). A cognitive–emotion–action sequence: Anticipated emotion consequences of causal attributions and reported communication strategy. *Developmental Psychology, 21,* 102–107.

Weiner, B., Russell, D., & Lerman, D. (1979). The cognition–emotion process in achievement-related contexts. *Journal of Personality and Social Psychology, 37,* 1211–1220.

Yuill, N. (1984). Young children's coordination of motive and outcome in judgments of justification and morality. *British Journal of Developmental Psychology, 2,* 73–81.

Yuill, N., & Perner, J. (1988). Intentionality and knowledge in children's judgments of actor's responsibility and recipient's emotional reaction. *Developmental Psychology, 24,* 358–365.

V

Social and Cultural Perspectives

10

The Development of Emotion from a Social Process View

K. Laurie Dickson, Alan Fogel, and Daniel Messinger

This chapter examines the definition of emotion and how emotions develop. Although many researchers speak of the development of emotion, there is neither consensus about what emotions are nor what it means to say that they develop. These issues have been the focus of an ongoing debate between differential (Izard, 1994; Izard & Malatesta, 1987), cognitive (Frijda, 1993; Lazarus, 1991; Lewis & Brooks-Gunn, 1979; Ortony, Clore, & Collins, 1988; Sroufe, 1979, 1984), and functional approaches to emotion (Barrett, 1993; Campos, 1994; Fischer, Shaver, & Carnochan, 1990). We examine these issues from the perspective of the social process view of emotion (Fogel et al., 1992).

First, we briefly describe current definitions of emotion and various conceptualizations of emotional development. Our review is by no means exhaustive; rather, it provides a sampling of the major theories in order to illustrate unique aspects of each perspective. Second, we present the social process theory regarding the definition and development of emotion. Third, in order to illustrate social process theory's propositions, data from two

K. Laurie Dickson • Northern Arizona University, Department of Psychology, Flagstaff, Arizona 86011. **Alan Fogel** • University of Utah, Department of Psychology, Salt Lake City, Utah 84112. **Daniel Messinger** • Departments of Pediatrics and Psychology, University of Miami, Miami, Florida 33101.

What Develops in Emotional Development? edited by Michael F. Mascolo and Sharon Griffin. Plenum Press, New York, 1998.

separate research projects are discussed. In conclusion, we attempt to describe the functions of emotional change for the psychological and social life of the child.

DEFINITIONS OF EMOTION

Differential emotion theorists (Ackerman, Abe, & Izard, Chapter 4, this volume; Izard, 1977, 1991; Izard & Malatesta, 1987) link facial expressions to proposed discrete emotion categories via a relatively unidirectional relationship between internal states and facial expressions. Emotions are "a particular set of neural processes that lead to a specific expression and a corresponding specific feeling" (Izard & Malatesta, 1987, p. 496). The development of emotion is accounted for by an innate core set of emotions that emerge primarily as a function of biological change, that is, central nervous system (CNS) maturation (Izard, 1990; Izard & Malatesta, 1987; Tomkins, 1962, 1981). A "fairly predictable" maturational timetable dictates the emergence of structured whole emotions, for example, sadness, anger, and fear (Izard & Malatesta, 1987). Izard (1994) believes that emotion experience is invariant. Thus, "the task of development becomes one of learning to control state fluctuations and modulate expressivity" (Izard, 1991, p. 13). Development involves the changing connection between invariant emotions and cognition. Although the emotion per se does not change, Izard believes that environmental influences and cognitive development play a role in how emotions are displayed and appraised.

Cognitive theorists focus on the evaluative element of emotion (Frijda, 1993; Lazarus, 1991; Lewis & Brooks-Gunn, 1979; Ortony et al., 1988; Sroufe, 1979, 1984). According to cognitive emotion theorists, cognitive development mediates emotional development. These theorists differ in their definition of emotion; however, they all assume that cognitions play a primary role in emotion. Although they assume that newborns are equipped with innate reflexive expressions triggered by physiological processes, they propose that emotions require cognitions that develop over the first year of life; that is, particular developmental milestones are required for the infant to appraise the innate physiological response (Lewis & Brooks-Gunn, 1979; Sroufe, 1979). For example, infants are unable to experience anger until about 7 months due to immature cognitive functioning (Sroufe, 1984). It can be inferred that young infants are incapable of certain emotions as a result of inadequate cognitive development. However, Cicchetti and Sroufe (1976) define the relationship between emotion and cognition as interdependent rather than causal.

Rather than placing primary emphasis on either CNS maturation or cognitive development, functionalists focus on the relationship between the organism and the environment. Emotions are viewed as "processes of establishing, maintaining, or disrupting the relations between the person and the internal or external environment, when such relations are significant to the individual" (Campos, Campos, & Barrett, 1989, p. 395). Functional theorists (Barrett, 1993, Chapter 5, this volume; Barrett & Campos, 1987; Campos & Barrett, 1984) emphasize the functional implications of "emotion" movements. Emotions exist to perform specific functions that are required due to the individual–environment interface, including social, internal, and behavioral regulation. They are not tied to specific neural programs as discrete emotions; rather, emotions comprise "emotion families." Emotion processes that comprise an emotion family involve similar person–environment relationships and serve similar regulatory functions. Physiological, facial, and vocal patterns are characteristic of certain emotion families (see Barrett, 1995; Barrett & Campos, 1987).

"Development does not cause emotions, as entities, to emerge at particular ages; rather, the developmental abilities of the organism influence which particular member of an emotion family will be displayed" (Barrett, 1993, p. 163). Barrett does not view emotions as entities; therefore, they cannot be present at birth as whole entities or emerge as whole entities at particular points in development. Emotions are processes that are affected by the situation, the person's competencies, abilities, personal attributes, and the person's previous relevant experiences, and so forth. The development of emotion involves multiple factors that influence the emotion process, including cognitive development, socialization, and motor development. Barrett has used the emotion family of sadness to illustrate her point. Sadness may exist at very young ages, though the form of sadness varies with development. Thus, sadness for an infant does not exist in all of the same forms that it will at later ages. The type of person–environment interactions that could initiate sadness during early infancy are very limited, given the cognitive and motor capabilities of the young baby and the baby's limited socialization experiences. If an infant does not display the expected emotion in a specific context, it is critical not to assume that the infant is incapable of that particular emotion. The complexity of the emotion process increases logarithmically as the person develops (K. C. Barrett, personal communication, January 24, 1996). According to this view, development involves changing functions of emotion families with respect to the environment.

In summary, for differential emotion theorists, the primary determinant of emotional development is biological maturation. For cognitive theorists, the primary element of early emotional development is cognitive development. The infant requires specific cognitive milestones to appraise innate physiological responses (Lewis & Brooks-Gunn, 1979; Sroufe, 1979). For functionalists, the primary focus is on the relationship between the organism and the environment. Thus, development involves the changing functions that emotions play due to person–environment interaction.

SOCIAL PROCESS THEORY OF EMOTION

The social process theory of emotion proposes that emotions are not states but self-organizing dynamic processes created by an individual's activity in a context. A large number of constituents are involved in emotion, including patterns of CNS activation, autonomic nervous system (ANS) arousal, actions of the face, body and voice, psychological processes (such as feelings, drives, motivations and evaluations), and processes related to the transaction between individual and environment. Emotions are not discrete entities encased in the individual, but are socially constructed, dynamically created out of the constituents' interaction (Fogel et al., 1992).

What makes a behavior an emotion constituent? Behaviors are emotional when they are related to other behaviors that reflect change and maintenance of significant ongoing relationships between an organism and its environment. There are several constituents that are traditionally viewed as emotional (smiles, laughs, racing heart), but the degree to which a behavior is emotional has to do with its role in maintaining and changing organism–environment relationships. Behaviors that are not typically viewed as part of emotion by other theories may be conceptualized as an emotion constituent according to the social process view. For example, a father's tickle may be emotional because of its relationship to the emerging smile, and the smile may be emotional because of its relationship with the anticipation of the tickle and the child's gaze behavior. Also, the tickle to both the father and infant is emotionally meaningful; the tickle means fun, stimulation, physical engagement, and so forth, and therefore must be considered a constituent. How heavy the individual is breathing and the degree of physiological activation may be emotional because of their relationship to other emotion constituents. Behaviors are not emotional because of what they are; rather, it is how they occur, organize, and are organized by other components that makes phenomena emotional. This dynamic interaction constitutes the emotion process.

Given that emotion is viewed as a continuous process, what makes the emotion process different from what we call cognitive processes or motivational processes, and so on? The primary distinguishing feature is that emotion is related to that which is significant or meaningful for the individual. One of the goals of our research is to interpret how the patterns we observe are organized into a pattern of significance. Examples from Dickson (1994) illustrate this point. Evidence suggests that the infant opens his or her mouth wide during tickling episodes. The significance could be interpreted as an approach–avoidance process; being tickled is exciting and maybe even surprising, but it also causes some cringing and withdrawal from the physical stimulation and intensity of the tickling, as illustrated by the physical struggling to remove the tickling. The significance of the process (the enjoyment of it) comes from the balance of the approach and withdrawal, wanting to be tickled and not wanting to be tickled. The dynamics and intensity can lead to an enjoyable process, a boring one, or an unpleasant one. Another example involves the significance of a surprise emotion pattern. The surprise pattern appears in various situations, including book reading, when the parent suddenly makes an animal sound or an exaggerated facial expression, or during a tickling episode, when the parent sneaks up on the child with a quick tickle to the infant's stomach. Both of these episodes can produce a favorable or enjoyable process if the balance between anticipation, startle, and security is maintained. Once again, the dynamics of timing and intensity, and the organization of the constituents influences the significance of the organism–environment relationship or the emotion process. Rather than deciding *a priori* which parts of a continuous stream of action are more salient or significant than others, "it makes more sense to talk about sequentially related phases in an emotional process, differences in intensity, variations in motivational attitude between the self and the environment, all from the perspective of how each of these variations makes a transition from one pattern to another" (Fogel et al., 1992, p. 133).

The social process theory of emotion employs dynamic systems tenets in its explanation of emotion and the development of emotion. The principle *self-organization* will be emphasized. The focus will be on the emergence of stable patterns of constituents that develop from the dynamic interplay of the constituents. Self-organization occurs as the contributing elements act together to constrain the multiple possible actions of other constituents so that the complex system organizes into recognizable patterns (Fogel & Thelen, 1987; Haken, 1977; Kugler, Kelso & Turvey, 1982). The coordinated patterns of preferred states are viewed as resulting solely from the interaction between contextual variables and component synergies, without the benefit of a central executive control agent (for a discussion see Camras, 1992; Fogel & Thelen, 1987). From the many forms of organization that are possible given a particular set of constituents, only a relatively small number of patterns emerge (Michel, Camras, & Sullivan, 1992; Thelen, Kelso, & Fogel, 1987) and result in organized and repeated emotion patterns.

The principle of self-organization applies to both real-time dynamics and ontological-time dynamics (Fogel & Thelen, 1987; Thelen, 1989); that is, emotion components arrange into coherent patterns during moment-to-moment interaction (real time) and over developmental time, as illustrated in the following examples. Emotion components, such as facial and body movements, motivation, and so on, create patterns of emotion that are unique to that dyad. The father and infant's behaviors are not controlled by an executive program; rather, their behaviors dynamically interact and organize into recognizable patterns. An example from Dickson (1994) illustrates a pattern in real time. As the infant rolls onto her back, the father lowers his head into her stomach saying, "I'm gonna get you." Her jaw drops while she is smiling as his face touches her stomach and she begins to laugh. Her vocalizations fluctuate at the same speed at which he is tickling her stomach with his face in a side-to-side fashion. Her laugh evens out in pitch as he lifts his head before tickling her with his fingers. The vocalizations' speed and fluctuation increase as the father speeds up his tickling. Her jaw closes into a basic smile as the father withdraws his physical stimulation. This emotion pattern is repeated several times, though it is not dictated by an executive control. The behaviors of the partners dynamically interact to create the emotion patterns' timing and intensity.

Related to ontological development, the dynamic systems perspective proposes that emotions need not emerge as structured wholes according to a maturational timetable. Emotion constituents, such as cognitive appraisal capabilities, action capabilities, self-regulation capabilities, and facial movements may develop heterochronically and over time be organized into emotion patterns. The social process theory assumes that when behavior develops, it is attributable to some change or alteration in the dynamic process by which the constituents interact. Development is conceptualized as changes in how a system's constituents influence each other. The resulting stable patterns are a product of all of the mutually constraining constituents, rather than implying the emergence of new executive controls (Fogel & Thelen, 1987; Thelen, 1989). In dynamic systems terminology (Fogel & Thelen, 1987; Kelso & Scholz, 1986), a control parameter is a component that catalyses a reorganization of the system. Reorganization of constituent patterns occurs when the control parameter reaches a critical value. The system may shift from one major coordination pattern to another because of a single critical component. Although a particular component may catalyze the change, it is no more important than any other component because the change is uniquely determined by all the constituents acting together. Development is too complex to afford one component sole responsibility for the change.

Another real-time example and an ontological example are presented to illustrate the control parameter concept. A horse's gait shifts from a trot to a gallop when the speed of locomotion increases past a critical threshold. The speed of locomotion functions as the control parameter that stimulates the reorganization of the system from a trot to a gallop; that is, the shift in patterns result from the dynamic interactions among the lower-level constituents rather than a command from a central program (Camras, 1991). Concentrating on ontological development, Thelen (1989) illustrates the potential value of the dynamic systems perspective in her analysis of the development of walking. Traditionally, similar to the development of emotion, walking was assumed to appear by autonomous changes within the organism reflecting a phylogenetic blueprint. Thelen found that walking occurs when the fat–muscle ratio in the leg changes so that the infant can lift its leg against gravity while in the upright position. The fat–muscle ratio catalyzes the reorganization of the system's components and a new developmental structure emerges; that is, when the ratio reaches a critical threshold, the constituents reorganize and walking emerges.

Similarly, the emotion process changes or develops as one emotion constituent (the control parameter) reaches a critical level. The reaching of a critical threshold by an obvious or noncentral constituent, for example, motor abilities or cognitive appraisal capabilities, may spur a reorganization of the emotion system resulting in a novel emotion pattern for that individual. Understanding the process of developmental change involves examining the continual interplay of newly formed constituents and their relationship to the ongoing history of the emotion system. Development is conceptualized as a reorganization of behaviors that results in a novel, stable pattern and reflects a change in the significance in the organism–environment relationship. It is not merely any change in behavior. Development may be the result of various changes within the system, such as the relative influences between constituents or alterations in one or more of the constituents themselves, for example, maturation of physical structures, neuromotor processes, and additions or deletions of the social context. It is unlikely that the same mutual influences are at work in the patterning of all emotions, or at all points in development.

Camras (1991) provides excellent examples of the developmental path for several emotion patterns. The surprise-expression pattern involved a distinct pattern of nonfacial behavior (i.e., soft panting and limb waving, suggesting arousal and excited attention) at 9 weeks of age. Developmentally, the non-facial components appeared to change in conjunction with motor development. For example, when directed reaching developed in the first 3 months, the surprise configuration was often observed during this activity. The context in which the surprise configuration was observed changed by 5 months; the surprise configuration often occurred during a reaching, grabbing, and mouthing of the object sequence. By the second year, the surprise pattern was not regularly observed during this context. A more frequent context at this age involved the infant imitating the adult's emblematic usage of the surprise expression. One interpretation is that motor development appears to function as a control parameter at about 3 months, with the development of directed reaching, and catalyzes the emotion constituents into a novel pattern, whereas the child's developing ability to imitate the adult's emblematic use of the surprise expression shifted the emotion pattern by the second year.

The social process theory makes no assumptions regarding the relative importance of any single constituent in influencing development. The social process theory of emotion affords no single emotion constituent primary responsibility. Given the focus on the dynamic relationship between emotion constituents, the emotion constituent that functions as the control parameter will vary depending on the relationship between the constituents involved. Each component that other perspectives afford primacy may take the role of control parameter at some point in development. For example, cognitive milestones, such as object concept, intentionality, and causality, may function as a control parameter for the development of the emotion pattern for anger at approximately 7 months, as Sroufe (1984) suggests. However, the emergence of other novel emotion patterns, such as sadness, may be due to other factors, including cognitive realization of the significance of the event, the person's motor-response repertoire, or the social context in which the infant is embedded. It is premature to say that one emotion component warrants credit for the development of emotion. This remains an empirical question.

According to the social process theory, emotion is the process that emerges from the interaction of emotion constituents that relate meaningfully to the organism–environment relationship. Constituents of interactive or behavior processes are emotional to the degree that they are involved in a process that is affecting and/or stemming from the ongoing significant relationship of an organism and its environment. This emotion process changes over time. The variability of patterning of emotion constituent or the social context specificity of various emotion constituents illustrates this change. Evidence for this position derives from research on infant emotion that illustrates the changing relationships among constituents over time (Demos, 1982; Dickson, Nwokah, Fogel, & Nelson, 1997; Dickson, Walker, Fogel, 1997; Holt, 1984, 1990; Jones & Raag, 1989; Messinger, 1994).

INFANT EMOTION EVIDENCE

In this section, we discuss two empirical studies that help illustrate some of the points discussed thus far. As dynamic systems developmentalists, we seek patterns in sequences of action in a context, in both real-time and developmental-time scales. In the first study, we (Dickson, Walker, et al., 1997) studied the context specificity of different smile types during infant–parent play, real-time interactions. In the second study, we (Dickson, Nwokah, et al., 1997) examined the relationship between different types of smiles and different types of laughter over the first year of life to illustrate the complex transformation of facial and vocal features of positive emotion, developmental time. Although the two studies we have chosen to discuss do not provide a critical test between theories, they illustrate the heuristic value of the social process view of emotions.

The Relationship between Smile Type and Play Type

Given the social process view of emotion, it is important to look for changing patterns in the relationship between emotion constituents, in this case, the relationship between different types of smiles and the social context.

Research suggests that there are several distinct types of smiles, and that these different types of smiles are context specific (Dedo, 1991; Dickson, 1994; Ekman, Davidson, & Freisen, 1990; Fox & Davidson, 1988; Holt, 1990; Messinger, Dickson, & Fogel, 1992a, 1992b). The different types of smiles that have been identified include basic, play, and Duchenne smiles (Dedo, 1991; Ekman et al., 1990; Fox & Davidson, 1988; Holt, 1990; Messinger et al., 1992a, 1992b). Facial expressions are coded according to action units (AU) that describe the specific muscle groups that are responsible for changing the facial features (Facial Action Coding System—FACS; Ekman & Friesen, 1978). A basic smile involves lip corner raises caused by a contraction of the zygomatic muscle (AU12). In play smiles, the jaw drops open and the lip corners are raised (AU12 and AU26/AU27). With a Duchenne smile, in addition to lip corner raises, the orbicularis oculi contracts and raises the cheeks and, in adults, crinkles the eye corners (AU12 and AU6).

Duchenne smiles are more often associated with pleasant stimuli and self-reports of pleasure in adults than are basic smiles (Ekman et al., 1990). In 10-month-old infants, Duchenne smiles are associated with mother approach, whereas basic smiles are associated with stranger approach. Infant Duchenne smiles are also differentially associated with left-hemisphere activation, as assessed by electroencephalogram recording (Fox & Davidson, 1988). Blurton-Jones (1972) reported a reliable association between three mouth positions and social context. During social exchanges, children most often displayed smiles with lips parted and teeth showing. Play-face smiles were associated with conditions of high excitement. Smiles with lips together tended to occur during solitary activities. Jones, Raag, and Collins (1990) also found with 17-month-old infants that different smile types were distributed differently between social and nonsocial targets. Bared-teeth smiles were more often directed toward the mother than an object; thus, they were more likely to occur in social versus nonsocial contexts.

Given the proposition that patterns emerge from the interaction of the emotion constituents, the goal of this study (Dickson, Walker, et al., 1997) was to identify regularities or patterns of emotion constituents in the play interaction. Although this study does not examine emotion development per se, it addresses the issue of how facial expressions, one constituent of emotion, dynamically interact with the social context, another emotion constituent. The focus is on the interaction of emotion constituents and how noncentral constituents of the system may alter the emotion process. This illustrates the utility of viewing emotion from a dynamic systems perspective.

This study explored the interactional process between parents and their infants by examining infant smiles during parent–infant play. The subjects consisted of 36 Caucasian families, with 17 female and 19 male 12-month-old infants. Each parent–infant dyad was videotaped playing at their home for 10 minutes. The videotaped sessions were coded continuously for smile type and play type. A coder certified in Ekman and Friesen's (1978) FACS and trained on the infant version, Baby FACS (Oster & Rosenstein, in press), coded infant smiles (basic, Duchenne, and play smiles) from videotapes that focused on the infant's face. The parent–infant interactions were categorized into play type (object play, physical play, vocal play, and book reading).

Loglinear analysis revealed that different types of smiles occurred during different types of play. This discussion focuses on several of the significant associations for co-occurring behaviors that were more likely to occur than expected by chance. Basic smiles were more likely to occur than expected by chance during book reading, whereas play smiles occurred during physical play more often than expected by chance (see Table 1).

Qualitative analyses were used to interpret the loglinear findings and to preserve the continuous nature of the communication process. The significant effects from the three-way association (Smile × Play × Parent Gender) in the loglinear model were elaborated by creating descriptive narratives of select play sequences. The associations that were more likely to occur than expected by chance for the three-way interaction guided the selection of the play sequences. Prior to examining the specific effects within the three-way association (e.g., the finding that Duchenne smiles were more likely to occur during vocal play for mother–infant dyads), the play sequences were selected on the basis of the following criteria in order to enhance the objectivity of the selection: To be selected for description, the infant's face was required to be in view of the camera for the entire sequence (between 15 and 20 seconds), and the infant had to smile at some point during the sequence, regardless of specific smile type. The six play sequences were chosen randomly from the 45 episodes that fit the criteria. The selected sequences included a play sequence from both mother–infant and father–infant dyads for physical play, object play, and book reading.

The descriptive narratives facilitated the interpretation of the finding that basic smiles occur during book reading. Basic smiles may occur during book reading because of the primary focus on visual attention. In the mother–infant book-reading sequence, the infant has a basic smile on his face while studying

Table 1. Percentages for Smile Type by Play Interaction Type from Loglinear Analysis

| Smile | Play | | | |
	Object	Physical	Vocal	Book reading
Basic	35.0	28.2	15.6	63.0
Duchenne	35.5	26.7	66.7	31.5
Play	29.5	45.1	17.8	5.6

the pictures. Also, in the father–infant book-reading sequence, the infant has a Duchenne smile as she raises her head to look at the camera. Her cheeks lower into a basic smile as she looks back at the pictures. Basic smiles were more likely to occur when the infant was studying the pictures, yet both Duchenne and play smiles were more likely to occur when the infant was gazing away from the book. Duchenne smiles, which involve cheek raises, may obscure the infant's vision and interfere with the activity; thus, Duchenne smiles may be more likely to occur when the infant is not focusing visual attention on the book. Visual attention on the task may function as a control parameter, thus playing a key role in the occurrence of basic smiles during parent–infant object play. Basic smiles may occur during book reading in which the communicative function of the smile is enjoyment of the activity, yet the infant can continue to attend and concentrate on the book.

The significance of visual attention and smile type could be implied in a Fox and Davidson study (1988). A study using 10-month-old infants found that Duchenne smiles occurred more often during mother approach, whereas non-Duchenne smiles occurred more often during stranger approach. One interpretation is that more visual attention may be required when an unfamiliar person approaches than when the familiar mother approaches, therefore, visual attention may be functioning as a control parameter in the creation of non-Duchenne smiles.

Two interpretations of the finding that play smiles were found to occur during physical play emerged from the descriptive narratives. First, infants may open their mouths into play smiles in order to increase their air intake during a physically stimulating activity. In the mother–infant physical play sequence, the infant's jaw drops into a play smile and a giggle erupts each time the mother shakes his body. As the movements become more vigorous, the infant's shoulders heave up and down as he breathes heavily. It appears that the infant's jaw drops simultaneously as the infant is inhaling deeply or breathing heavily, which may help explain the occurrence of play smiles during physical play.

Second, there is evidence that tactile stimulation may help create play smiles. In the father–infant physical play sequence, the infant's jaw drops into a play smile as the father's face touches her stomach. She begins to laugh as he tickles her stomach with his face in a side-to-side motion. Her vocalizations fluctuate at the same speed as his tickling. Her jaw closes into a basic smile as the father withdraws his physical stimulation. Depending on how the emotion constituents organize, either tickling or inhaling deeply may function as a control parameter at 1 year of age during parent–infant play.

An example from the mother–infant object play sequence may help illustrate the idea that tactile stimulation alone does not cause play smiles in a linear manner. The mother and infant lean toward each other with basic smiles on their faces as the mother lies on the floor. The infant watches as the mother lowers her head. The infant's cheeks raise into a Duchenne smile as the mother makes rumbling sounds. Then, the infant's jaw drops into a play smile just as the mother shakes her head against the infant's stomach. The infant pats the mother's head with her hand a couple times. The infant's face changes to a neutral expression just as the mother raises her head away from the infant's stomach. The infant looks past the mother. Then, the mother leans into the infant's face and neck, and pretends to bite the infant's neck while making chomping noises. Before the mother pulls back, the infant looks at a toy that is beside her. The mother quickly buries her face into the infant's stomach as she did moments before, yet the infant does not smile. The mother attempts again to stimulate the infant's stomach, though the infant's attention remains focused on the block that she is now holding. The mother then pulls back and watches the infant play with the block.

Close examination reveals that various components must be present in order for the interaction to include a smile. The pattern that organizes depends on the components involved in the interaction. It appears that tactile stimulation functions as the control parameter in the creation of the play smile at the beginning of this narrative; however, when the components are organized differently, tactile stimulation does not function as a control parameter for this pattern. Other components in the system, such as the infant's increased desire to engage with the block, overstimulation from the tactile component, the mother's facial expressions, the timing or intensity of the tickle, and so forth, may play a key role in the interactions that did not result in a play smile. Given that tactile stimulation does not cause or elicit play smiles, regardless of other components, affords credence to the notion that other components in the system must interact to create the smile types. The principle of self-organization can be used as a heuristic to better understand this phenomenon. There does not appear to be a linear relationship between the environment and the facial expression, via an innate emotion program. The dynamic constituents involved in the emotion process interact to create the facial expression that is part of the emotion process. Thus, smiles emerge from the interaction of all the communicative components rather than being elicited or caused by a specific behavior.

This study examined the interaction of emotion constituents in real time to illustrate the utility of the social process perspective. The findings suggest that emotion constituents, in this case, different types of smiles, are created by the interaction of the different emotion constituents, including visual attention, tactile stimulation, vocalizations, and so forth. Recall that behaviors are considered emotion constituents when they are related to other behaviors that reflect change and maintenance of significant ongoing relationships between an organism and its environment. Smile types do not appear to be dictated by one specific component, such as feeling states, tactile stimulation, or cognition. There is no evidence that emotions or facial expressions are the result of a sole determinant. A more plausible explanation lies in the principle of self-organization. Different smile types may partially be determined by the reaching of a critical point by a control parameter, such as tactile stimulation and the formation of play smiles. However, a particular configuration of the other constituents of the system is also necessary. Next, we examine the principle of self-organization with respect to developmental time.

The Relationship between Laughter Types and Smile Types

This exploratory study (Dickson, Nwokah, et al., 1997) examined the changing relationship between smile type and laughter type (emotion constituents) over the first 2 years of life. Different types of smiles and laughs are not emotions; they are motor and vocal constituents of the emotion system. Recall that no one behavior is considered an "emotion." Related behaviors that organize into coherent patterns relative to the organism–environment relationship constitute the emotion process. According to the social process theory, the development of emotion can be described as the systematic change in the relationship between emotion constituents. Attention was paid to nonobvious emotion constituents that may be functioning as control parameters in the changing relationship between these emotion constituents.

Via acoustic analysis, Nwokah, Hsu, Dobrowolska, Fonte, and Fogel (1990) have found that laughter can be categorized into eight distinct types, and these laughter types appear to be context specific in the first 2 years of life. Three laughter types were examined in this study. The comment laugh is characterized by a single vocal peak with an explosive and aspiration quality. Comment laughter tends to occur during play; the child may reference the mother visually or it may be in response to mother's vocalizations. Comment laughs are often breathy and occur during conversation. The chuckle has two vocal peaks. The chuckle laugh tends to occur following an accomplishment by the infant or in response to the mother's behavior. The rhythmical laugh is characterized as a multiple laugh sequence of varying intensity. Rhythmical laughter tends to occur when there is an element of teasing, such as the infant dropping a toy and looking at the mother to see her reaction.

Eleven infants, 6 males and 5 females, were videotaped weekly when they were between 1 and 12 months of age and bimonthly during the second year. Each time the infant laughed, it was classified according to laughter type generated by the acoustical analyses (see Nwokah, Davies, Islam, Hsu, & Fogel, 1993). Each time laughter occurred, the infant facial expression was coded (basic, Duchenne, and play smiles) using FACS, as discussed previously (Ekman & Freisen, 1978).

To examine whether there is a systematic relationship between these emotion constituents for each mother–infant dyad, configural frequency analysis with smile type and laughter type was used. One subject was omitted due to low frequency of all types of laughter. Consistent with previous laughter research (Nwokah, Hsu, Dobrowolska, & Fogel, 1994), the data were aggregated into two time blocks (4–32 and 33–103 weeks) to assess developmental change. Nine months was employed as the boundary due to the reorganization of the babbling phonatory–articulatory–auditory mechanism.

The findings of this study illustrate a systematic relationship between smile type and laughter type and that this relationship changes over the first 2 years of life. Two major developmental trends emerged from the data. First, for 67% of the dyads before 9 months, play smiles were more likely to occur with comment laughter than expected by chance, whereas after 9 months, basic smiles were more likely to occur with comment laughter for 78% of the dyads. Second, for 33% of the dyads before 9 months, basic smiles were more likely to occur during rhythmical laughter, whereas after 9 months, Duchenne smiles were more likely to accompany rhythmical laughter for 56% for the dyads.

Speculations regarding potential control parameters are discussed for the changing developmental patterns of these emotion constituents. Although the factors we discuss have not been studied in relation to these variables, they may help explain the dynamic relationship between the constituents. In the first 6 months of life, the infant's tongue is still quite large, filling most of the mouth. The infant's epiglottis is in contact with the palate and restricts the range of vocalizations. Major anatomical changes during the first year allow air to flow in and out of the infant's mouth more effectively (Kent, 1981). In order to make a comment laugh before 6 months, the infant may need to drop the jaw in order to allow sufficient intake of air to create the explosive peak. As the physical structure of the infant's head and neck change, the relationship between the emotion constituents (i.e., gaze behavior, physiological reactions) may change, which allows the infant to create a comment laugh without the jaw drop. In other words, given that the infant has sufficient air intake without opening the mouth wide, the infant can create an explosive peak (comment laugh) without the jaw drop, which results in the comment laugh–basic smile pattern that appears after 9 months. Thus, the physical changes may function as a control parameter in the changing relationship between the emotion constituents.

Another possible interpretation involves the dyad's social interactions. Basic smiles occurring during comment laughter make intuitive sense, because the comment laugh is used as a conversational enhancer by adults and children (Nwokah et al., 1990; Provine, 1993). Informal observations indicate that adults in everyday conversations often make a comment laugh accompanied by a basic smile to acknowledge their ongoing interest in the conversation. The infant may be imitating the mother's use of a basic smile during comment laughter, and this pattern becomes more frequent after 9 months of face-to-face interaction. Recall that this aspect of the interaction was not examined in this study; the discussion is speculative in nature. The mother–infant interaction may help create the emotion pattern of the comment laughter accompanying a basic smile, thus functioning as a control parameter.

Rhythmical laughter is a multiple-sequence laughter of varying intensity and has been categorized as "real laughter" in adults. Ekman et al. (1990) suggest that Duchenne smiles signal enjoyment in adults and infants (Fox & Davidson, 1988). Given that rhythmical laughter has been categorized as "real laughter" and Duchenne smiles have been linked to intense enjoyment, it is hypothesized that Duchenne smiles may be more likely to occur during rhythmical laughter. It may be through mother–infant interaction that the infant's emotion constituents form patterns that are similar to adult emotion patterns.

The main findings are that specific types of smiles occur during specific types of laughter, and that these relationships change developmentally. These findings suggest that there may be an increasing match between infant and adult organization of emotion constituents, even before the age of 2 years. Rather than assuming a hardwired relationship between emotion constituents, the social process theory looks for nonobvious factors of the emotion system, such as physical growth and social interaction, that may be influencing the development of emotion. Dynamical systems mechanisms provide a procedure for the systematic search for critical elements that help explain development and interaction. Although we only examined one relationship among the many interactive emotion elements, these findings lend support for the social process theory's proposal that changing relationships among emotion elements over time help explain the development of emotion. Future research will examine a wider range of emotion constituents and experimentally test the hypothesis that specific emotion constituents are functioning as control parameters in the development of emotion.

CONCLUSION

One concern of this volume is the functions of emotional change for the psychological and social life of the child. We have chosen to address this issue in two parts. First, do emotion processes have specific functions? Second, what function is served by emotional development?

According to the social process theory, there is no set or specified function for different emotions; rather, the function of the emotion process emerges from the dynamic interaction of the emotion constituents. For example, anger does not have the specific function of serving as a social motive, regardless of context. The function of anger may be to regulate one's own physiological reaction to a situation, or it may be to force others to change their behavior. The functionalist perspective (Barrett, 1993) proposes that functions mediate the display of emotions. The adaptive functions that emotions serve include intrapersonal regulation, behavior regulation, and social regulation. The social process theory supports the notion that emotions serve these functions as well. However, we would argue that the function of the emotion acts as one of the many emotion constituents that interact with other constituents to determine which emotion pattern is created. The function of the emotion does not directly dictate the display of emotion. The emotion process that emerges from the interaction of the constituents determines the function of the emotion. The function of emotion emerges from the situation and the capabilities of the individuals involved.

Although emotion processes do not have specific, nonvarying functions, various functions are served by emotion processes as dictated by the organization of the constituents. The emotion process also involves a communicative function. This function has been discussed previously by emotion theorists; however, we stress that the communicative function emerges from the interaction of constituents, including the social context, rather than solely as a by-product of the individual. The focus is the changing communicative function for the relationship and how the function influences further relationships among emotion constituents, not on how an emotion *within* an individual changes functions over time. Emotion patterns and the communicative function build upon the cumulative patterns of prior interactions. These patterns are simultaneously influenced by and contribute to the emergent emotion process that has a communicative function. The function of emotion could be thought of as either intentionally or unitentionally communicating the significance of the interaction whether it is pleasant, unpleasant, embarrassing, and so forth.

Another function of emotion processes involves a way to organize and interpret experiences. As emotional processes develop, the way in which we interpret and organize experiences changes. For example, the emotion process of flailing arms, furrowed brow, narrowed eyes, clinched fists, and shaking head ("anger" for a 12-month-old) may function as opposition or as a request for assistance in withdrawing from the precipitating agent of the anger, whereas the emotion process of attacking with flailing arms, clinched firsts, and wide-open mouth and eyes ("anger" for a 25-year-old) may function to eliminate or scare the precipitating agent of the anger. Thus, the function of the emotion reflects the organization of the available emotion constituents. The 12-month-old's emotion process involved more limited motor and cognitive abilities, and differing motivations. The 25-year-old's motivation may have been to conquer the precipitating agent and might have been partially created because of the older individual's physical ability to achieve that goal. As evidenced by this example, emotion processes involve individual differences that are influenced by the available constituents of the individual, whether that is dictated by development or individual variation in situation and/or ability. The pattern of available constituents functions to organize and interpret experiences.

In conclusion, we discuss the relationship between function and the development of emotion. As discussed, emotional development is predicated by the development of various components, including cognitive and physical development, and interpersonal experience. As these components change and develop, their interactions organize into patterns of behavior. With these increasing competencies, the individual is able to interpret and organize experiences in more complex ways. For example, the development of an emotion process for anger involves the interaction of cognitive and physiological development. With this increased understanding of anger and increased ability to cope with anger, the significance of the experience is more complex. The primary functions of emotional change for the psychological and social life of the child involve the increased ability to organize and interpret experiences, and the increased ability to regulate intrapersonal, behavioral, and social interaction. These functions, as emotion constituents, are influenced by and influence the emotion process.

REFERENCES

Barrett, K. C. (1993). The development of nonverbal communication of emotion: A functionalist perspective. *Journal of Nonverbal Behavior, 17*(3), 145–169.

Barrett, K. C. (1995). A functionalist approach to shame and guilt development. In J. Tangney & K. Fischer (Eds.), *Self-conscious emotions: The psychology of shame, guilt, embarrassment, and pride* (pp. 25–63). New York: Guilford.

Barrett, K. C., & Campos, J. J. (1987). Perspectives on emotional development: II. A functionalist approach to emotions. In J. Osofsky (Ed.), *Handbook of infant development* (2nd ed., pp. 555–578). New York: Wiley.

Blurton-Jones, N. G. (1972). Non-verbal communication in children. In R. A. Hinde (Ed.), *Nonverbal communication* (pp. 271–296). Cambridge, UK: Cambridge University Press.

Campos, J. J. (1994, Spring). The new functionalism in emotion. *SRCD Newsletter*, pp. 1–14.

Campos, J. J., & Barrett, K. C. (1984). Toward a new understanding of emotions and their development. In C. Izard, J. Kagan, & R. Zajonc (Eds.), *Emotions, cognition and behavior* (pp. 229–263). New York: Cambridge University Press.

Campos, J. J., Campos, R. G., & Barrett, K. C. (1989). Emergent themes in the study of emotional development and emotional regulation. *Developmental Psychology, 25*, 394–402.

Camras, L. A. (1991). Conceptualizing early infant affect: View II and reply. In K. Strongman (Ed.), *International review of studies on emotion* (pp. 16–28, 33–36). New York: Wiley.

Camras, L. A. (1992). Expressive development and basic emotions. *Cognition and Emotion, 6*, 269–283.

Cicchetti, D., & Sroufe, A. (1976). The relationship between affective and cognitive development in down's syndrome infants. *Child Development, 47*, 920–929.

Dedo, J. Y. (1991). *Smiling during later infancy: Relationships among facial expressions, contexts and other communicative behaviors.* Doctoral dissertation, Purdue University, West Lafayette, IN.

Demos, E. (1982). Facial expressions of infants and toddlers: A descriptive analysis. In T. Field & A. Fogel (Eds.), *Emotion and early interaction* (pp. 127–160). Hillsdale, NJ: Erlbaum.

Dickson, K. L. (1994). *The parent–infant communication system: Infant smiles in relation to play type and gaze direction.* Doctoral dissertation, University of Utah, Salt Lake City, UT.

Dickson, K. L., Nwokah, E., Fogel, A., & Nelson, C. (1997). *Developmental analysis of the relationship between laughter type, smile type, and social context.* Manuscript in preparation.

Dickson, K. L., Walker, H., & Fogel, A. (1997). The relationship between smile type and play type during parent–infant play. *Developmental Psychology, 33,* 925–933.

Ekman, P., Davidson, R. J., & Friesen, W. V. (1990). The Duchenne smile: Emotional expression and brain physiology II. *Journal of Personality and Social Psychology, 58,* 342–353.

Ekman, P., & Friesen, W. (1978). *The Facial Action Coding System.* Palo Alta, CA: Consulting Psychologists Press.

Fischer, K. W., Shaver, P. R., & Carnochan, P. (1990). How emotions develop and how they organize development. *Cognition and Emotion, 4,* 81–127.

Fogel, A., Nwokah, E., Dedo, J. Y., Messinger, D., Dickson, K. L., Matusov, E., & Holt, S. A. (1992). Social process theory of emotion: A dynamic systems approach. *Social Development, 1,* 122–142.

Fogel, A., & Thelen, E. (1987). Development of early expressive and communicative action: Reinterpreting the evidence from a dynamic systems perspective. *Developmental Psychology, 23,* 747–761.

Fox, N. A., & Davidson, R. J. (1988). Patterns of brain electrical activity during the expression of discrete emotions in ten-month-old infants. *Developmental Psychology, 24*(2), 230–236.

Frijda, N. H. (1993). The place of appraisal in emotion. *Cognition and Emotion, 7,* 3–4, 357–387.

Haken, H. (1977). Some aspects of synergetics. In H. Haken (Ed.), *Synergetics* (pp. 1–17). New York: Springer-Verlag.

Holt, S. A. (1984, September). *The morphology and social context of toddler smiles: An ethological study.* Paper presented at the British Psychological Society, Developmental Section Meeting, Lancaster, UK.

Holt, S. A. (1990, April). *Toddler smile characteristics: Type and context similarities, sex and age differences.* Poster presented at the International Conference on Infant Studies, Montreal, Canada.

Izard, C. E. (1977). *Human emotions.* New York: Plenum Press.

Izard, C. E. (1990). Facial expressions and the regulation of emotions. *Journal of Personality and Social Psychology, 58,* 487–498.

Izard, C. E. (1991). *The psychology of emotions.* New York: Plenum Press.

Izard, C. E. (1994). Intersystem connections. In P. Ekman & R. J. Davidson (Eds.), *The nature of emotion: Fundamental questions* (pp. 356–372). New York: Oxford University Press.

Izard, C. E., & Malatesta, C. Z. (1987). Perspectives on emotional development I: Differential emotions theory of early emotional development. In J. Osofsky (Ed.), *Handbook of infant development* (2nd ed., pp. 494–554). New York: Wiley.

Jones, S. S., & Raag, T. (1989). Smile production in older infants: The importance of a social recipient for the facial signal. *Child Development, 60,* 811–818.

Jones, S. S., Raag, T., & Collins, K. (1990). Smiling in older infants: Form and maternal response. *Infant Behavior and Development, 13,* 147–165.

Kelso, J. A. S., & Scholz, J. P. (1986). Cooperative phenomena in biological motion. In H. Haken (Ed.), *Synergetics of complex systems in physics, chemistry and biology* (pp. 124–149). New York: Springer.

Kent, R. D. (1981). Articulatory–acoustic perspectives on speech development. In R. Stark (Ed.), *Language development in infancy and early childhood* (pp. 105–106). New York: Elsevier.

Kugler, P. N., Keslo, J. A. S., & Turvey, M. T. (1982). On the control and coordination of naturally developing systems. In J. A. S. Keslo & J. E. Clark (Eds.), *The development of movement control and coordination* (pp. 5–78). New York: Wiley.

Lazarus, R. S. (1991). Progress on a cognitive–motivational–relational theory of emotion. *American Psychologist, 46,* 819–834.

Lewis, M., & Brooks-Gunn, J. (1979). *Social cognition and the acquisition of self*. New York: Plenum Press.

Michel, G. F., Camras, L. A., & Sullivan, G. (1992). Infant interest expressions as coordinative motor structures. *Infant Behavior and Development, 15*, 347–358.

Messinger, D. (1994). A dynamic systems perspective on the development of infant smiling. Doctoral dissertation, University of Utah, Salt Lake City, UT.

Messinger, D., Dickson, K. L., & Fogel, A. (1992a, March). *The development of infant Duchenne and play smiles*. Paper presented at the meeting of the Southwestern Society for Research in Human Development, Tempe, AZ.

Messinger, D., Dickson, K. L., & Fogel, A. (1992b, May). *Infant and mother interactive smiles: Morphological and temporal characteristics*. Paper presented at the International Conference on Infant Studies, Miami, FL.

Nwokah, E., Davies, P., Islam, A., Hsu, H. C., & Fogel, A. (1993). Vocal affect in three-year olds: A quantitative acoustic analysis of child laughter. *Acoustical Society of America, 94*(6), 3076–3090.

Nwokah, E., Hsu, H., Dobrowolska, O., & Fogel, A. (1994). The development of laughter in mother–infant in communication: Timing parameters and temporal sequences. *Infant Behavior and Development, 16*, 23–25.

Nwokah, E., Hsu, H., Dobrowolska, O., Davies, P., Fonte, P., & Fogel, A. (1990, April). *Variations in the acoustic and contextual features of infant laughter*. Paper presented at the International Conference on Infant Studies, Montreal, Quebec.

Ortony, A., Clore, G. L., & Collins, A. (1988). *The cognitive structure of emotions*. New York: Cambridge University Press.

Oster, H., & Rosenstein, D. (in press). *Baby FACS: Analyzing facial movement in infants*. Palo Alto, CA: Consulting Psychologists Press.

Provine, R. R. (1993). Laughter punctuates speech: Linguistic, social and gender contexts of laughter. *Ethology, 95*, 291–298.

Sroufe, A. (1979). Socioemotional development. In J. Osofsky (Ed.), *Handbook of infant development* (pp. 462–516). New York: Wiley.

Sroufe, L. A. (1984). The organization of emotional development. In K. Scherer & P. Ekman (Eds.), *Approaches to emotion* (pp. 109–128). Hillsdale, NJ: Erlbaum.

Thelen, E. (1989). Self-organization in developmental processes. Can systems approaches work? In M. Gunnar (Ed.), *Systems in development: The Minnesota Symposium in Child Psychology, 22*, Hillsdale, NJ: Erlbaum.

Thelen, E., Keslo, J. A. S., & Fogel, A. (1987). Self-organizing systems and infant motor development. *Developmental Review, 7*, 39–65.

Tomkins, S. (1962). *Affect, imagery and consciousness* (Vol. 1). New York: Springer.

Tomkins, S. (1981). The quest for primary motives: Biography and autobiography of an idea. *Journal of Personality and Social Psychology, 41*, 306–329.

11

The Analysis of Emotions
Dimensions of Variation

Nico H. Frijda and Batja Mesquita

THE NATURE OF EMOTIONS

Emotional development implies that some things in emotions can differ from one age period to another. Which could these things be? To answer that question, it may be useful to look at emotions from the point of view of individual or cultural variation. The aspects of emotion that vary between individuals or groups may also be among the aspects that vary in an individual between different moments of its life span.

We survey emotions from this vantage point. Our orientation comes from exploring cultural variations (Mesquita & Frijda, 1992), because the perspective that showed itself useful there may profitably be applied to the study of emotional development. That perspective consists of a functional as well as a componential approach to emotions (Frijda, 1986; Lang, 1977; Lazarus, 1991; Ortony & Turner, 1990; Scherer, 1984). We summarize the main points of our theoretical perspective.

First, emotions are considered to be an individual's response to events appraised as relevant to his or her concerns: his or her motives, values, and emotional sensitivities. Appraisal of event relevance is one of the major

Nico H. Frijda • Department of Psychology, University of Amsterdam, Roetersstraat 15, 1018 WB Amsterdam, Netherlands.   Batja Mesquita • Department of Psychology, Wake Forest University, Winston Salem, North Carolina 27106.

What Develops in Emotional Development? edited by Michael F. Mascolo and Sharon Griffin. Plenum Press, New York, 1998.

functions of the emotion process. Relevance is signaled by affect, that is, by feelings of pleasure or pain. The central place of concerns in the arousal of emotions implies that emotions are tied to the individual's motivation.

Second, emotions are functional processes. They seek to deal with relevant events for the sake of the concerns (Campos, Mumme, Kermoian, & Campos, 1994; Frijda, 1986; Oatley, 1993). This is their second major function. They seek to do so by changes in action readiness and in energy mobilization, the physiological arousal changes. They seek to do so when the relevant event cannot be dealt with in a routine way. That is what emotions are for, at least in principle, because not all emotional phenomena are functional: Situations may be impossible to deal with, or resources may be exhausted, as in apathy.

Third, emotions are *interactional* processes rather than (only or mainly) intraindividual states or feelings (Campos et al., 1994; Frijda, 1986; Lazarus, 1991). This means that emotions are always "about" something, as the philosophers say (e.g., Kenny, 1963). Emotions are never disembodied *qualia*, not even when the aboutness is vague or the emotion is in search of an object, as in rage of neuropathological origin. It also means that emotions are best viewed as inclinations or disinclinations for engaging (or not engaging) in a particular form of interaction with the real or imagined object or person that is the source of relevance. They involve the aim or goal of changing or maintaining the relationship, or an explicit absence of a goal for relational change (as, again, in apathy).

Fourth, and implied in the foregoing, emotions always have to do with a call for action. They are processes that tend to control behavior and thought. They involve what we call "control precedence." They tend to interfere with other activities including thought, interrupt ongoing behavior, and they block the influence of stimuli having to do with other goals. When angry, angry goals (e.g., getting even with the antagonist) seek to take precedence over other concerns; that is, angry impulse, angry behavior, and/or angry thoughts seek to take precedence over other activities. Emotions, in other words, represent a goal shift of the individual, or a clinging to the current goal in the face of obstacles and distractions.

Emotions are sometimes viewed as cognitive states, as representations of the world or the self, or of desirable goals. This view misses the major point of control over action. Emotions are, first of all, action dispositions, regardless of whether actual action follows and whether, on occasion, the disposition is for inaction.

Fifth, emotions are multicomponential responses of which the components are only moderately correlated. Each response component has its own particular functions and determinants and thus may show its own independent development. The determinants include specifics of the emotion-eliciting situation and the prevailing state of the organism (e.g., fatigue, mood). The fact of moderate correlation between components is well established. Blaming someone for a harmful event, angry facial expression, other angry behavior, and increase in blood pressure, for instance, do not always co-occur. Moreover, when they do, their intensity does not always match (see Lang's "three-system theory"; Lang, 1977). Components may occur in many different combinations; there is happy experience with relaxation as well as with high motor activation, for instance. However, not all possible combinations occur due to the functional relationships between the components (e.g., strong action-tendency is unlikely with weak physiological arousal). What binds the various components together is the goal or aim of establishing, changing, or maintaining a particular relationship with the emotional object in the specific situation. If the goal is to be close or to possess, the action impulse is to approach, the appraisal includes appraisal of the possibilities to do so in the given situation, and the arousal matches the effort expected under the circumstances at hand.

The componential view conflicts with the view that all emotions are variants of a small set of "basic emotions." It assumes that the various components of each basic emotion are solidly welded together, vary simultaneously, and form characteristic patterns. Standard patterns for joy, sadness, fear, anger, surprise, and disgust are supposed to exist. In fact, names such as "joy" and "sadness" are supposed to refer to such patterns. In contrast, in the componential view, emotion names are related to emotion concepts that are fuzzy and probabilistic (Fehr & Russell, 1984), and refer to one or more emotion components (response components as well as process components, e.g., the antecedent event); when used to refer to one component, emotion words do not guarantee presence of the others. In several Western languages, the components that contribute most to the distinction of emotion concepts are appraisal outcome ("anger" as the experience of having been subject of a blameworthy action), action readiness ("fear" as impulse to avoid), and kind of emotion antecedent ("jealousy" as the negative response, whatever its further nature, elicited by a triangular rivalry situation).

The variability of component relationships and the fuzziness of emotion concepts make verbal emotion categories less suitable as a starting point for cross-cultural or developmental comparisons; it is preferable to focus directly on the emotion components. This allows one to locate differences or developments in each of the components. It makes it possible to describe the elicitors of respective components, the conditions that stimulate or hinder the appearance of each of them. It also enables one to focus on their consequences, such as their effects upon social interaction, upon the individual's self-image, and upon cognitive functioning. We follow the usage of referring to emotions by name but will put in efforts to specify which components we thereby have in mind.

Our final point is that this view implies that emotional experience is just one of the emotion components among others. The subjective experience of emotion is not what emotion is all about: The other components such as appraisal, action readiness, behavior, physiological response, and belief changes may exist without one being aware of them. In fact, emotional experience is where all components may come together. Focus upon emotional experience, however, may obscure the fact that such experience is the experience of these other response components.

We give an operational definition of what we mean by "emotion." Such a definition is needed, for instance, to enable discussing the development of emotional sensitivity to a particular kind of event (say, "jealousy" events, or "shameful" events) without confounding it with a discussion of what the emotion itself (jealousy or shame) consists of.

An emotion, then, is an event-elicited response set that involves one's relationship to some object or person (possibly the self), and that involves control precedence.

EMOTION COMPONENTS

Emotions are processes that involve several process components: perception of some event (the antecedent event), appraisal of that event in terms of its relevance for the individual's concerns, and activation of the various response components. The response components give rise to other components that, in turn, influence them: significance of the emotion for the subject, and emotion regulation. We summarize the components in Figure 1.

It should be emphasized that the sequence of components in the diagram is merely a logical one. It is not necessarily the sequence in which the

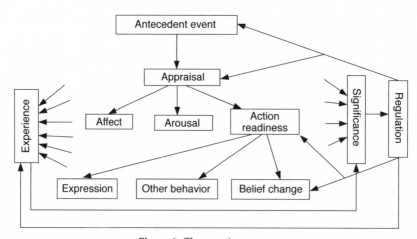

Figure 1. The emotion process.

components actually occur. In fact, emotions are nonlinear processes. Outcomes feed back to influence the processes that gave rise to them. Furthermore, each component may itself change over time: Appraisals of a given event may change as time goes on and attention wanders; action readiness may change when exhaustion sets in; availability of particular forms of action readiness or behavior may influence appraisal. Finally, the results of previous emotions may drastically alter the response to a given encounter (see also Dickson, Fogel, & Messinger, Chapter 10, this volume; Lewis & Douglas, Chapter 7, this volume).

The following sections discuss the various components from the point of view of their possible cultural or developmental variations. We will not discuss the component of affect, although the role of basic hedonic processes is essential in emotion. However, no cultural or developmental differences in this regard are known to us. Of course, there do exist individual differences in propensity for positive and negative affect (Watson & Tellegen, 1985), as well as for affective intensity generally (Diener & Larsen, 1993), but it is not clear how these are to be understood.

ANTECEDENT EVENTS

Emotion elicitation has to be examined from various angles.

Antecedent Events as Such

The specific kinds of events that elicit emotions show differences between individuals and groups. One reason is that they live in different ecologies. In violent environments, fear, anger, and grief have a different place than in peaceful environments, for instance (Osofksy, 1995). Conversely, certain antecedents for particular emotions are more prominent in some environments than in others. For instance, for members of minority groups, discrimination is a major antecedent for anger (Mesquita, 1993); among Japanese subjects, fear of strangers occurs less frequently than elsewhere, presumably because in many regions of Japan, strangers are few (Scherer, Walbott, & Summerfield, 1986). Human development brings obvious ecological changes as the child grows to move in different and increasingly wider social and material circles.

Different environments may also offer drastically different classes of antecedents because of more explicitly cultural factors. Social-status distinctions and the rules of respect that they prescribe are considerably stronger in one culture than in another, and educational rules differ in strictness, thus providing for different numbers of occasions for shyness, shame, and fear, and for satisfaction upon smooth conformity. Religious and supernatural beliefs and practices of magic provide other instances that are emotionally important also in that they may form occasions for experiences of belonging-ness (Baumeister & Leary, 1995) and self-loss (Baumeister, 1991), as well as particular forms of threat (Levy, 1973).

The degree of difference in emotion antecedents between individuals or groups depends strongly upon their level of description. Considered at some higher level of abstraction, emotion antecedents tend to show remarkable cross-cultural agreement, as has been established in a series of questionnaire studies in which university students from several West European countries, Israel, the United States, and Japan were asked to describe a situation or event that had caused them to feel each of the four emotions: sadness, anger, fear, and happiness (e.g., Scherer et al., 1986; Scherer, Walbott, Matsumoto, & Kudoh, 1988). The antecedents were grouped into general categories, such as good and bad news, problems with relationships, feeling rejected, permanent separation, birth and bereavement, success and failure in achievement situa-tions, obtaining desired objects or outcomes, harm to physical welfare, and threat and overcoming threat. The more important antecedents for the four emotions were virtually the same in the different groups, for instance, separa-tion and bereavement generally leading to sorrow, birth and success to joy, and so on. Similar results were obtained by Boucher and Brandt (1981) with American and Malaysian subjects. Certain types of events thus appear to be highly general, if not universal, both as events with emotional charge and as elicitors of particular emotions. At the same time, when described at some more specific level, strong differences appear. For example, what makes one feel rejected, or what precisely are the situations of achievement may differ cross-culturally. Something similar may hold for different ages: The general antecedent themes may remain similar, whereas the specific incidents of those themes may vary across developmental stages.

It should be emphasized that different antecedents for particular emo-tions, even if falling in the same general class, may have importantly different emotional implications. They may differ vastly in the occasions that they provide for social interaction and resulting further emotions, and in norm conformity. For instance, although most causes of amusement and joy can be interpreted as situations that provide varied stimulation, it makes consider-able difference whether that varied stimulation comes from reading, perform-ing sports, gang fighting, or vandalism, or from watching public executions. Particular attributes of antecedent events may further modify their emotional implications. For instance, belief in magic not only provides threats but also threats that are ever-present and difficult to detect. Fear of magic spells thereby implies the emotionally important appraisal aspect of uncontrolla-bility (to follow). Dominance of particular antecedents for a particular type of emotion may thus have consequences for the structure of that emotion as a whole; it may render one person's fear, shame, or joy, almost incomparable to other instances of these emotions. Differences may be so extensive that they lead particular cultures to produce specific emotion labels that have no equivalent elsewhere. For example, Utku Inuits have different words for sadness depending on the precise eliciting condition (Briggs, 1970).

Concerns

Because emotions result from events appraised as relevant for one or more of the individual's concerns (motives, values, and sensitivities), these concerns are among the emotion antecedents.

Concerns vary from one individual or culture to another (Schwartz, 1992; Schwartz & Sagiv, 1995). For instance, concerns for smooth relationships with close others are vastly more important in Japan than in North America, and emotions related to possible gain or loss in such relationships are more frequent and prominent there; Japanese has emotion concepts in the relational domain that have no equivalent in English (Markus & Kitayama, 1991).

Conversely, given events differ with regard to the concerns for which they are appraised as relevant; that is, they differ in meaning between individuals and groups. In Western cultures, signs of marital infidelity are primarily felt as threats to the relationship; in Mexico, they are seen as threats to trust in the partner (Hupka et al., 1985). Whereas academic success meant to Dutch people in one of our studies that they reached the goal they set out for themselves, Turkish people also tended to see success as a tribute to their family's honor (Mesquita, 1993). Illness may represent a threat to health; it may be seen as the result of black magic used by other people (called *wisi* among African Surinamese people; Wooding, 1979), or it may express the wrath of a divine power who was not given appropriate attention (Lienhardt, 1961). Southerners in the United States have been reported more likely to interpret insults as a damage to their strength and masculinity than Northerners (Nisbett & Cohen, 1996); among Turkish and Surinamese respondents in one of our studies, insults were more readily taken to be damaging for the respectability of the family than among the Dutch respondents (Mesquita, 1993).

Although concerns and their prominence differ from one group to another, basic and important concerns appear to be rather similar across cultures. Here, again, what is different at one level of analysis may be similar at a higher level, and again, analogous relationships may hold between developmental stages.

APPRAISAL

The term *appraisal*, as used in this chapter, refers to the information processes that link perception of an event to emotional meaning. Events presumably elicit emotions when, and only when, they are *appraised* as relevant to some concern ("relevance" or "primary" appraisal). The type of emotion elicited is assumed to depend largely upon the appraisal of one's possibilities or difficulties in dealing with the event ("context" or "secondary" appraisal).

The appraisal process can be conceptualized as applying a series of checks to the perceived event; each check involves one from a set of "appraisal dimensions." The resulting pattern of dimension values determines whether an emotion is elicited, and which kind of emotion.

Appraisal Dimensions

There is a fair amount of agreement in the literature on the appraisal dimensions that account for emotion differentiation in terms of verbal categories and modes of action readiness (Frijda, 1986; Lazarus, 1991; Ortony, Clore, & Collins, 1988; Roseman, Antoniou, & Jose, 1996; Scherer, 1988). Those most frequently mentioned dimensions are given in Table 1.

Different patterns of values on these appraisal dimensions should correspond to different emotions; to the extent that the subject is aware of them, they should represent an important aspect of the experience of particular emotions. Empirical studies have amply corroborated this hypothesis with regard to self-reported emotional experience (e.g., Frijda, Kuipers, & Terschure, 1989; Roseman et al., 1996; Smith & Ellsworth, 1985). There is accumulating evidence that the appraisal dimensions are cross-culturally relevant and explain a fair amount of variance in emotion labeling in different cultures (Frijda, Markam, Sato, & Wiers, 1995; Mauro, Sato, & Tucker, 1992).

At the same time, cross-cultural research has yielded clear evidence of differences in the propensity to apply certain appraisal dimensions. The dimensions of controllability and the agency of other people in unpleasant events are considerably more important for American than for Chinese and Japanese subjects; in American subjects, they explain more of the variance in

Table 1. Major Appraisal Dimensions

Positive/negative valence
Novelty/familiarity
Goal consistency/inconsistency
Controllability/difficulty
Expectedness/unexpectedness
Certainty/uncertainty about implications
Causal agency self/someone else/circumstances
Fairness/unfairness
Modifiability/definitiveness
Involves well-being of someone else

---

emotion differentiation (Mauro et al., 1992). Among the Semai of Malaysia, the tendency to blame (attribution of other's agency) has been shown to be weak or absent, and by consequence, frustration elicits *pehunan*, a state of fear and the perception of grave danger, rather than anger (Robarchek, 1977). Unfairness is a much less important anger antecedent for Japanese than for American and European subjects (Scherer et al., 1988). By contrast, the easy anger in honor societies (e.g., Miller, 1993) and in violence subcultures (Wolfgang & Ferracuti, 1969) suggests a high propensity for blame attribution in these cultures.

Appraisal and Cognitive Processes

The word *appraisal* may evoke the suggestion of deliberation or conscious awareness, which is emphatically not what is meant. What is meant is that cognitive processes intervene in the elicitation of most emotions. They do not always do so. Relevance appraisal sometimes consists of nothing but arousing the automatic, prewired affective effects of a particular stimulus; some stimuli just hurt, feel pleasant, or satisfy a desire. In such cases, there obviously is appraisal but no cognitive process. However, most emotion antecedents are appraised as relevant because they signal affective outcomes rather than directly causing them, or because they disagree with, or confirm, expectations.

The cognitive processes involved vary in kind and degree of complexity. Simple, and sometimes unconscious, associative learning and conditioning (Merkelbach, 1989; Öhman, 1993), as well as simple cognitive matches and mismatches (Murphy & Zajonc, 1993), are at the less complex extreme. Social modeling, such as in food aversions and disgust reactions (Rozin, Haidt, & McCauley, 1993) and cognitive anticipations, integration of pertinent cues, symbolic processes, and imagination (as with the fears aroused by spirits and black magic) are more complex forms of cognition. In other words, elementary cognitive capabilities are responsible for many emotional appraisals, and complex cognitive capabilities are responsible for many others. This has obvious implications for developmental changes in emotional sensitivities: Emotional sensitivities are likely to grow as complex cognitive abilities develop.

The processes involved in context appraisal likewise vary in complexity. Detection of most appraisal features indicated in Table 1 involves quite elementary cognitive operations. The operations are part and parcel of general processes of perception and recognition. For instance, novelty detection, which is a condition for attentional arousal or surprise, is just the output of a failed cognitive assimilation operation, just as familiarity assessment is nothing but the output of, or the feeling contingent upon, successful assimilation. Agency attribution is rooted in the perception of causality and of intentionality, both of which seem to belong to the elementary perceptual categories (Mandler, 1992; Michotte, 1946; Stern, 1995; current work of, e.g., Meltzoff and Moore, 1979). The formation and disconfirmation of expectations likewise develop early and, thus, are cognitively elementary (Parrott & Gleitman, 1989). Uncontrollability appraisal can be understood as the result of the failure of available coping resources and, in more developed form, as the anticipation of such failure. Difficulty appraisal thus is just the result of finding oneself without available means to cope with the particular situation, just as controllability appraisal rests upon the opposite contingency. Probably, only dimensions such as fairness and morality–immorality are intrinsically more cognitively complex or representational.

However, out of these elementary cognitive processes grow more complex or elaborate ones. Appraisal often uses more complex information than perceptual cues. Expectations can build upon complex chains of subtle signs, cognitive schemas, and imagery. Some causal attributions are based upon suppositions of black magic or merely suspected evil intent, instead of upon perceived causality. Causal attribution to the "self" or to properties of the self (as in guilt feeling, social rejection, and the nonmoral shame that results) probably is an extension of the elementary awareness of being the cause of one's actions and of effects in the environment that motivates circular reactions (Piaget, 1935), and, in turn, is extended in notions of the self as involving norms and norm transgression. The degree of cognitive extension of the cues for a given appraisal dimension may well be a source of variation in propensity to use the dimension, and cultures, individuals, and age groups may all differ in this regard.

It seems worthwhile to study the development of appraisal dimensions and of their elaborations. Such development may be responsible for changes in appraisal of given events. One may also derive developmental hypotheses from the supposition that some appraisal dimensions are intrinsically more complex than others. Such a hypothesis has been advanced by Scherer (1984). Novelty assessment, for instance, may well be intrinsically simpler than the assessment of goal conduciveness, since the former merely requires matching, whereas the latter requires integration of an event, a goal, and the implications of the former for progress toward the latter.

AROUSAL

Cross-cultural research, so far, has produced no evidence for systematic differences in physiological arousal responses to stimuli that produce otherwise similar emotional reactions. The only finding we know of concerns evidence for a stronger propensity for high-blood-pressure responses to frustrations among black Americans (Harburg et al., 1973).

It may be useful to mention that, so far, no solid evidence exists of specific relationships between particular emotions and particular patterns of physiological response (Cacioppo, Klein, Berntson, & Hatfield, 1993; Stemmler, 1989); the evidence that has been produced is unreliable. By consequence, no group differences can be assessed, and no age differences can be expected. Surprisingly, very clear-cut and cross-culturally stable relationships do exist between self-reports of bodily response patterns and particular emotions (Rimé, Phillipot, & Cisamolo, 1990); their origin is unclear.

ACTION READINESS

The notion of "action readiness" refers to readiness or lack of readiness to entertain or modify some form of relationship with the environment. Note the emphasis upon the relational content of this central emotion component. Major forms of action readiness correspond to major goals in the interaction with the social or nonsocial environment. They include moving toward, moving away, moving against, dominance and submission, hyperactivation or exuberance, hypoactivation or apathy, and inhibition (Davitz, 1969; Frijda, 1986). The major forms of action readiness map fairly clearly and distinctly onto major emotion categories, such as exuberance onto joy and moving against onto anger (Frijda et al., 1989; Roseman, Wiest, & Swartz, 1994). The mappings appear to hold cross-culturally (Frijda et al., 1995; Scherer & Wallbott, 1994).

Forms of action readiness are defined by their aims or goals in establishing or changing a particular kind of relationship (Roseman et al., 1994): moving toward aims at access, moving away at diminishing harm, moving against at removal of an offender, exuberance at increasing interaction generally, and so on. They are best understood as the activation of behavioral systems in the sense that term is used in ethology, that is, of sets of behaviors sharing a common aim. Which of these behaviors is actually shown depends upon particulars of the situation and the individual's response repertoire.

Forms of action readiness can be described at different levels of abstraction. The forms distinguished in the preceding paragraphs form the higher level. They probably form a universal and basic set; at least, most of them turned up as factors in the action readiness factor analyses of the three cultural groups (Dutch, Indonesian, Japanese) included in our cross-cultural study (Frijda et al., 1995). However, the contribution to variance explained by the factors identified in all three groups differed drastically from one group to the other. For instance, "moving away" was twice as important for the Dutch than for the other two groups in distinguishing the 16 emotions, whereas the reverse held for "moving toward." Propensity for the various emotional impulses, even if universally present, thus appears sensitive to cultural variables.

Moreover, forms of action readiness may also be described at a more specific level, such as the level of the individual items of the action readiness questionnaire. At this more concrete level, there may be variance across individuals, cultural groups, or developmental stages. The more specific forms of action readiness can be regarded as different ways to achieve a given relational aim as described at the higher level. For instance, one can distinguish between readiness to shut oneself off, to retreat, to escape, and to avoid, as different forms of readiness to "move away," or between hostile tendency and the tendency to turn away and break off contact as forms of "moving against." The more specific forms in fact describe drastically different forms of the "same" emotion. Anger involving an impulse for hostile behavior is a different anger from one that turns away and breaks contact. In our cross-cultural study (Frijda et al., 1995), important group differences were indeed found in the importance of particular action-readiness items (e.g., aggressive impulse vs. "boiling inwardly" within the category of "anger").

Finally, there is some evidence of cultural influences on the forms of emotional action readiness evoked by particular types of events. For example, in one study, Dutch, Surinamese, and Turkish people living in the Netherlands were asked how they had reacted in situations in which they had behaved improperly toward an intimate other. Surinamese and Turkish subjects reported that they did not dare to look the other person in the face and had the desire not to be noticed or seen; the Dutch reported no such tendencies (Mesquita, 1993).

BEHAVIOR: EXPRESSIVE BEHAVIOR

We only discuss facial expression. There is strong evidence for universality of a set of seven or eight facial-expression patterns that have more or less distinct relationships with the emotion classes labeled in English as happiness or joy, sadness, fear, anger, surprise, disgust, and interest, and perhaps contempt (Ekman, 1994; Izard, 1994). Also, there is evidence that many or most of these facial-expression patterns already occur in early childhood (e.g., Izard & Malatesta, 1987).

However, it is not immediately clear what these findings mean. First, the universal expressions are not invariably accompanied by the emotions they seem to signal; that is, they are not always accompanied by other components of those emotions such as the emotional experience, nor do they invariably follow antecedent events that might have elicited such emotions (Fridlund, 1994; Russell, 1994). Second, the universality of facial-expression patterns says little about the practice of their occurrence, that is, about their connection with the emotions they may seem to show. Most occurrences of particular emotions are in fact not accompanied by the expressions that recognition experiments suggest show those emotions. Moreover, many facial expressions occur with other states than the ones they are theoretically linked to, including nonemotional states such as fatigue and effort. The relevant evidence is reviewed by Fridlund (1994) and by Frijda and Tcherkassof (1997). For instance, viewing films appraised as amusing often does not lead to laughter or smiling (Fridlund, 1994), and winning an Olympic contest may evoke laughter or smiling no earlier than that the winner faces the public (Dols, 1997).

The data indicate that facial expressions do not have a strict and unique relationship with particular emotions. At least two alternative views on facial expressions have been advanced. One is that facial expressions implement states of action readiness. In need of reorientation, one interrupts behavior and opens the eyes widely (the "surprise" expression). And when desiring to protect oneself, one frowns, narrows the eyes, and draws the head backward as far as one can (the "fear" expression) (Frijda, 1986; Frijda & Tcherkassof, 1997). This action-readiness interpretation of facial expressions gives a functional interpretation of the components of the facial expressions in terms of enabling, facilitating, or hindering one's relations with the environment. The components, in turn, can be linked to specific dimensions of appraisal (Scherer, 1992; Smith, 1997).

The second alternative view considers facial expressions as social signals conveying intentions, commands, and requests. The smile (or many smiles) can be understood as an appeasement request or as signaling approach with nonhostile intent; angry expressions can be seen as threat displays (Fridlund, 1994; Frijda, 1986). The two views are compatible in that the social signals usually serve to achieve the aims of some emotional action-tendency, even if somewhat indirectly.

These interpretations suggest that facial expressions can be read as cues to the prevailing readiness or unreadiness in the social or nonsocial interaction, regardless of the emotion category applied. Smile variants, for instance, differ in the social receptivity that they imply and the social response that they invite (Bloom & Beckwith, 1989). Variations in expressions during anger likewise represent differences such as those between fierce threat and withdrawal from contact.

Display Rules and Social Dynamics

Cultural differences in the ecology of facial expression have been explained by Ekman and Friesen (1969), by what they coined as *display rules*. Cultures may differentially suppress, attenuate, or enhance facial expressiveness or particular expressions. Display rules are often context-specific. For instance, explicit rules existed in traditional China with regard to the frequency and magnitude of weeping as a function of one's relationship to the deceased (Granet, 1922). Display rules do not account for all cultural differences in facial expression but they can be considered a major source of variation.

The term *display rules* does not always do justice to what actually makes expressions vary as a function of social norms. Cultural variations in which facial expressions are shown are often not due to the rules of expression per se but to rules of proper conduct and respect or, more generally, to the social implications of particular expressions. Among the Japanese, for instance, facial expressions of displeasure in face-to-face contact, rather than being suppressed, tend to be overruled by the expression corresponding to polite intercourse: the smile (Lebra, 1976). The smiling may also help the individual to focus on the interaction, thereby drawing his or her attention away from the source of discontent. Due to differences in social implications, particular facial expressions may have appreciably different meanings in different contexts, even when their basic emotional message is similar. A smile may be an expression of pleasure or friendliness always and everywhere, but showing friendliness may be insolent in one cultural context, a reason for distrust in another, and may fit the interaction rules or emotional climate in a third.

OTHER BEHAVIOR

Appraisals and relational action-tendencies motivate social behaviors, including investigative behavior, proximity seeking, withdrawal behavior, and aggression. Particular emotions (e.g., particular appraisals and action-tendencies) motivate particular kinds of social behavior. Guilt feelings (that is, the appraisal of having caused harm) may lead to solicitous caregiving and public atonement. Shame (that is, appraisal of having caused threat of social rejection or of being treated as inferior) may lead to submissive and hiding behavior, to leaving one's job, and to suicide, as well as to aggression aimed at undoing the inferiority.

Kind and range of social behaviors vary considerably across individuals and cultures. Angry behavior is not tolerated in one culture, has to be limited to scolding in another, and only involves turning away, falling silent, and breaking contact in a third. For instance, absence of violence appears to characterize the everyday life of the Utku Eskimos and the Tahitians. In both cultures, hostility is mostly restricted to "small acts" such as gossip, teasing, or coolness (Levy, 1973), or sulking, being silent, and withdrawal (Briggs, 1970). Grief behavior in Western cultures, is almost restricted to silent sobbing and apathy but may involve loud wailing in public ceremonies in black-Surinamese and probably other cultures. Affiliative behavior such as embracing, seeking support, and maintaining a bond regardless of controversy, shows very large cultural differences, as the much greater emphasis on proximity seeking is apparent in differentiating emotions in Japanese and Indonesian subjects than in the Dutch (Frijda et al., 1994).

Social behaviors often elicit reactions from the environment, and differences in behaviors thus cause differences in repercussions. Retaliation in response to anger displays, social acceptance or reacceptance in the case of shame displays, and anger attenuation in the case of manifest guilt, are cases in point. The way the social environment reacts may itself feed back to the emotion. The repercussions may prolong or enhance the emotional situation's impact or may cause environmental compliance and help. Also, the more extreme the emotional behavior, the more serious the subsequent transaction can be expected to be. Extremity, in turn, is influenced by social norms and the outcomes of previous transactions.

Emotional behavior may also exert strong retroactive effects upon the emotion process as a whole. Aggression may enhance anger and thus reinforce itself (Frijda, 1995). In general, performing social behaviors tends to induce one to seek justifications for it, thereby amplifying the underlying appraisal, thereby also amplifying action-tendencies and arousal.

All preceding outcomes of emotional behavior may enter what we will discuss as the "significance" of the emotion and thereby become part of emotional experience. The feeling connected with an impulse or action that has drastic social consequences is different from one that only remains internal or a mere facial grimace.

BELIEF CHANGES

Emotions, that is, appraisal processes and states of action readiness, may also engender beliefs. The way an object or person is appraised in emotion— as the agent of evil in anger, or as a creature with gentleness and beauty in infatuation—may be generalized beyond the content of the emotional event and turned into an attribution of stable characteristics that persists and outlives the emotion. Appraisals may thus be turned into an emotional attitude or sentiment with regard to the object or person. Anger, for instance, may lead to a sentiment of hate; that is, the appraisal of someone having performed a blameworthy act may lead to the belief in the bad nature of that person. Likewise, an emotion of fear may turn into a phobia, that is, into the belief that the object is evil and will continue to elicit fear (Frijda, Mesquita, Sonnemans, & Van Goozen, 1991).

Beliefs not only result from generalization, but also from elaboration of the appraisals that gave rise to the emotion or that emerged in the process. Emotions often instigate elaboration of appraisals in order to find a reason or a justification for them, or to support actions to cope with the event. For instance, the belief that what one is ashamed of deserves shame—a frequent element in shame feelings—probably is construed for the sake of counteracting the felt or feared rejection (one at least agrees with the rejecting others; Frijda, 1993); the hatred–belief is often construed to justify one's anger.

The extension of emotional appraisal into a fixed belief, and the extremity of that belief, are dimensions of variation of emotions. They are, it seems, influenced by cultural habits as well as by individual inclination. Distinct group differences have been found in this regard. For instance, Surinamese subjects tend more strongly to change their beliefs about a person (for instance, a friend) who treated them badly than autochtonous Dutch subjects do (Mesquita, 1993).

SIGNIFICANCE

Specific emotional experiences, individual emotion components, and kinds of emotions usually possess a "significance." By "significance" we mean the evaluation of the experience, component, or kind of emotion for the subject him- or herself. One may feel that it is good, or bad, to experience a particular emotion, to feel impelled to a particular kind of behavior, or show a particular physiological response such as blushing or wetting one's pants. One may feel it is childish, or cowardly, or immoral, or refined. One may be proud or ashamed of it.

Several kinds of significance can be distinguished: significance with respect to one's self-image and self-esteem, with respect to external effects such as eliciting help or retaliation, and with respect to one's social position (Frijda, 1986, p. 445ff.).

Cultures differ widely in the significance attached to given emotions or emotion instances in specific situations. Anger is condemned by the Utku Eskimos (Briggs, 1970) and applauded as manifesting masculine dignity by the Kaluli bushmen (Schieffelin, 1983). Among the Awlad 'Ali Bedouins, the expression of some emotions, such as love, sadness, and despair, is restricted to occasions when one is in the company of intimates who are one's equals, because they are considered to be "weak" emotions (Abu-Lughod, 1986). Expressing weak emotions would, in other contexts, show one's dependence and therefore damage one's honor.

Significance can be the source of having other emotions contingent on having the significant emotion and arising simultaneously with them: shame, distress, confusion, pride, and joy, for instance. Those latter emotions blend with the former, or color them; an accepted emotion and one that elicits shame presumably feel differently. Cultural norms, again, are among the factors that decide about the significance and the resulting emotions that accompany the initial one.

REGULATION

Regulation refers to attenuation or inhibition of emotions caused by anticipated adverse effects of uncontrolled emotion, as well as to enhancement of emotion because of anticipated advantageous effects. The negative and positive effects that trigger regulation may be external (e.g., retaliation, profit), internal (e.g., pangs of conscience), or purely intrapsychic (e.g., discomfort). The adverse and advantageous effects are those just described as emotion significance. Emotion significance is the major motor for emotion regulation. Presumably, negative emotion significance is the basis for emotion control, and positive significance is the basis for enhancement of its expression or for seeking its occurrence. The regulating effects may come from internalized social norms as well as from actual or anticipated repercussions in the given social situation.

Regulation can affect all emotion components. It may lead to avoiding or seeking out situations that might elicit particular emotions, to appraising a situation in such a way that a particular emotion will not arise (as in deciding not to take an insult seriously), or to suppressing an action-tendency and attenuating a facial expression. Regulation thus may affect the very arousal and experience of an emotion, and not merely its outward expression.

Regulation of emotions has consequences beyond having or showing the emotion. Because emotions usually have social consequences, regulation of emotions affects social interactions. The taboo among the Orissa in India on touching a menstruating woman probably affects the freedom of the mother–child interaction, because a child who approaches the mother during her period is vehemently pushed back (Shweder, 1993). The social rule against free expressions of joy among the Ifaluk leads to reprimanding a child who behaves exuberantly, as well as an adult who might encourage such behavior by smiling, thus toning down the entire interaction (Lutz, 1988). Regulation of sexual emotions, of course, deeply affects interpersonal interactions and emotions in a large domain.

EMOTIONAL EXPERIENCE

Emotional experience consists of the awareness of some or all other components. Emotional experience is composed of affect, awareness of the emotion antecedent as appraised and of emotion-generated beliefs, awareness of one's state of action readiness, of one's physiological response, of the emotion's significance, and of the various effects of regulation. We think that emotional experiences are also colored by the awareness of the social and other consequences of what one feels impelled to do or to leave undone. Experience, as we said before, is where all components may come together, and to which all can contribute. But although they may, not necessarily do they. At its most elementary, emotional experience is entirely unreflective and consists of nothing but the experience of an event as appraised, with "affect" as its perceived attractiveness or aversiveness (Frijda, 1986). Reflectiveness is not part of the definition of experience.

Emotional experiences change over time as attention wanders over the various aspects of the emotional situation and, reflexively, over one's pattern of reaction, the unreflected perceptual awareness included. This need not surprise, since reflexive experiencing is an act, an activity superimposed upon "having" whatever it is that is experienced: the results of the cognitive processes of appraisal, action readiness, arousal, regulation. It thus is a product of separate development, largely independent of the development responsible for emotional sensitivity, the articulation of appraisal, and the progressive differentiation in modes of action readiness and forms of emotional behavior, that is, emotion itself.

Our approach makes it obvious that we consider the hypothesis of basic emotional *qualia* (e.g., Izard, 1977) to be unfruitful. Indeed, we think the hypothesis untestable, incompatible with cross-cultural differences in emotion taxonomies (Mesquita, Frijda, & Scherer, 1997; Russell, 1994), and unnecessary. There is ample material to make an experience of, say, anger different from one of fear. The only *qualia* are those of affect: the experiences of pleasure and pain.

Identifying one's emotion and emotion labeling are not the core of emotion, as little as reflexive experience is. Emotion labeling, too, is an extra activity. Like consciously identifying one's emotion and being aware of it, it presupposes a reflexive act that is unnecessary for the other components to occur. Labeling appears to rest upon drastically different developmental conditions.

Categorizing or labeling one's experience may take awareness of any of the components of the emotion as its starting point. An experience may be called "fear" by the subject because there is experience of threat, or because there is a felt impulse to withdraw. In fact, emotion words differ with respect to which components are central to their meaning. Also, different languages may favor different components. Some languages favor eliciting events (as is the case with "jealousy" in our languages); others favor moral viewpoints, that is, significance (as *song* in the Ifaluk language, since it translates as justified anger; Lutz, 1988).

Yet, identifying or labeling one's emotion may influence one's emotional response, experience included. It may direct one's attention toward event features and, thus, to one's appraisal, and it provides access to emotional significance and thereby affects regulation. Only empirical research can indicate when and where this actually takes place and how influential labeling is; it should not be taken for granted.

CONCLUDING REMARKS

We have reviewed the sources of interindividual variation in emotions. Our points of departure were the functional and componential approaches to emotion and the evidence on emotion variations obtained from cross-cultural research.

We have argued that emotion labels form a poor starting point for developmental study of emotions. It is confusing to discuss the development of a given emotion without specifying which component or components are meant, or what criterion is used to study the development of a given kind of emotion. When studying the development of shame, for instance, does one study the development of emotional responsiveness to a given type of event (e.g., real or anticipated social rejection), regardless of the kind of response involved, or a given type of response such as blushing or hiding, a given type of appraisal such as self-blame, or the use of the word "shame" by the subject?

Emotions can vary in very many regards, intraindividually and cross-culturally, as well as developmentally. The differences can be profound. They cannot satisfactorily be captured by saying that the same basic emotions may show variations in detail in different individuals or groups. The differences in components accompanying a common core that leads one to compare two emotions, as two "angers" may be so different that the common core dwindles in importance in the face of the differences. The pattern of appraisal, the concerns that a given event touches upon, modes of social embedding, significance, mode of action readiness at some lower level, and dominant mode of social or other behavior may make two kinds of "anger" almost incomparable. The two kinds may involve two kinds of response to the appraisal of being the subject of someone's blameworthy action, such as hostile impulse and breaking off contact. They may involve two different concerns, and result, for instance, from appraised harm to the concern for goal achievement or for self-esteem. They may differ in significance: hostile impulse with full internal approval versus hostility within a dominant orientation toward interpersonal harmony. In this same vein, a particular kind of emotion, as defined in some way, may radically change its nature over development.

In addition, emotional processes may change with development. There probably will be changes in articulation or complexity of appraisals. More concerns may become involved in the relevance of a given event, more or different appraisal aspects may become simultaneously operative, and the role of cognitive variables will change, as may the roles of emotion significance and emotion categorization and labeling.

Also, the role and structure of emotional experience may change, from nonreflective experience of an event as appraised and as affect merely influencing action readiness and physiology, to articulate and reflective awareness of the various components and their being "one's own."

Our thesis in this chapter has been that whatever in emotions can vary cross-culturally can also vary developmentally. It in fact represents a lower bound of possible developmental variability. There are aspects of emotion that are more or less stable cross-culturally but that may vary developmentally for biological reasons. But the main point we hope to bring across is that developmentally, emotions can vary in many more respects than the age at which they begin to manifest themselves, the age at which individuals begin to understand or use their names, and the kinds of events that elicit them.

REFERENCES

Abu-Lughod, L. (1986). *Veiled sentiments*. Berkeley: University of California Press.

Barrett, K. S., & Campos, J. J. (1987). Perspectives on emotional development II: A functionalist approach to emotions. In J. D. Osofsky (Ed.), *Handbook of infant development* (2nd ed., pp. 555–578). New York: Wiley.

Baumeister, R. F. (1991). *Escaping the self: Alcoholism, spirituality, masochism, and other flights from the burden of selfhood*. New York: Basic Books.

Baumeister, R. F., & Leary, R. M. (1995). The need to belong: Desire for interpersonal attachment as a fundamental human motivation. *Psychological Bulletin, 118*, 497–529.

Bloom, L., & Beckwith, R. (1989). Talking with feeling: Integrating affective and linguistic expression in early language development. *Cognition and Emotion, 3*, 313–342.

Boucher, J. D., & Brandt, M. E. (1981). Judgment of emotion: American and Malay antecedents. *Journal of Cross-Cultural Psychology, 12*, 272–283.

Briggs, J. L. (1970). *Never in anger: Portrait of an Eskimo family*. Cambridge, MA: Harvard University Press.

Cacioppo, J. T., Klein, D. J., Berntson, G. G., & Hatfield, E. (1993). The psychophysiology of emotion. In M. Lewis & J. Haviland (Eds.), *Handbook of emotions* (pp. 119–143). New York: Guilford.

Campos, J. J., Mumme, D. L., Kermoian, R., & Campos, R. G. (1994). A functionalist perspective on the nature of emotion. In N. A. Fox (Ed.), The development of emotion regulation: Biological and behavioral considerations. *Monographs of the Society for Research in Child Development, 59*, 284–303.

Davitz, J. R. (1969). *The language of emotion*. New York: Academic Press.

Diener, E., & Larsen, R. (1993). The experience of emotional well-being. In M. Lewis & J. M. Haviland (Eds.), *Handbook of emotions* (pp. 405–416). New York: Guilford.

Ekman, P. (1994). Strong evidence for universals in facial expression: A reply to Russell's mistaken critique. *Psychological Bulletin, 115*, 268–287.

Ekman, P., & Friesen, W. V. (1969). The repertoire of nonverbal behavior: Categories, origins, usage and coding. *Semiotica, 1*, 49–98.

Fehr, B., & Russell, J. A. (1984). Concept of emotion viewed from a prototype perspective. *Journal of Experimental Psychology: General Section, 113*, 464–486.

Fernández-Dols, J. M., & Ruiz-Belda, M. A. (1997). Spontaneous facial behavior during intense emotional episodes: Artistic truth and optical truth. In J. A. Russell & J. M. Fernández-Dols (Eds.), *The psychology of facial expression* (pp. 255–274). Cambridge, MA: Cambridge University Press.

Fernández-Dols, J. M., & Carroll, J. M. (1997). Is the meaning perceived in facial expression independent of its context? In J. A. Russell & J. M. Fernández-Dols (Eds.), *The psychology of facial expression* (pp. 275–294). Cambridge, UK: Cambridge University Press.

Fridlund, A. J. (1994). *Human facial expression: An evolutionary view.* New York: Academic Press.

Frijda, N. H. (1986). *The emotions.* Cambridge, UK: Cambridge University Press.

Frijda, N. H. (1993). The place of appraisal in emotion. *Cognition and Emotion, 7,* 357–388.

Frijda, N. H. (1995). Passions: Emotions and socially consequential behavior. In R. D. Kavanaugh, B. Zimmerberg, & S. Fein (Eds.), *Emotion: Interdisciplinary perspectives* (pp. 1–28). Mahwah, NJ: Erlbaum.

Frijda, N. H., Kuipers, P., & Terschure, E. (1989). Relations between emotion, appraisal, and emotional action readiness. *Journal of Personality and Social Psychology, 57,* 212–228.

Frijda, N. H., Markam, S., Sato, K., & Wiers, R. (1995). Emotion and emotion words. In J. A. Russell, J.-M. Fernandez-Dols, A. S. R. Manstead, & J. Wellenkamp (Eds.), *Everyday conceptions of emotion* (pp. 121–144). Dordrecht: Kluwer.

Frijda, N. H., Mesquita, B., Sonnemans, J., & Van Goozen, S. (1991). The duration of affective phenomena, or emotions, sentiments and passions. In K. Strongman (Ed.), *International review of emotion and motivation* (pp. 187–225). New York: Wiley.

Frijda, N. H., & Tcherkassof, A. (1997). Facial expression and modes of action readiness. In J. A. Russell & J. M. Fernández-Dols (Eds.), *Facial expression: New directions in theory and method* (pp. 78–102). Cambridge, UK: Cambridge University Press.

Granet, M. (1922). Le langage de la douleur en Chine [The language of mourning in China]. *Journal de Psychologie, 19,* 97–118.

Harburg, E., Erfurt J. C., Hauenstein, L. S., Chape, C., Schull, W. J., & Schork, M. A. (1973). Socioecological stress, suppressed hostility, skin-color and black–white male blood pressure. *Detroit Psychosomatic Medicine, 35,* 276–296.

Hupka, R. B., Buunk, B., Falus, G., Fulgosi, A., Ortega, E., Swain, R., & Tarabrina, N. V. (1985). Romantic jealousy and romantic envy: A seven nation study. *Journal of Cross-Cultural Psychology, 16,* 423–446.

Izard, C. E. (1971). *The face of emotion.* New York: Appleton-Century-Crofts.

Izard, C. E. (1994). Innate and universal facial expressions: Evidence from development and cross-cultural research. *Psychological Bulletin, 115,* 288–299.

Izard, C. E., & Malatesta, C. Z. (1987). Perspectives on emotional development I: Differential emotions theory of early emotional development. In J. D. Osofsky (Ed.), *Handbook of infant development* (2nd ed., pp. 494–554). New York: Wiley.

Kellman, P. J., Spelke, E. S., & Short, K. R. (1986). Infant perception of object unity from translatory motion in depth and vertical translation. *Child Development, 57,* 72–86.

Kenny, A. (1963). *Action, emotion and will.* London: Routledge & Kegan Paul.

Lang, P. J. (1977). Physiological assessment of anxiety and fear. In J. D. Cone & R. P. Hawkins (Eds.), *Behavioral assessment: New directions in clinical psychology* (pp. 178–195). New York: Brunner/Mazel.

Lang, P. J., Bradley, M. M., & Cuthbert, B. N. (1990). Emotion, attention, and the startle reflex. *Psychological Review, 97,* 377–395.

Lang, P. J., Greenwald, M. K., Bradley, M. M., & Hamm, A. O. (1993). Looking at pictures: Affective, facial, visceral, and behavioral reactions. *Psychophysiology, 30,* 261–273.

Lazarus, R. S. (1991). *Emotion and adaptation.* New York: Oxford University Press.

Lebra, T. S. (1983). Shame and guilt: A psychocultural view of the Japanese self. *Ethos, 11,* 192–209.

Levy, R. (1973). *Tahitians: Mind and experience in the Society Islands.* Chicago: University of Chicago Press.

Lienhardt, G. (1961). *Divinity and experience: The religion of the Dinka.* Oxford, UK: Oxford University Press.

Lutz, C. (1988). *Unnatural emotions: Everyday sentiments on a Micronesian atoll and their challenge to Western theory.* Chicago: University of Chicago Press.

Mandler, J. M. (1992). How to build a baby: II. Conceptual primitives. *Psychological Review, 99,* 587–604.

Markus, H. R., & Kitayama, S. (1991). Culture and the self: Implications for cognition, emotion, and motivation. *Psychological Review, 98,* 224–253.

Mauro, R., Sato, K., & Tucker, J. (1992). The role of appraisal in human emotions: A cross-cultural study. *Journal of Personality and Social Psychology, 62,* 301–317.

Meltzoff, A. N., & Moore, M. K. (1979). Interpreting "imitative" responses in early infancy. *Science, 205,* 217–219.

Merkelbach, H. L. G. J. (1989). *Preparedness and classical conditioning of fear: A critical inquiry.* Maastricht: University of Limburg, Ph.D. Thesis.

Mesquita, B. (1993). *Cultural variations in emotions. A comparative study of Dutch, Surinamese and Turkish people in the Netherlands.* Ph.D. thesis, University of Amsterdam, Amsterdam, Holland.

Mesquita, B., & Frijda, N. H. (1992). Cultural variations in emotion: A review. *Psychological Bulletin, 112,* 179–204.

Mesquita, B., Frijda, N. H., & Scherer, K. R. (1997). Culture and emotion. In P. R. Dasen & T. S. Saraswathi (Eds.), *Handbook of cross-cultural psychology* (Vol. 2, pp. 255–298). Boston: Allyn & Bacon.

Michotte, A. E. (1946). *La perception de la causalité.* Louvain: Editions de l'Institut Supérieur de Philosophie.

Miller, W. I. (1993). *Humiliation.* Ithaca: NY: Cornell University Press.

Murphy, S. T., & Zajonc, R. B. (1993). Affect, cognition, and awareness: Affective priming with optimal and suboptimal stimulus exposures. *Journal of Personality and Social Psychology, 64,* 723–739.

Nisbett, R. E., & Cohen, D. (1996). *Culture of honor: The psychology of violence in the South.* Boulder: Westview Press.

Oatley, K. (1993). *Best-laid schemes.* Cambridge, UK: Cambridge University Press.

Öhman, A. (1993). Fear and anxiety as emotional phenomena: Clinical phenomenology, evolutionary perspectives, and information-processing mechanisms. In M. Lewis & J. M. Haviland (Eds.), *Handbook of emotions* (pp. 511–536). New York: Guilford.

Ortony, A., Clore, G., & Collins, A. (1988). *The cognitive structure of emotions.* Cambridge: Cambridge University Press.

Ortony, A., & Turner, T. (1990). What's basic about basic emotions? *Psychological Review, 97,* 315–331.

Osofsky, J. D. (1995). The effects of exposure to violence on young children. *American Psychologist, 50,* 782–788.

Parrott, W. G., & Gleitman, H. (1989). Infants' expectations in play: The joy of peek-a-boo. *Cognition and Emotion, 3,* 291–312.

Piaget, J. (1935). *La naissance de l'intelligence.* [The origins of intelligence in the child.] Neuchatel: Delachaux & Nietslé. London: Routledge & Kegan Paul, 1953.

Rimé, B., Phillipot, P., & Cisamolo, D. (1990). Social schemata of peripheral changes in emotion. *Journal of Personality and Social Psychology, 59,* 38–49.

Robarchek, C. (1977). Frustration, aggression, and the nonviolent Semai. *American Ethnologist, 4,* 762–779.

Roseman, I. J., Antoniou, A., & Jose, P. E. (1996). Appraisal determinants of emotions: Constructing a more accurate and comprehensive theory. *Cognition and Emotion, 10,* 241–278.

Roseman, I. J., Wiest, C., & Swartz, T. S. (1994). Phenomenology, behaviors, and goals differentiate discrete emotions. *Journal of Personality and Social Psychology, 67,* 206–221.

Rozin, P., Haidt, J., & McCauley, C. R. (1993). Disgust. In M. Lewis & J. M. Haviland (Eds.), *Handbook of emotions* (pp. 575–594). New York: Guilford.

Russell, J. A. (1994). Is there universal recognition of emotion from facial expression? A review of the cross-cultural studies. *Psychological Bulletin, 115,* 102–141.

Scherer, K. R. (1984). Emotion as a multicomponent process: A model and some cross-cultural data. In P. Shaver (Ed.), *Review of personality and social psychology* (Vol. 5, pp. 37–63). Beverly Hills: Sage.

Scherer, K. R. (1988). Criteria for emotion-antecedent appraisal: A review. In V. Hamilton, G. H. Bower, & N. H. Frijda (Eds.), *Cognitive perspectives on emotion and motivation* (pp. 89–126). Dordrecht, The Netherlands: Kluwer.

Scherer, K. R. (1992). What does facial expression express? In K. T. Strongman (Ed.), *International review of studies of emotion* (Vol. 2, pp. 139–165). New York: Wiley.

Scherer, K. R ., & Walbott, H. G. (1994). Evidence for universality and cultural variation of differential emotional response patterning. *Journal of Personality and Social Psychology, 66,* 310–328.

Scherer, K. R., Walbott, H. G., Matsumoto, D., & Kudoh, T. (1988). Emotional experience in cultural context: A comparison between Europe, Japan, and the United States. In K. R. Scherer (Ed.), *Facets of emotions* (pp. 5–30). Hillsdale, NJ: Erlbaum.

Scherer, K. R., Walbott, H. G., & Summerfield, A. B. (1986). *Experiencing emotions: A cross-cultural study.* Cambridge, UK: Cambridge University Press.

Schieffelin, E. D. (1983). Anger and shame in the tropical forest: An affect as a cultural system in Papua New Guinea. *Ethos, 11,* 181–191.

Schwartz, S. H. (1992). Universals in the content and structure of values: Theoretical advances and empirical tests in 20 countries. *Advances in Experimental Social Psychology, 25,* 1–65.

Schwartz, S. H., & Sagiv, L. (1995). Identifying culture-specifics in the content and structure of values. *Journal of Cross-Cultural Psychology, 26,* 92–116.

Shweder, R. A. (1993). The cultural psychology of the emotions. In M. Lewis & J. Haviland (Eds.), *Handbook of emotions* (pp. 417–433). New York: Guilford.

Smith, C. A. (1997). In J. A. Russell & J. M. Fernández-Dols (Eds.), *Facial expression: New directions in theory and method.* Cambridge, UK: Cambridge University Press.

Smith, C. A., & Ellsworth, P. C. (1985). Patterns of cognitive appraisal in emotion. *Journal of Personality and Social Psychology, 48,* 813–838.

Stemmler, D. G. (1989). The autonomic differentiation of emotions revisited: Convergent and discriminant validation. *Psychophysiology, 26,* 617–632.

Stern, D. (1995). *The motherhood constellation: A unified view of parent–infant psychotherapy.* New York: Basic Books.

Watson, D., & Tellegen, A. (1985). Towards a consensual structure of mood. *Psychological Bulletin, 98,* 219–235.

Wolfgang, M. E., & Ferracuti, F. (1967). *The subculture of violence.* New York: Barnes and Noble.

Wooding, C. (1979). Winti: Een Afroamerikaanse godsdient in Suriname [*Winti: An Afro-American religion in Surinam*]. Meppel, The Netherlands: Krips Repro.

12

The Narrative Construction of Emotional Life

Developmental Aspects

James C. Mancuso and Theodore R. Sarbin

INTRODUCTION

> William, an 11-year-old child, receives a gift from his aunt, who prompts him to
> open the package in her presence. He does so and looks upon a sweater that he
> regards as singularly ugly. Notwithstanding, he enacts an emotional display that
> causes his aunt to appear "pleased." Sarah, a seven-year-old child endures a similar
> gift presentation of an "ugly" sweater. Unlike William, Sarah offers an emotional
> display that offends her aunt. Later that day, Sarah's mother tries to educate Sarah
> in "appropriate" ways of conducting her emotional life.

Will Sarah eventually learn one of life's more important lessons? With
further experience, will she no longer "feel sad and disappointed" when
others fail to meet her expectations? Traditional students of emotional life
might ask: Has William been socialized into suppressing his "true emotions,"
thus making him a candidate for a life of tension-ridden inauthenticity?

Such questions about "true emotions" are futile. More productive are
questions of this sort: What skills underlie the performance of recounting

James C. Mancuso • Department of Psychology, State University of New York, Albany, New
York 12222.   **Theodore R. Sarbin** • University of California–Santa Cruz, Carmel, California
93923.

What Develops in Emotional Development? edited by Michael F. Mascolo and Sharon Griffin.
Plenum Press, New York, 1998.

socially acceptable stories about emotional life? How did William develop the skills required to understand his own emotional life? Which skills facilitate his inference making about his emotional display causing his aunt to enact the emotion display he had predicted?

In this chapter, we offer propositions that relate the child's acquisition of knowledge about emotional life to facility with narrative syntax. Our major thesis may be expressed as follows: As children acquire skill in using narrative syntax, their "understandings of emotion" gain social validation; that is, as children elaborate their knowledge of the social construction, *story*, they become more and more adept at constructing forward-predicting narratives about the emotional life involved in interacting with their social worlds (Mancuso, 1986; Mancuso & Sarbin, 1983).

Our objective is to account for the psychological changes that accompany observed alterations in children's understanding of emotional life, as illustrated by the vignettes in the lives of William and Sarah. Note our use of the term "emotional life, rather than the term *emotions*. Our linguistic preference reflects our rejection of traditional constructions of "emotions"—constructions that have risen from a commitment to the psychophysiological symbolism that has prompted scholars to assign thing-like qualities and causal properties to "specific emotions" (Averill, 1986). The metaphor *emotional life* directs us to observe our friends and neighbors as actors involved in multipersoned plots that are identified as anger, fear, pride, envy, joy, and so on.

To advance our overall goal, we discuss four topics:

1. We examine the widespread belief that emotions are embodied—that the actor involved in an emotional experience perceives the activation of sensory systems within the physical body. Some observers regard the reported "feelings" as accompaniments of "the emotion," others as constitutive (Averill, 1986).
2. To support our major propositions, we examine published studies of children's development of the construction: *story*.
3. We analytically review relevant studies that illuminate our view of the development of children's "understandings of emotion."
4. At the end of the chapter, we briefly note some of the consequences of adopting the narrative perspective on emotional life.

ON THE EMBODIMENT OF EMOTION CONSTRUCTS

The etymology of the term *emotion* reminds us that our ancestors borrowed a word for *move* or *movement* to refer to motions within the body. Early (and now obsolete) usages referred to physical movements or agitations, as in descriptions of foul weather. In was not until the seventeenth century that *emotion* was treated as a figurative expression to refer to internal mental states.

In the nineteenth century, *emotion* lost its metaphorical moorings and was given literal and ontological status as a faculty of the mental apparatus, coordinate with cognition and conation. Statements about emotion could then begin from a proposition implicating motions or movements within the body cavity. For example, when hearing the spoken word, *emotion*, listeners will form or reform a construction that centers on sensory or quasi-sensory inputs arising within the body. Psychologists continue the centuries-old practice by remembering constructions of emotion that implicate interoceptive or proprioceptive events occurring within the boundaries of the discoursers' skins.

Calling such views into question, social constructionist discourses on emotional life (see Harré, 1986; Sarbin, 1995) have focused on data showing that, when asked to define emotion, people ordinarily define emotion by employing psychophysiological language. Yet when asked to provide an example of "emotions," the same people tell multipersoned stories involving moral features. Doing so, they give little evidence of having considered the features of their psychophysiological definitions of discrete emotions. These puzzling findings have done little to influence those theorists who discuss emotional life by referencing, for example, the physiological symbolism associated with discrete emotions. By leaning on the authority of Darwin's formulations (Darwin, 1965/1872), theorists continue to support the contested view that emotional life is determined by motions from within. Caroll Izard (1993), for example, regularly evokes evolutionary imagery.

> I present evidence and arguments in support of discrete-emotions concepts and variables ... [by answering] two questions about a sample of specific emotions. First, does this discrete emotion have functions that can be readily understood as providing an adaptive advantage in evolution? Second, does this specific emotion continue to serve functions that facilitate development, adaptation and coping? (p. 633)

Izard goes on to provide the following illustrations:

> In the course of evolution, grief, by strengthening communal bonds, increased the probability of surviving.... A unique function of sadness is its capacity to slow the cognitive and motor systems.... The sadness-induced slowing of mental and motor activity can have adaptive effects. The slowing of cognitive processes may enable a more careful look for the source of trouble. (p. 634)

Such appeals to the rhetoric of Darwinism do not obviate the assertion that thorough understandings of everyday emotional life involves *social* and *moral contexts* that includes far more than the corporeal residues of eons of evolutionary adaptation.

On the Reports of Experienced "Feelings"

An extensive literature on varieties of specific emotions has led to one firm conclusion: No valid basis has been established to support the widely held belief that specific, physiologically differentiable emotions occur when a person is exposed to one or another kind of stimulus event (see, e.g., Cacioppo, Klein, Bernston, & Hatfield, 1993; Ortony & Turner, 1990). We refrain, therefore, from the tedious process of identifying support for, or contradiction of, this traditional position, and we proceed to outline our alternative perspective.

Elsewhere (Mancuso, 1996; Mancuso & Adams-Webber, 1982; Mascolo & Mancuso, 1990; Sarbin, 1995), we have developed the parsimonious motivation-explaining proposition that psychological processes are directed constantly toward creating and validating *anticipatory constructions*—models that aid in anticipating or preparing for a personally involving sequence of actions. Our choice of the term anticipatory construction alerts the reader to focus on the person's proactive constructional activity. Persons build anticipatory constructions in millisecond-by-millisecond sequence and then monitor the "match" between such anticipatory constructions and continued sensory events.

In short, we subscribe to the foundational postulate that persons are ever proactive beings who direct their activity toward "knowing" the world of occurrences that are assumed to be associated with inputs. (Let it be clear that here the term *input* denotes sensory activity.) When persons fail in their effort to know, that is, when persons fail to build a construction that gains validation, they prepare for effort. Consider 13-year-old Carlo, proudly demonstrating his newly mastered soccer moves to his grandfather. Grandpa asks, sardonically, "Will that improve your speed when we pick the beans tomorrow morning?" His query, the precursor to complex auditory inputs and Carlo's construction processes, provides social invalidations of Carlo's self-constructions (reflected in his prideful demonstration) as a budding soccer star. Thereupon, Carlo must put atypical effort into "doing something." He might, for example, silently relegate Grandpa to the category of "outmoded old fogey," or he might vow to convince Grandpa that his aspiring to soccer stardom does not constrain his development as a skillful bean harvester, or he might essay to demean and intimidate Grandpa through a display of "anger."

At this point, we propose a shift in terms. Henceforth the term *discrepancy resolution* stands as a generic term. The term signifies the conduct of a person who has encountered evidence that his or her constructions do not anticipate the world of occurrences: that he or she does not know a part of the world. *Discrepancy resolution* denotes the psychological activity (motoric and/or cognitive) whereby one expends effort to bring about a correspondence between the flow of inputs and the internal models of the distal ecology variously referenced as anticipatory constructions (Kelly, 1955/1991), situation models (van Dijk & Kintsch, 1983); schemas (Mandler, 1984), or modules (Sarbin, Taft, & Bailey, 1960).

Other theorists have offered parallel propositions, but they appeal to *direct* instigation of arousal processes. Mandler (1992), for example, has written,

> The theory proposes two basic underlying processes, autonomic (sympathetic) nervous system arousal and evaluative cognitions. In addition, it suggests that the majority of occasions for sympathetic nervous system (SNS) arousal come about by occurrence of discrepancies in perception, action, and thought. (p. 103)

Stein and Levine (1991) address the same phenomenon when they write: "When new information is detected in the input, a mismatch occurs, causing an interruption in current thinking processes. With the attentional shift comes arousal of the autonomic nervous system." (p. 46).

Our emphasis centers on discrepancy and preparation for effort, with the resulting alterations of the functioning of a number of anatomical and physiological systems. With preparation for effort, the person's interoceptive and proprioceptive systems provide additional sensory input; that is, following a person's failure to produce a valid anticipatory construction, the physiological and anatomical system changes (that occur during heightened efforts to act) activate sensory endings to produce inputs. Supports from their surrounding cultural and linguistic worlds encourage persons who process those inputs to claim that their active efforts to reduce discrepancy were *caused* by their "feelings." Carlo (the aspiring soccer star) might tell his friends, "When the old man said that, very powerful feelings of anger rose up in me, and I just couldn't restrain my outburst."

We hold that through participating in many sequences entailing social validation—that is, no discrepancy results from applying the assembled construction—persons will master the social constructions to be used in construing their emotional lives. If the act of attributing his or her displays to "feelings" receives social validation, he or she will continue to affirm cause-and-effect connections in which the vocabulary of "feelings" is central. The sequence may be represented as follows: (1) anticipatory construction (constructions with a future reference, entailing beliefs and values); (2) a mismatch between input from the world of occurrences and the anticipatory construction; (3) preparation for effort to reduce the discrepancy; (4) interoceptive and proprioceptive sensory inputs arising from heightened effort; (5) labeling such sensory inputs as "feelings;" (6) intentional acts to reduce discrepancy; and (7) attributing (misattributing?) the cause of the intentional acts to "feelings."

Following this formulation, when Carlo attributes his emotional-life experiences to feelings, he engages in an unrecognized use of metonymy: The *effect*—the effort related internal changes—takes the place of *cause* in the episode. In our view of emotional life, the registering of mismatch and the subsequent increase in preparation for action are more direct antecedents to conduct that might be labeled *emotional enactment*—the animated enactment of an emotion story that entails the singular motive: discrepancy resolution. The interoceptive and proprioceptive data associated with the preparation for effortful action are *adjuncts* rather than the *causes* of a particular enactment and display. The enactment and display occur in a context that includes the person's socially constructed knowledge about emotional-life stories.

NARRATIVE CONSTRUCTION: THE EPISTEMIC PROCESSES OF EMOTIONAL LIFE

The development of children's understandings of emotional life proceeds in tandem with their progressive mastery of narrative structures. Such mastery then provides the framework for building increasingly complex, socially validated emotion stories. To advance to our goal, we note briefly the construction *narrative grammar*. How a person develops epistemic structures that define the narrative grammar has been addressed by a number of writers (see, e.g., Britton & Pellegrini, 1990; Mancuso, 1986; Mancuso & Sarbin, 1983; Stein & Glenn, 1979; Sutton-Smith, 1986).

Narrative grammarians (e.g., Mandler, 1984; Thorndyke, 1977) generally agree that an emplotted story (material in brackets, which follows) entails the use of six "parts of speech," as follows: (1) establishing the setting of a story [e.g., The children were taking turns being pushed on the playground swing]; (2) the initiating event of a narrative episode, which places the protagonist in a position to react, thus creating a cause [Johnny was to have the next turn, but Billy refused to get off the swing]; (3) goal setting, including internally set goals and ascribed internal experiences [Johnny wants his turn on the swing and becomes angry]; (4) descriptions of goal-directed conduct and an outcome of the conduct [Johnny grabs the swing seat and pulls it out from under Billy, tumbling him to the ground]; (5) an ending, which sets the outcome in a broader context [The child-care worker reprimands Johnny: "When boys become angry, they must control their anger, otherwise they might hurt other people"]; (6) a global ending, particularly if the episode is to be coalesced with other episodes [Johnny felt very sad because he had done something that might have hurt Billy]. A child who develops the social construction that allows the distinction between *random text* and *emplotted story* learns that a "good" story contains, in proper sequence, these six elements (see Mancuso, 1986). When the story plot describes emotional-life incidents, as in the foregoing bracketed material, the child also has instruction in how such occurrences are to be constructed.

We now proceed to reinterpret the studies reported by mainline investigators to buttress our propositions about the relationships between children's increasing skill in using the construction *emplotted story* and their development of understandings of emotion life.

Infant Development of Narratives about Emotional Life

Protonarrative in Infants' Emotional Life

Investigators (e.g., Fogel & Thelan, 1987; Trevarthen, 1993) have provided illustrations of the ways in which infants develop their skills in holding dialogues about emotional life, and the ways in which the behavior of infants serves as text, that is, sources of complex input, to be construed by other persons in the discourse. Here, we speak of behavior as text, in that any behavior can function as does written or spoken text by providing inputs that a dialogue partner must process (see Mancuso, 1996).

The first, most salient, postnatal signs of discourse about emotional life are those produced by infants showing signs of heightened preparation for effort in the presence of discrepant inputs. We draw attention to the evidence (DeCasper & Fifer, 1980; DeCasper & Spence, 1986) suggesting that a neonate has developed constructions even before parturition. DeCasper and Fifer (1980) have demonstrated "that a newborn infant younger than 3 days of age not only can discriminate its mother's voice but also will work to produce her voice in preference to the voice of another female" (p. 1175). We take this demonstration as evidence that while *in utero*, these neonates had developed constructions to integrate inputs provided by their mothers' vocalizations. We are also encouraged to assume that the infant had developed other constructions during the last 4 months of its *in utero* development, that is, during the prenatal period following the appearance of a well-developed neural system. Those constructions would have developed to integrate the steady-state temperature of uterine life, the relatively regular inputs from blood nutrient levels, the constant supply of blood oxygen, and so on. Thus, in early postnatal life, when related inputs vary, the already-formed constructions cannot subsume the variations, and a discrepancy situation will set up the conditions calling for heightened effort.

A mother can readily detect the ways in which her behavior causes responses in the infant (Cohn & Tronick, 1987; Murray & Trevarthen, 1985), and can quickly discover that she can take control of the infant's sensory systems by providing those inputs—from her vocalizations, gentle rocking, and so on—that the neonate can readily assimilate through the use of its existing construction system. Such knowledge would be particularly useful when the mother judges that the infant shows signs of preparation for effort.

When preparing for effort, the infant shows his or her expending above-standard levels of effort when its usual limb and head movements turn into intensive thrashing about. The infant's heightened inspiration and exhalation produces the sounds that caretakers construe as crying. Trevarthen (1993) notes other reactions, and concludes, "In short, orientation of any of the special receptors that are important ... in exploration of objects ... offer a mother critical evidence about the pace and direction of information-seeking by the baby" (p. 135). Highly energized reactions are generally unwanted by caretakers who instigate dialogues that aim either to reduce discrepant inputs or to introduce a variety of masking inputs. If the caretaker construes the infant's text as hunger, he or she might first divert the infant by cooing or speaking (i.e., providing inputs that readily access the infant's anticipatory construction processes). Then, the delivery of food serves to cut off the inputs that are discrepant from those *in utero*-developed constructions with which the infant processed its steady state of nutrition. Overall, "the behaviors of a mother seeking contact with her baby match, complement, and confirm the information-seeking efforts of the baby" (p. 135).

Caretakers observing a sleeping newborn infant see signs of near total absence of preparation for effort. More significantly for emotion-story development, protosmiles occur during the infant's rapid-eye-movement sleep. Thus, one may conclude that the newborn has in its action repertory a signal that caretakers eventually can take as a sign of minimal preparation for effort.

By coordinating the child's behavior-in-context with his or her own constructions (see Fogel, 1993; Fogel & Thelan, 1987), the infant's caretaker can quickly adapt the context of the continually varied interactions. By the end of several weeks, the infant will smile regularly on hearing familiar voices and sounds. By 2 months, the infant will produce a smile in face-to-face social situations. The infant's discourse partners, of course, construe such smiles as evidence that the infant has attained a state of pleasure.

The mother or another caretaker, having taken the infant's action as a positive reaction, then gives behavioral signals that she, too, has achieved confirmation of the anticipatory constructions that guided her actions in the context. Such caused actions of a mother, particularly if they are vocal, can be detected by infants as young as 2 months of age, who then show efforts to imitate (Papousek, Papousek, & Bornstein, 1985). Furthermore, these young infants show an ability to imitate in order "to cause" the dialogue partner to continue to vocalize.

Such, then, are the occasions in which the basics of a narrative syntax are constructed and become connected to emotion-life plots. The child can locate him- or herself as a protonarrative's protagonist who has been exposed to inputs from the distal ecology that create discrepancy-producing inputs (narrative grammar element 1, the setting), thus defining a cause for the child/ protagonist reactions (narrative grammar element 2, the cause), leading to definition of and actions to achieve goals (e.g., crying; element 3), whereupon the child's behavior, in turn, results in caretaker's intercession (element 4). The episode (a narrative in miniature) concludes when the actions of the caretaker achieve a resolution (element 5). Note well that, according to our account, both actors take turns in assuming agency.

The Infant's Use of Social Referencing to Guide Its Emotion Protonarratives

Stenberg and Campos (1990) studied whether restrained 4-month-old infants would show a reaction that fits "the specific anger template" (p. 262). Though the results, relative to the investigators' major hypothesis, allow much equivocation, one intriguing result evoked further analysis and a search for an explanatory framework. Twelve of the 16 four-month-old infants continued to look at the source of the restraint after the first signs of a "negative expression." Fourteen of 16 of the more developed 7-month-old infants instead gaze at the mother.

Another team investigated this *social referencing* by exposing 38 infants (aged 12–23 months) to "surprise" situations. During play with an experimenter, a remotely controlled robot appeared from its hiding place. The toddlers saw the experimenter show one of two reactions: (1) "fear" expression or (2) smiling toward the robot. The children's emotional display emulated that of the experimenter, allowing the conclusion that the infants had used a relatively strange adult as a model for their emotion enactments (Klinnert, Emde, Butterfield, & Campos, 1986, p. 431).

The process of social referencing was further analyzed by Cohn and Tronick (1987), who collected records of infants (3–9 months) in face-to-face interactions with their mothers. Generally, with 3-month-old infants, the mother begins the interaction by obtaining the infant's attention and then proceeds to show "pleasant" responses. The infant then shows similar behavior. By 9 months, the infant is more likely to show "positive" behavior before the mother does. Thus, we would expect that 9-month-old Bettina would have learned to construe her self as happy when she enters into a face-to-face interaction; that is, she "knows" that she can construct a "happy self" and that her future-defining narrative will be validated by the dialogue partner showing reciprocal "pleasant" behavior that is caused by enactments associated with her "happy self."

From our perspective, we make use of these observations to support the claim that infants enact the protagonist's role in a protonarrative about emotional life—that they can frame such stories on the basis of the narrative plots they develop through observing an adult dialogue partner. With the later development of language skills, narratives, heretofore composed of interactive gestural and motoric sequences, may be told as stories.

The Consequences of Providing Infants and Caretakers with Disconfirmations of the Utility of a Narrative Construction

One can explain the ways in which emotional-life protonarratives function by observing infants who have developed the rudiments of the construction *emplotted narrative,* but then encounter failure in their efforts to create a forward-predicting narrative. Murray and Trevarthen (1985) have reported studies of the consequences of discrepancy-laden mother–infant emotion-life dialogue. In one illustrative study, 4 infants (between 6 and 12 weeks) and their mothers engaged in play situations. Each mother had been instructed to make two kinds of breaks in the play: (1) to attend to the experimenter who had interrupted the play; and (2) to continue to look at the infant, presenting a blank face. Both breaks were 30 seconds in duration.

During standard play, the infants displayed "typical positive" actions. Furthermore, the emotion enactments of the mother and the infant were in close correspondence. During the experimenter interruption, the infant showed signs indicating heightened preparation for effort but no evidence of "distress." On the other hand, during the blank-face interruption, the infant's actions signified both distress and heightened effort to reinstate the flow of the standard play episodes, and, by diverting its gaze, tried to shut off the disconfirming text provided by the mother's face.

This demonstration strengthens the more general conclusion that infants show heightened effort to cut off or to alter the flow of inputs that invalidate the anticipatory constructions that they can build to understand the world of occurrences. Specifically, infants show heightened efforts when their proto-narratives about emotional life do not anticipate effectively.

Language and the Codevelopment of Narrative Structure and Understanding of Emotional Life

A sampling from the numerous published studies provides insights into the acquisition of skills in employing "positive emotion terms" and "negative emotion terms" for use in emotional-life narratives.

Learning the Language of Discourse on Emotional Life

That emotional-life discourses are learned in interactional sequences is amply demonstrated in Fivush's (1993) report of her studies. She paired mother–child and father–child dyads, and then instructed parents to talk with their child about significant events that they had experienced together. When speaking with daughters, contrasted to when speaking with sons, parents more frequently provide frames for standard emotional-life terms and place emotion terms in a social–relational framework. When speaking with girls, for example, parents talk more frequently about sadness. Mothers focus more on elaborating the narratives surrounding sadness and show more concern about resolving a sadness episode through adult comfort and reassurance. Mothers focus more on others causing the child's sadness. Mothers less frequently frame events as anger, and tend to focus on restoring relationships damaged through anger enactments. Additionally, when mothers discourse about fear, they seem more concerned about fear in sons.

These observations, an embarrassment for theorists who rely on evolutionary biology to account for the beginnings of gender differences in understanding "discrete emotions," clearly demonstrate the early social shaping of emotional-life scenarios.

Brody and Harrison (1987) had reported on a grand-scale study of age and gender differences in the matching and labeling of 19 different emotion situations. Children of two age categories participated in the study (preschoolers and third and fourth graders). Following a procedure typical for this genre of studies, the investigators first collected brief emotional-life stories. They then ascertained that adults could name the "emotion" label that would characterize each story. Two different stories were created for each emotion situation. The researchers then presented the stories to the participating children. The stories used "you" as the protagonist (e.g., to recount a tale of jealousy, the investigator told the child, "You want a bicycle. Your friend gets one and rides it all the time."). The participating children then were asked to name the emotion that they would ascribe to their own reaction had they been the protagonist in the two stories (presented in proximal sequence). In a variation of the task, the children were asked to indicate which of two comparison stories "made them feel the same way as [did the protagonist in] the target story" (p. 352).

We pointedly note that the children who participated in this study were directed to react to the stories in terms of specific emotions. Like other investigators who conduct similar studies under similar assumptions, Brody and Harrison tried to determine whether the children were "capable of accurately labeling the emotions depicted" (p. 360). The investigators apparently had overlooked the linguistic boundaries they had placed on the children's responses, and they had implicitly imposed their own ontological assumptions on the children.

In general, the Brody and Harrison study shows that children have not yet learned to use emotion names that closely match the emotion names that adults employ to categorize the emotion narratives. The children's designations, however, were more like those of adults when labeling those stories intended to chronicle happiness, sadness, anger, and disgust. On these four types of stories (story types that frequently enter early parent–child dialogues about emotional life), the name-matching skills of the older children exceeded those of the younger children. Age-related improvement in matching adult labels also appears when the children work with stories intended to depict fear, embarrassment, gratitude, pride, worry, nervousness, embarrassment, and frustration. The children performed particularly poorly on the task of producing those adult-endorsed emotion names that are less well grounded in emotional-life narratives—surprise, relief, hope, guilt, jealousy, tenderness, and satisfaction.

Barden, Zelko, Duncan, and Masters (1980) reported an illustrative study

of the development of consensus in labeling the presumed "emotion consequences" in emotional-life scenarios. From our perspective, we conclude
that Barden et al. have shown that 4- to 5-year-old children can construe
achieving success and receiving nurturance as the grammatical elements of
happiness stories. Barden et al. also replicated the finding that young children, unlike older children (age 9 years and beyond) and adults, are more
likely to construe an unjustified punishment episode using the *sad* narrative
rather than the *mad* narrative. Younger children, more than older children,
showed high consensus in using the construction *sad* to label the emotional-
life story that portrays self-as-failure. Older children showed little agreement about whether such situations would evoke either the *sad, mad, scared,*
or *neutral* stories. Thus, rather than having moved toward "greater accuracy
in identifying specific emotions," the older children reflect the society's lack
of consensus about which emotion-life story is appropriate in failure situations.

Other studies corroborate the evidence for the growing concordance of
children and adult's emplotments of emotional life. Strayer's (1986) results
show that older children more frequently place interpersonal and achievement events in the "causes" slots of narratives, particularly to explain anger
and sadness. Denham, Cook, and Zoller (1992) found that when mothers
construed and labeled emotional life in socially validated ways (i.e., were
more "accurate"), their children (mean age 3 years, 8 months) tended to use
the same constructions to label the emotion situations.

Formal studies, then, readily support the conclusion that with developing competence in the use of narrative syntax, children can approximate the
adult use of the vocabulary used in emotion-story plots. Interindividual
differences in using adult emotion terms, then, may be ascribed to differential skill in using narrative syntax to frame the linguistic signs to construct
socially valid emotional-life stories.

*The Social Construction of Cause-and-Effect Formulation for Use in Emotional-
Life Narratives*

Perusing Dunn and Brown's summarizing review (1991), one can conclude that by the time that he or she reaches age 24 months, the average child
can adeptly use language to discourse about discrepancy-producing inputs.
Verbalization of causes of attributed emotions becomes solidified during the
average child's third year, particularly in cases where the child seeks another's help in reducing discrepancy-producing inputs. Corroborating other
studies that show that young children know a great deal about distress
enactments, Dunn and Brown found that more than half of the children's
causal conversational turns were focused on distress. Only a small proportion
were focused on the theme of pleasure or liking.

Additionally, during their third year, children readily display the ability to frame the behavior-as-text of others into cause-and-effect constructions. To illustrate, Dunn and Brown give an example of a child of 30 months building an anticipatory construction that is based on understandings of cause and effect in anger situations. The young child had observed his mother reprimanding his older brother, who had poked the mother. Later, having observed her younger child kicking his brother, the mother enacted a behavior/text that the younger child could interpret as an anger display. Revealing his understanding of complex causal relationships in anger narratives, the boy attempted to show that justified anger had motivated the retaliatory kick: "Don't! Don't hurt me, Len!" (p. 95).

Miller and Sperry (1994) have chronicled the ways in which children might receive schooling in the use of this "justified anger" narrative. They observed 3 girls (aged around 2 years at beginning of study) within the family context, focusing particularly on the emotion narratives told by the mothers and children. While in the presence of their youngsters, the mothers frequently structured, verbalized, and enacted narratives on themes of anger, violence, and aggression. Miller and Sperry reach a number of conclusions from their observations, such as the following:

1. "The narrator's anger is taken to be valid to the extent that she links it to a convincing cause, that is, to an intentional, unwarranted transgression" (p. 14).
2. Though a mother who had been the target of her child's aggressive act might reprimand her child, such acts were encouraged "when they were performed teasingly, often at the mother's own instigation" (p. 17). The mothers believed that such teasing pretense schooled the child to defend him or herself so that he or she would not be regarded as a "sissy," or "spoiled."
3. False accusation, which occurred in one child at age 23 months, "suggests that the children had some understanding that they needed to justify their anger/aggression" (p. 25).

Concluding another study, Dunn and Brown (1993) deduced that the earliest emotional-life discourse of young children (33 months) centers on emotion causality when seeking to gain satisfaction of their wants. In the terms of this chapter, children's first socially valid emotion narratives serve to resolve discrepancies between the anticipatory construction *myself-as-satisfied* and the inputs that are discrepant with that self-construction. By being able to articulate the cause of the discrepancy in a "good" emotional-life narrative, a child can better convince his or her mother to concur with his or her construction. We would expect, then, that a father would be quite likely to change the course of a stroll when his early-verbalizing child would say. "That big doggie (cause) on that street scares me (effect)."

Skills in Inferring the Inner States of Others and Changes in Emotional-Life Narratives

Children who have passed their fourth birthday begin to show a newly developed skill in their telling of tales. They can make inferences from their construing another person's construction system. This skill allows them to make judgments about the ways in which another person's particular past experience will affect that person's current emotional-life enactment. If, for example, 5-year-old Bruno knows that Roseanne has been nipped by a dog, or if he has seen her protest vigorously at a dog's approach, he will infer that she will enact a fear display if another dog were to appear. Working from the premise that "predicting another person's emotional reading requires inferring that person's appraisal of an object or event and applying that understanding to the person's current situation" (Gnepp, 1989, p. 282), Gnepp demonstrated the working of inferencing skill. She studied three samples of children (mean ages about 6 years, about 8 years, and about 11 years). The participants heard stories about children in emotion-life situations. One episode, for example, told of a child accompanying his or her family on a walk in a park. The child in the story became hot, was scratched, and sustained sore feet. At another point in the story, the protagonist's mother again suggests a walk in the park. To assess inference-making skills, the participants were asked,"How do you think [the protagonist] felt?" A child would demonstrate having made a "result inference" (Frederiksen, 1979) by reporting that the protagonist would "feel sad" about the suggested outing; that is, the respondent would have overcome the propensity to regard a walk in the park as pleasurable. The respondent would have inferred that the protagonist, due to previous experiences, would construct a self-narrative in which the protagonist would enact sadness. The participants in Gnepp's (1989) study, as well as the children in other studies (e.g., Hadwin & Perner, 1991), clearly showed an age-related acquisition of skill applying this kind of inference making to predict outcomes in emotional-life narratives. William, the protagonist in our introductory vignette, had constructed a self-guiding narrative that was based on his reading of his aunt's anticipatory constructions. Sarah, on the other hand, constructed a story that reflected her poor skills in construing the constructions of others.

Bamberg and Damrad-Frye (1991) have further demonstrated the progression of a related skill—reading "the landscape of consciousness" (Feldman, Bruner, Renderer, & Spitzer, 1990). Participants (mean ages of three sets of 12 children: 5 years, 7 months; 9 years, 8 months; college age) in the Bamberg and Damrad-Frye study were given a picture book containing 24 pictures that could serve as illustrations for a complete story involving a dog and a boy trying to find a pet frog that has escaped from its container. The

5-year-old children were able to use evaluative clauses describing frame of mind, but, unlike some of the older participants, they showed no strong preference for that type of clause.

Bamberg and Damrad-Frye also showed that the older children and the adults use inferences to explicate the flow of the action, particularly to explain causal relations. Such inferences frequently revealed the child's knowledge of socially valid cause-and-effect configurations in emotion-life sequences. For example, at one point, the dog was implicated in smashing a jar. An ensuing picture shows the boy holding the dog, his face drawn so as to depict an expression that can be taken as anger. The dog appears to be licking the boy's face. The younger children focus on the boy and the anger caused by the breaking of the jar. Older children, however, recognize that the overall story—the successful search for the frog—can best proceed if there is a resolution of the boy's anger. Most adults offer two different frame-of-mind clauses—one for the boy, and one for the dog.

Thus, inference-making skills facilitate incorporating into stories both "the landscape of consciousness" and "the landscape of action" (Feldman et al., 1990) into his or her stories. An average child older than 6 years would take into account the emotional-life stories constructed by others in order to explain the causes of their overt conduct, that is, that function as element three of our proposed narrative grammar (goal setting, including internally set goals and internally ascribed experience).

THE CONSEQUENCES OF REGARDING EMOTIONAL LIFE AS ENACTMENT OF NARRATIVE

We have tried to frame contemporary knowledge of the development of emotional-life understanding in terms of children's advances in skill to manipulate narrative grammar. Those skills function in the service of construing those varied contexts in which children mobilize effort to reduce discrepancies. Our perusal of the literature on the development of emotional-life discourse has increased our awareness of the typical investigators' reluctance to explore the benefits of a straightforward "narrative approach." Fivush (1993) came tantalizingly close to paraphrasing our position: "If children are learning the canonical narrative forms for recounting and representing their past in early-adult guided conversations, they may also be learning the emotional framework for evaluating events in their conversations" (p. 44). She proceeds: "Both the adult and the child, in discussing a past emotion are simultaneously interpreting that emotional reaction" (p. 46). Fivush indicated that she will be obligated to respond to concerns about "reality/mind relationships," and she anticipated questions about "how accurate parents are in attributing emotions to their children" (p. 65). An advocate of a narrative approach can appreciate her very cogent retort: "It is not so much a question of accuracy as one of interpretation of emotional experience" (p. 65).

The implications of Stein and Levine's (1991) discussion of children's use of narrative syntax support the proposition that children "make sense" of emotional life in direct proportion to their ability to form adequate emotion stories. The authors note, for example, "the prototypic context in which both emotions [anger and sadness] *are expressed* is one of loss, where the loss is brought about by intentional harm" (p. 67, emphasis ours), allowing the reader to infer that Stein and Levine regard sadness and anger as discursive displays. Nevertheless, rather than following through on the narrative framework, they revert to the traditional notions of reaction and action being dependent on stirrings from within: "The effects of happiness on subsequent thinking is that ..." (p. 59) "negative emotions might well facilitate performance on a task" (p. 59); "aversive events indeed prime anger, irritation, and hostility across a variety of contexts" (p. 69), and so on.

This reluctance to replace a construction anchored to "stirrings from within" with contextually based constructions of emotional-life enactments persists despite cogent observations and conclusions like those reported by Sherman (1927a, 1927b) 70 years ago. Sherman showed that medical students, nurses, freshman, normal school students, psychology graduate students, all alike, could not agree on the "specific emotions" being shown by infants who had received various discrepancy-producing stimulation. For example, psychology graduate students were shown films of the behavior of infants, several days old, who had been suddenly dropped about 2 feet onto a soft mattress. The students did not see the stimulating condition. Fourteen of the 32 participating students reported that the infant had shown *anger*. Six reported that the infant had shown *hunger*, whereas 5 reported having seen *fear*. Of the 42 medical students who watched the "dropped infant" film, 7 reported that the infant had shown anger, 11 that the infant had shown effects of colic, and 11 that the infant had been awakened from sleep.

In a variation of these studies, medical students were shown an emotional-life drama created by splicing a scene showing an infant being restrained onto a segment of a film of the reaction resulting from the infant having been dropped. Thirteen of the 30 medical students who saw this emotional-life episode reported that they had seen anger (which the behaviorists had asserted to be the "natural" reaction to restraint), whereas 4 reported having seen a fearful infant. When those filmed sequences were reversed, so that the medical student viewers watched a sequence showing the infant being dropped spliced on to a film of the infant's reaction to restraint, 10 of 25 reported having seen fear, whereas 7 reported having seen anger.

Though Sherman's studies attracted widespread attention immediately after their publication, few investigators followed their promise of parsimonious alternatives to the prevalent explanations based on psychophysio-logical metaphors. As a result, completed studies of the ways in which members of different social groupings construct and promulgate the stories that are to be enacted in particular contexts (e.g., Shweder, 1993) provide a scant base from which to disrupt the 100-year-old debates about "basic emotions," "neurological emotion centers," and so on.

We recognize, as well, that constructions based on the narrative approach can stand as disjunctive from not only the emotion constructions of mainline investigators, but also from laypersons' common sense about "emotions." In this vein, consider the Brody and Harrison (1987) study discussed earlier. We take that study to be illustrative of the ways in which scholars unwittingly contrive to guide the social construction of emotional-life stories. Recall that the children who participated in the study were asked to think about "emotion stories" and to react to them in terms of specific emotions. When mainline investigators draw their conclusions about children's "accuracy" in labeling emotions, they divert attention from the observation that children and others are taught to attend to the social context to determine which emotional-life story is appropriate to various discrepancy situations. The conclusions of such mainline studies eventually appear in standard personality psychology textbooks. There, they add credibility to the everyday emotional-life dis-course that incorporates metaphors connoting specific stirrings from within.

One must also consider the ideological support of the notion of emotions as stirrings from within. Averill (1992) has noted the widespread belief that a person in touch with his or her feelings is capable of expressing an authentic view of social norms and values. Such an ideology, for example, validates "justified anger" at terrorist bombers. More benignly, in our introductory example, Sarah's authentic expression of sadness—her "true feelings" to-ward an aunt who lacks valid aesthetic vision—would justify her having made a sadness display that was unexpectedly contrary to and thus invalidat-ing to her aunt's "good intentions."

The narrative approach would redirect efforts to explain the develop-ment of children's understanding of emotional life. Instead of seeking to explain children's acquisition of skill in identifying "accurately" their "emo-tions," the narrative approach focuses on how children understand multiper-soned emotional-life plots. Eventually, parents and teachers (and investiga-tors of emotional life) would prompt children to recognize the important goal of achieving a resolution of discrepancy between the flow of inputs and anticipatory constructions. They would see, for example, that an anger dis-play represents one of many routes to the goal of modulating a source of inputs that does not match a self-defining anticipatory construction. Social constructions would develop to replace the belief that "an 'angry' (or 'griev-ing,' or 'fearful') person must let it all out." Societies could improve instruc-tion techniques that prompt skills in conducting dialogues based on the recognition that all participants seek to validate the anticipatory constructions that they create in the interaction. Investigators who study a child like Sarah will inquire into how she, like William, could enact an emotional-life story that brings her own anticipations into line with the flow of inputs, without unnecessarily invalidating the anticipatory constructions of the giver of the "unattractive" gift.

REFERENCES

Averill, J. R. (1986). The acquisition of emotions during adulthood. In R. Harré (Ed.), *The social control of emotion* (pp. 98–118). New York: Basil Blackwell.

Averill, J. R. (1992). The structural bases of emotional behavior: A metatheoretical analysis. In M. S. Clark (Ed.), *Emotion* (pp. 1–24). Newbury Park, CA: Sage.

Bamberg, M., & Damrad-Frye, R. (1991). On the ability to provide evaluative comments: Further explorations of children's narrative competencies. *Journal of Child Language, 18*, 689–710.

Barden, R. C., Zelko, F. A., Duncan, S. W., & Masters, J. C. (1980). Children's consensual knowledge about the experiential determinants of emotion. *Journal of Personality and Social Psychology, 39*, 968–976.

Britton, B. K., & Pellegrini, A. D. (Eds.). (1990). *Narrative thought and narrative language.* Hillsdale, NJ: Erlbaum.

Brody, L. R., & Harrison, R. H. (1987). Developmental changes in children's abilities to match and label emotionally laden situations. *Motivation and Emotion, 11*, 347–365.

Cacioppo, J. T., Klein, D. J., Bernston, G. G., & Hatfield, E. (1993). The psychophysiology of emotion. In M. Lewis & J. M. Haviland (Eds.), *Handbook of emotions* (pp. 447–460). New York: Guilford.

Cohn, J. F., & Tronick, E. Z. (1987). Mother-infant face-to-face interaction: The sequence of dyadic states at 3, 6, and 9 months. *Developmental Psychology, 23*, 68–77.

Darwin, C. (1965). *The expression of emotions in man and animals.* Chicago: University of Chicago Press. (Original published 1872)

De Casper, A. J., & Fifer, W. P. (1980). Of human bonding: Newborns prefer their mothers' voices. *Science, 208*, 1174–1176.

DeCasper, A. J., & Spence, M. J. (1986). Prenatal maternal speech influences newborn's perception of speech sounds. *Infant Behavior and Development, 9*, 133–150.

Denham, S. A., Cook, M., & Zoller, D. (1992). "Baby looks very sad": Implications of conversations about feelings between mother and preschooler. *British Journal of Developmental Psychology, 10*, 301–315.

Dunn, J., & Brown, J. R. (1991). Relationships, talk about feelings, and the development of affect regulation in early childhood. In J. Garber & K. A. Dodge (Eds.), *Cambridge studies in social and emotional development* (pp. 89–108). New York: Cambridge University Press.

Dunn, J., & Brown, J. R. (1993). Early conversations about causality: Content, pragmatics and developmental change. *British Journal of Developmental Psychology, 11*, 107–123.

Feldman, C. F., Bruner, J., Renderer, B., & Spitzer, S. (1990). Narrative comprehension. In B. K. Britton & A. D. Pellegrini (Eds.), *Narrative thought and narrative language* (pp. 1–78). Hillsdale, NJ: Erlbaum.

Fivush, R. (1993). Emotional content of parent–child conversations about the past. In C. A. Nelson (Ed.), *Memory and affect in development. The Minnesota Symposia on Child Psychology* (26, 39–77). Hillsdale, NJ: Erlbaum.

Fogel, A. (1993). *Developing through relationships: Origins of communication self, and culture.* Chicago: University of Chicago Press.

Fogel, A., & Thelan, E. (1987). Development of early expressive action from a dynamic systems approach. *Developmental Psychology, 23,* 747–761.

Frederiksen, C. H. (1979). Discourse comprehension in early reading. In L. N. Resnick & P. A. Weaver (Eds.), *Theory and practice of early reading* (Vol. 1, pp. 155–186) Hillsdale, NJ: Erlbaum.

Gnepp, J. (1989). Personalized inferences of emotions and appraisals: Component processes and correlates. *Developmental Psychology, 25,* 277–288.

Hadwin, J., & Perner, J. (1991). Pleased and surprised: Children's cognitive theory of emotion. *British Journal of Developmental Psychology, 9,* 215–234.

Harré, R. (Ed.). (1986). *The social control of emotion.* New York: Basil Blackwell.

Izard, C. E. (1993). Organizational and motivational functions of discrete emotions. In M. Lewis & J. M. Haviland (Eds.), *Handbook of emotions* (pp. 631–641). New York: Guilford.

Kelly, G. A. (1991). *The Psychology of Personal Constructs.* New York: Routledge. (Original work published 1955).

Klinnert, M. D., Emde, R. N., Butterfield, P., & Campos, J. J. (1986). Social referencing: The infant's use of emotional signals from a friendly adult with mother present. *Developmental Psychology, 22,* 427–432.

Mancuso, J. C. (1986). The acquisition and use of narrative grammar structure. In T. R. Sarbin (Ed.), *Narrative psychology: The storied nature of human conduct* (pp. 91–110). New York: Praeger.

Mancuso, J. C. (1986). Constructionism, personal construct psychology, and narrative psychology. *Theory and Psychology, 6,* 47–70.

Mancuso, J. C., & Adams-Webber, J. R. (1982). Anticipation as a constructive process: The Fundamental Postulate. In J. C. Mancuso & J. R. Adams-Webber (Eds.), *The construing person* (pp. 8–32). New York: Praeger.

Mancuso, J. C., & Sarbin, T. R. (1983). The self-narrative in the enactment of roles. In T. R. Sarbin & K. Scheibe (Eds.), *Studies in social identity* (pp. 233–253). New York: Praeger.

Mandler, J. M. (1984). *Scripts, stories, and scenes: Aspects of a schema theory.* Hillsdale, NJ: Erlbaum.

Mandler, G. (1992). Emotions, evolution and aggression: Myths and conjectures. In K. T. Strongman (Ed.), *International review of studies of emotion* (pp. 97–116). New York: Wiley.

Mascolo, M. F., & Mancuso, J. C. (1990). The functioning of epigenetically evolved emotion systems. *International Journal of Personal Construct Psychology, 3,* 205–220.

Miller, P., & Sperry, L. L. (1994). The socialization of anger and aggression. *Merrill–Palmer Quarterly, 40,* 1–31.

Murray, L., & Trevarthen, C. (1985). Emotional regulation of interactions between two-month-olds and their mothers. In T. Field & N. Fox (Eds.), *Social perception in infants* (pp. 177–197). Norwood, NJ: Ablex.

Ortony, A., & Turner, T. J. (1990). What's basic about basic emotions? *Psychological Review, 97,* 315–331.

Papousek, M., Papousek, H., & Bornstein, M. (1985). The naturalistic vocal environment of young infants: On the significance of homegeneity and variability in parent speech. In T. Field & N. Fox (Eds.), *Social perception in infants* (pp. 269–297). Norwood, NJ: Ablex.

Sarbin, T. R. (1995). Emotional life, rhetoric, and roles. *Journal of Narrative and Personal History, 5,* 213–220.

Sarbin, T. R., Taft, R., & Bailey, D. E. (1960). *Clinical inference and cognitive theory.* New York: Holt, Rinehart & Winston.

Sherman, M. (1927a). The differentiation of emotional responses in infants: I. Judgments of emotional responses from motion picture views and from actual observation. *Journal of Comparative Psychology, 7,* 265–284.

Sherman, M. (1927b). The differentiation of emotional responses in infants: II. The ability of observers to judge the emotional characteristics of the crying of infants and of the voice of an adult. *Journal of Comparative Psychology, 7,* 335–351.

Shweder, R. A. (1993). The cultural psychology of emotions. In M. Lewis & J. M. Haviland (Eds.), *Handbook of emotions* (pp. 419–433). New York: Guilford.

Stein, N. L., & Glenn, C. G. (1979). An analysis of story comprehension in elementary school children. in R. O. Freedle (Ed.), *New directions in discourse processing* (Vol. II, pp. 53–120). Norwood, NJ: Ablex.

Stein, N. L., & Levine, L. J. (1991). Making sense out of emotion: The representation and use of goal-structured knowledge. In W. Kessen, A. Ortony, & F. I. M. Craik (Eds.), *Memories, thoughts, and emotions: Essays in honor of George Mandler* (pp. 295–322). Hillsdale, NJ: Erlbaum.

Stenberg, C. R., & Campos, J. J. (1990). The development of anger expressions in infancy. In N. L. Stein, B. Leventhal, & T. Trabasso (Eds.), *Psychological and biological approaches to emotion* (pp. 247–282). Hillsdale, NJ: Erlbaum.

Strayer, J. (1986). Children's attributions regarding the situational determinants of emotion in self and others. *Developmental Psychology, 22,* 649–654.

Sutton-Smith, B. (1986). Children's fiction making. In T. R. Sarbin (Ed.), *Narrative psychology: The storied nature of human conduct* (pp. 91–110). New York: Praeger.

Thorndyke, P. W. (1977). Cognitive structures in comprehension and memory of narrative discourse. *Cognitive Psychology, 9,* 77–110.

Trevarthen, C. (1993). The self born in intersubjectivity: The psychology of an infant communicating. In U. Neisser (Ed.), *The perceived self: Ecological and interpersonal sources of self-knowledge* (pp. 121–173). Cambridge, UK: Cambridge University Press.

van Dijk, T. A., & Kintsch, W. (1983). *Strategies of discourse comprehension.* New York: Academic Press.

VI

Conclusion and Integration

Alternative Conceptions of Emotional Development
Controversy and Consensus

Michael F. Mascolo and Sharon Griffin

ALTERNATIVE APPROACHES TO EMOTIONAL DEVELOPMENT

The contributors to this volume have put forth a variety of perspectives addressing the nature, development, and functions of emotion. These models can be usefully understood in terms of four general categories. These include characterizations of emotions as (1) discrete states, (2) multicomponent processes, (3) emergent coordinations of self-organizing systems, and (4) constructed modes of experience. Consistent with the recent trends in emotion theory reviewed in the introductory chapter, the approaches to emotion represented in this volume differ with respect to the number of component systems invoked to define or explain emotion, as well as in the relations among those proposed systems. In what follows, for each general approach to emotional development, we examine the ways in which the concept of emotion is defined, what about emotion undergoes developmental change, and the proposed functions of emotional processes.

Michael F. Mascolo • Department of Psychology, Merrimack College, North Andover, Massachusetts 01845.   Sharon Griffin • Frances Hiatt School of Education, Clark University, Worcester, Massachusetts 01845.

What Develops in Emotional Development? edited by Michael F. Mascolo and Sharon Griffin. Plenum Press, New York, 1998.

Emotions as Discrete States

Proponents of discrete emotion theory define emotions as distinct, neurobiological processes (Ackerman, Abe & Izard; Panksepp, Knutson, & Pruitt; and to an extent, Lewis & Douglas). Panksepp et al. define emotion in terms of a set of distinct "operating systems in the brain [that] orchestrate a variety of changes in behavior, various automatic bodily functions, as well as subjectively experienced affective states" (p. 54). Ackerman et al. define particular emotions in terms of innate, encapsulated sets of neurochemical processes, expressive behavior, and subjective feeling states. In their dynamic systems approach to emotional development, Lewis and Douglas also define emotion in terms of nonreducible affective states. From these views, distinct emotional states reflect the activation of hardwired biological systems that are largely independent of cognitive and other psychological processes. Specific instances of any given emotion are discrete in the sense that they are distinguishable from other particular emotional states. As such, basic emotional states such as anger, joy, or sadness are defined in terms of patterns of neurochemical activity, emotional expression, and subjective feeling that are distinguishable from each other.

In support of this view, Panksepp et al. describe research that is beginning to link particular classes of emotion (desire/seeking; anger/attack; fear/freezing) and socioemotional behavior in animals (separation distress, rough-and-tumble play, sexuality, nurturance, dominance) to the activity of specific brain structures and neurochemical processes. For example, Panksepp et al. link angry attack to stimulation of the central medial amygdala and to different patterns of dopaminergic and serotonergic activation. Ackerman et al. draw upon the research of Izard and others to demonstrate discreteness of emotion-related facial expressions during the first year of life and their evocation in emotion-typical situations. For example, Izard et al. (1995) reported that among 2- and 9-month-olds observed in face-to-face dyadic play, full-faced expressions of anger, interest, and joy predominated over partial and blended expressions of these emotions. Such findings are consistent with the proposition that emotions exist as encapsulated neurophysiological states or systems.

In speaking of the nature of emotional development, discrete state theorists suggest that the emergence of emotional states is governed by a maturational timetable. For example, Panksepp et al. show that the ontogenesis of emotional behaviors such as separation distress, rough-and-tumble play, sexual behavior, nurturance, and dominance follows a predictable ontogenetic course in mice and other animals (see Chapter 3, Table 1). Panksepp et al. cite evidence that links changes in these behaviors to the maturation of specific anatomical and neurochemical changes. For example, Panksepp et al. describe the ways in which dominance and angry attack rise upon puberty in male rats and upon lactation in female rats. In rats, nurturant behavior (e.g., nest building and cleaning) begins just prior to the birth of offspring and has been linked to hormonal changes in progesterone and estrogens. Changes in levels of oxytocin as well as other hormones and peptides are linked to a suite of emotion-relevant processes in mother rats (e.g., milk production, nursing), which are postulated to prepare mothers for the care of their pups. Panksepp et al. suggest that neurochemically induced affective states may well underlie such behaviors.

Discrete state theory generally proceeds from the premise that as non-reducible affective states, basic emotions per se do not undergo developmental transformation subsequent to their emergence in ontogenesis. For example, Ackerman et al. demonstrated that basic emotional expressions show considerable stability during the first year of life. Expressions of interest, joy, sadness, and anger emerge from the first weeks to 2–4 months of life, whereas fear expressions begin to emerge between 7 and 9 months. Once they emerged, the pattern of interest, joy, anger, and sadness expressions was stable when assessed at 2.5 and 9 months in the context of dyadic play. Such data are consistent with the proposition that basic emotional states exhibit stability throughout ontogenesis.

According to discrete state theorists, although core emotions per se do not change, peripheral aspects of emotional processes change in ontogenesis (e.g., the decoupling of emotion from expression, the regulation of emotion, understanding emotion). For example, with socialization and the development of volitional control, children learn to regulate their emotional expressions. The main source of emotional development, however, occurs through the formation of links between emotion and cognition. Whereas Ackerman et al. call such links *affective–cognitive structures*, Lewis and Douglas call them *emotional interpretations*. Through the formation of links between cognition and affect, cognition-dependent emotional experiences such as disappointment or pride can emerge. However, according to Ackerman et al., affective–cognitive structures result in the formation of new emotionally charged experiences in development, but these emergent experiences are not themselves new emotions. Interactions between affect and cognition do not transform emotional feelings states; rather, they "connect invariant feelings with changing images and thoughts. Thus, the emotion feeling is the stable component of an affective–cognitive structure" (p. 93).

From a discrete state, view, emotional states are inherently functional. The activation of discrete neurochemical process underlies the production of different classes of emotional behavior. Panksepp et al. have demonstrated ways in which developmental changes in neurochemical production play a role in activating different classes of emotional behavior (e.g., acetylcholine in rough-and-tumble play; biogenic amines such as dopamine in aggressive behavior). According to Ackerman et al., differential emotions theory "assumes that feeling states are evolutionary distillates and thereby *inherently adaptive*" (p. 87, italics in original). Specific emotions motivate specific classes of behavior: "Interest motivates orienting and exploration, fear motivates avoidance, and anger motivates removal of a goal obstruction" (p. 88). Beyond the motivating functions of local emotions, through the formation of affective–cognitive structures, emotion acts as the primary motivational system for the human organism. The affective–cognitive structures "forms a fundamental building block of mental life and self" (p. 86). This point will be explored further in our discussion of Lewis and Douglas's dynamic systems model of the development of cognitive-emotion links.

Emotions as Multicomponent Processes

Several contributors have defined emotions as multicomponent processes organized around a functional core (Barrett; Frijda & Mesquita; Kozak & Brown). Such approaches proceed from the assertion that emotions are best conceptualized as evolving *processes* rather than as discrete states. Componential theorists maintain that many aspects of organismic functioning are relevant to the emotion process." For example, Barrett states that "emotions are not specific 'expressive' or other behaviors; not specific cognitions, or specific feelings; each of these elements is *a part* of the emotion process' (p. 110, emphasis in original). Furthermore, Frijda and Mesquita assert that the various components of the emotion "are only moderately correlated" (p. 274). Thus, any particular instance of any given emotion category (e.g., anger, joy, sadness) can take on myriad different forms, and no single component constitutes a necessary or sufficient condition for the attribution of emotion. For this reason, Barrett (this volume) speaks of the production of emotion *families* rather than discrete emotion states.

Even though instances of particular emotion families show variability from event to event, emotion families are defined by *inclinations toward action* or by the *functions they serve* for the organism within a given context. For Barrett, one can attribute a particular emotion to an organism to the extent that the organism's evoked behaviors serve a particular set of functions for the organism relative to its ongoing relationship with the environment. For Frijda and Mesquita, instances of various emotion categories (e.g., anger, joy) call forth emotion-typical control precedences—action-tendencies that serve particular functions for the fate of the organism's concerns. For example, according to Barrett and Campos (1987), anger involves an event-appraisal that there exists an obstruction to obtaining one's goals. Anger involves action-tendencies to move forward to eliminate the obstacle functions in the service of the motives and goals implicated the initial event appraisal. Thus, "[w]hat binds the various components together is the goal or aim of establishing, changing or maintaining a particular relationship with the emotional object in the specific situation" (Frijda & Mesquita, p. 275). Thus, for functionalist approaches, although instances of particular categories of emotion are characterized in terms of correlated configurations of concerns, appraisals, bodily reactions, action-tendencies, and the like, they are nevertheless organized around a common set of functions or control precedences. Such a view differs markedly from discrete state theory. For example, Ackerman et al. hold that

> a core tenet of DET [differential emotions theory] is that the emotion experiences or feelings states associated with discrete expressions are also stable and unchanging over time. Once an infant reliably displays an emotion, the motivational feeling state of the specific emotion is invariant; fear is fear is fear. Thus, a fear expression is always linked with the same motivational state, which energizes the same type of behavior: escape or harm avoidance across development. (p. 89)

Although functional theorists would agree that a specific function of all instances of "fear" would involve something like "escape or harm avoidance," they would disagree with an assertion such as "fear is fear is fear." For example, Barrett distinguishes "fear that no one will find one's theory compelling" with the infant's fear of heights. According to Barrett, these two fear-family members would differ markedly in the age of display, the patterning of facial and physiological activity, the action-tendencies displayed, and in the overall fear experience. Barrett concludes that "few would suggest that these two forms of fear are the same" (p. 116). In addressing this issue, one might suggest that Ackerman et al. would conceptualize "fear that no one would find one's theory compelling" as an affective–cognitive structure composed of an invariant feeling state coupled with a particular thought. Thus, according to differential emotions theory, the feeling state of fear would be the same in both cases, although other elements of the affective–cognitive structure would be different.

Like discrete state theorists, functionalists argue for some stability in the development of emotions. However, unlike discrete emotions theorists, it is the general *functions and action precedences* associated with a particular emotion process that remains invariant in ontogenesis, rather than underlying states or subjective experiences. All other elements in the emotion—including emotional experiences—exhibit variation as a result of development, situation, or culture.

Barrett illustrates this principle in her analysis of the development of social standards that mediate the production of pride and shame in infants and young children. For example, Barrett suggests that one can identify an instance of pride to the extent that the child's behaviors serve a particular set of functions: (1) decreasing distance between self and other; (2) showing others that one has met a desired standard; (3) highlighting standards for the self. If the child's behavior exhibits these functions, then, regardless of the child's age or the precise behaviors observed, one might say that pride is present. Barrett also suggests that for pride to occur, a child must be able to appreciate that he or she has met some type of rule or standard. However, the production of pride is not defined or caused by any particular level of cognitive awareness. As such, it may be possible that even a rudimentary awareness of goal-related standards is sufficient to evoke pride-like behaviors in children. For example, Barrett presents evidence that even 12-month-old infants are able to represent simple standards and, as such, may be able to exhibit pride or pride-relevant responses in appropriate circumstances. Subsequent to their early emergence, there are both quantitative and qualitative changes in pride-relevant processes, including changes in the number and complexity of self-relevant standards and goals, the significance of such standards to the child, the representation of self as agent and object, specific pride behaviors, and the situations in which such behaviors occur. Thus, the development of pride-relevant processes is characterized by both wide variation and functional continuity.

Functionalist models also hold that the experience of emotion changes in ontogenesis. This assertion marks a second important difference between functionalist theory and discrete state approaches. For discrete state theory, discrete emotional states involve a distinct subjective feeling state that remains invariant in ontogenesis (Izard & Malatesta, 1987). Frijda and Mesquita, for example, explicitly reject the idea of emotion-specific *qualia*. With respect to the development of subjective experience, they write:

> At its most elementary, emotional experience is entirely unreflective and consists of nothing but the experience of an event as appraised, with "affect" as its perceived attractiveness or aversiveness (Frijda, 1986). Reflectiveness is not part of the definition of experience.... Emotional experiences change over time as attention wanders over the various aspects of the emotional situation and reflexivity, over one's pattern of reaction, the unreflected perceptual awareness included.... [Emotional experience] thus is a product of separate development, largely independent of the development responsible for emotional sensitivity, the articulation of appraisal, and the progressive differentiation of modes of action readiness and forms of emotional behavior, that is, emotion itself. (p. 290)

Part of the disagreement between differential emotions theory and functionalist theory may concern the meaning of the terms *experience* and *feeling state*. Functionalists assert that the *experience* of any given emotion undergoes developmental change; differential emotions theorists maintain that what is invariant in development is the *feeling state* that accompanies any given emotion. However, differential emotions theorists agree with functionalist theorists that feelings are but one aspect of a more encompassing emotional experience (Izard, personal communication, April 25, 1997). Thus, although some functionalist theories reject the idea that discrete emotions are accompanied by any specific *qualia* (Frijda & Mesquita), at least part of the distance between differential emotions theorists and functionalist theories may be diminished if one grants that it is possible that some emotional *feelings* may remain invariant even as the broader *experience* of a given emotion changes in ontogenesis.

Kozak and Brown also differentiate between affect, feeling, and value structures on the one hand, and emotions on the other. For Kozak and Brown, although emotional reactions involve feelings, feelings are fundamentally different processes than emotions. Feelings accompany all adaptive and deliberative activity and function to select ideas and action. Kozak and Brown write: "Cognitively, [individuals] may be able to rule out relatively small numbers of simple courses of actions ... but in the end, all of the great human decisions involve so many degrees of freedom that objectivity and certainty are unachievable. In such cases, feelings decide" (p. 148–149). On the other hand, emotion "is a particular form of reaction that occurs only in conjunction with adaptive malfunction" (p. 149). Whereas feelings are "the conscious manifestation of evaluative activity," emotional reactions "serve the function of restoring adaptive order, even if only of a lower level, when adaptation fails" (p. 150). As value structures and thus feelings undergo developmental change, adaptive activity becomes more successful. As a result, emotional reactions, as responses to maladaptation, decrease in both frequency and intensity.

Kozak and Brown maintain that most contemporary emotion researchers have generally failed to discriminate between the study of "affective in general" (feelings, values, evaluative activity) on the one hand, and emotion on the other. Regardless of whether one accepts this criticism, Kozak and Brown's chapter contains much of importance for those interested in "affectivity in general," as well as for those concerned about the nature of cognition and mind. In suggesting that feelings play a central role in decision making, Kozak and Brown make a case for the fundamental inseparability of affect and cognition in everyday human activity. If feelings function to select ideas and actions, cognition simply cannot function without the participation of affect, and vice versa. In making this assertion, Kozak and Brown challenge approaches that characterize the mind as a primarily rational entity or process. Furthermore, if feelings play a central role in all adaptive activity, there must be important ontogenetic changes in affectivity and its role in cognitive and behavioral activity. A developmental analysis of the role of affect and valuation in cognition and action remains largely uncharted territory.

Whereas Panksepp et al. describe epigenetically canalized aspects of emotional development, Frijda and Mesquita's descriptions of cultural variations in emotional components illustrates plasticity in emotional development. Frijda and Mesquita describe cultural variations in virtually every emotion component they examine (i.e., antecedent events, concerns, appraisals, action readiness, beliefs, regulation, etc.). Cultural differences in goals and concerns prompt differences in the meaning that is assigned to various emotion-relevant antecedent events. For example, whereas academic success indicates attainment of personal goals among the Dutch, it is seen as homage to familial honor among Turkish people. Furthermore, despite their stability in explaining variability among emotional experiences across cultures, there are nonetheless important differences in the significance of various appraisal dimensions for creating emotional experience. For example, the tendency to blame is attenuated among the Semai of Malaysia, who respond to frustration with *pehunan*—a state of fear following an expectation of serious danger—rather than anger. Finally, even modes of action readiness—which Frijda and Mesquita argue are the primary basis for the differentiation of emotion—also show cultural influence. For example, "moving away" is a more important dimension for discriminating among the varieties of emotional experience for Dutch than for Indonesian and Japanese participants. In Frijda and Mesquita's analysis, the only emotion component that does not yield evidence of cross-cultural variability is physiological arousal. However, they also suggest that "no solid evidence exists of specific relationships between particular emotions and particular patterns of physiological response" (p. 283). The theorists thus conclude that

> Emotions can vary in very many regards, intraindividually and cross-culturally, as well as developmentally.... They cannot satisfactorily be captured by saying that the same basic emotions may show variations in detail in different individuals or groups. The differences in components accompanying a common core that leads one to compare two emotions, as two "angers" may be so substantial that the common core dwindles in importance in the face of the differences. (p. 291)

Thus, unlike differential emotions theory, functionalist researchers suggest that emotions and their components undergo nontrivial change in ontogenesis. The ontogeny of emotion is characterized by quantitative as well as qualitative changes in individual members of any given emotion family (see Barrett's comment about the development of fear, discussed earlier). However, in their endorsement of the view that emotions change in ontogenesis, functionalist theorists generally do not embrace a model of development defined in terms of structural transformation. For example, Barrett defines emotions in terms of functions that are invariant in ontogenesis and explicitly rejects the notion that emotional processes may develop in a series of steps defined in terms of the organization of emotional components. As such, Barrett appears to focus on continuity rather than discontinuity in the development of emotion.

Finally, as indicated throughout this discussion, functionalist theorists agree with discrete state theorists that emotions are inherently functional processes serving internal, behavioral, and socially adaptive functions. However, advocates of the functionalist perspective depart from discrete emotions theory by making an additional claim. Specifically, functionalists assert that emotional processes and their functions are evoked with reference to appreciations or appraisals of events in terms of salient motives and concerns; that is, although emotions motivate, they are also motivated. As such, their form and function are dependent upon multiple systems of organismic functioning.

Emotions as Emergent Coordinations of Component Systems

Several theorists in this volume have advanced systems perspectives on the nature of emotion (Dickson, Fogel, & Messinger; Lewis & Douglas; Mascolo & Harkins; Mascolo & Griffin). The systems approaches represented in this volume are similar to functionalist models in many ways. Both depict emotional events as processes assembled from the activation of multiple component systems; both link the production of emotional processes to changes in the organism's relationship to personally meaningful environmental events; both maintain that feeling is but one part of a larger emotion process; both assert that particular classes of emotional responding serve adaptive functions for the organism. The views differ mainly with respect to their representation of the processes by which emotional elements come together to form emotional constellations that display both stability and fluidity in ontogenesis.

Although functions and event-appraisals are important aspects of the emotion process, from a systems approach, no single emotion component is privileged in the organization or definition of an emotional experience, including functions, appraisals, control precedences, or felt experiences. Rather, particular emotional constellations *emerge* through the *self-organization* of interacting components within a social context. Within this view, various component systems (e.g., motivational, appraisal, action, experiential, etc.) mutually influence, constrain, and regulate each other throughout the course of any given emotional episode. As such, systems perspectives predict both stability and flexibility in the production of emotional processes. On the one hand, because emotional constituents can combine in many possible ways, the number of possible emotional states is large. On the other hand, mutually regulating emotion-relevant subsystems have a tendency to settle into a finite number of generally stable patterns, sometimes called attractors. Thus, without postulating fixed emotion programs in the brain, systems approaches provide a framework for understanding the ways in which emotional constituents combine to form general patterns with a virtually infinite number of minor variations. Moreover, although we may be able to refer to many such patterns with existing emotion names (e.g., anger, pride, humiliation), systems approaches suggest that there will also be many emergent patterns that are unnamed by the existing emotion lexicon.

If emotional processes are emergent products of the interaction of multiple-component systems, what is it that makes an emotion process emotional? How can one differentiate emotional processes from psychological functioning in general? Systems theorists differ in their responses to this question. For example, Dickson et al. and Mascolo and Harkins argue for the interdependence of the various systems that produce feeling and emotional behavior. Emotional experiences emerge out of intersystemic interactions following changes in an individual's relationship to his or her environs. As such, what makes a psychological process emotional is the patterned transformation of component systems as a result of personally significant changes in one's world. In their version of dynamic systems model of emotional development, Lewis and Douglas invoke Izard's (Ackerman et al., this volume; Izard, 1977) definition of emotion as discrete, physiologically based affective states. In Lewis and Douglas's approach, separate cognitive and emotional systems dynamically interact with each other to form dynamic structures called *emotional interpretations* (Izard's affective–cognitive structures). Thus, to Lewis and Douglas, what makes a process emotional is the participation of affective states in a larger dynamic process. Still others advise caution in attempts to define the concept of emotion as an independent state. For example, Mascolo and Harkins note that the concept of emotion has its origins in everyday understanding and is invoked to refer to multiple aspects of human behavior. As such, it would be a mistake to assume that "emotion" refers to a singular, bounded, or extant entity. Additional theoretical and empirical work is needed to construct more precise theoretical constructs to differentiate and/ or otherwise clarify the diverse ways in which the concept of emotion is used by laypersons and theorists alike (see Mancuso & Sarbin for an extended analysis of this point).

In addressing the issue of the nature of emotional development, systems perspectives stand in contrast to traditional approaches that "round off the immense variability in real behavior, extract a generalized description, and then show the universality of that description" (Lewis and Douglas, p. 159). Systems theory is an approach that embraces the notions of both determinacy and indeterminacy in development. Because self-organizing systems tend toward stable patterns within any given context, systems approaches predict the production of more or less stable patterns of emotional processes in development. However, because social context exerts a direct role in the production of emotional behavior, proponents of systems approaches suggest that nontrivial transformations in a given category of emotional processes can occur as a function of changes in social context. Furthermore, system theorists generally endorse the view that emotional states and experiences can undergo structural transformation in ontogenesis. In defining emotion in terms of relations among multiple-component processes, systems theorists generally maintain that emotional states and experiences can undergo qualitative transformation as their components undergo developmental change and reorganization in relation to each other.

Dickson et al. illustrate several of these principles in their analysis of contextual and developmental variations in smiling and laughter. Dickson et al. maintain that rather than following as an expression of a fixed feeling state or genetic program, smiling emerges within social contexts as a result of interactions among multiple emotional constituents. For example, Dickson et al. demonstrate that different types of smiles are more likely to occur in different types of infant–adult interactions. Basic (upturn of the lips), Duchenne (upturn of the lips and cheeks) and play (open jaw) smiles were more likely to occur in joint book reading, vocal activities, and physical interactions, respectively. Furthermore, relations between smiling and laughter changed over the course of infancy. For example, prior to 9 months, comment laughter was more likely to co-occur with play smiles, whereas after 9 months, comment laughter occurred more often with basic smiles. The researchers suggested that developmental variation in smiling and laughter follows changes in *control parameters* that catalyze the reorganization of multiple emotional constituents. For example, decrements in the size of the infant's tongue over the first year of life may make it easier for the infant to inhale when engaging in comment laughter. As a result, a nonobvious factor such as changes in tongue size may act as (but one) control parameter that prompts a developmental shift in the type of smiles that accompany comment laughter over the first year of life, that is, from play to basic smiles. Thus, from this view, smiling self-organizes in development and thus cannot be seen as a simple product of the unfolding of a genetic plan or affective state.

Similarly, Mascolo (Mascolo & Harkins; Mascolo & Griffin) suggested that emotional episodes and experiences undergo quantitative and qualitative transformation with changes in emotion-relevant component systems and their intercoordinations. Mascolo and Harkins described developmental changes in the complexity of pride behaviors in children between 1 and 3 years of age, both as a function of cognitive development and social context (e.g., the amount of emotional scaffolding provided by socialization agents). Unlike Barrett, for example, who rejects the idea of developmental levels when applied to self-evaluative emotion, Mascolo and Harkins propose a series of steps in the development of pride-relevant appraisals and behaviors. Similarly, Mascolo and Griffin propose that anger episodes and experiences undergo qualitative transformation along multiple pathways as anger-relevant appraisals shift from "want violations" to qualitatively different types of "ought violations."

Lewis and Douglas build on Izard's differential emotions theory in their dynamic systems approach to the development of cognitive–emotional interactions. Lewis and Douglas define emotion and cognition as partially independent systems that interact to produce emotional interpretations, which are similar to Izard's affective–cognitive structures. As such, Lewis and Douglas's approach can be seen as a type of rapprochement between discrete state and systems approaches to emotional development. Lewis and Douglas propose that cognitive and emotional systems self-organize to produce emotional interpretations such as pride, humiliation, and anxiety. Such emotional interpretations function as attractors and repellors in both real time and in development, and function as basic building blocks in the development of cognition, personality, and self. Lewis and Douglas's model of the self-organization of defensive reactions illustrates the role of emotion in personality formation. For example, Lewis and Douglas suggest that a painful event prompts the elaboration of emotional interpretations such as anxiety or a wish to escape the situation. The cognitive–emotion system undergoes a "phase shift" in order to escape the painful event. Repeated instantiations of these processes leads to stabilization of a defensive pattern into an emotional attractor, which can thus function as a dynamic personality structure. Lewis and Douglas's analysis of the formation of defensive patterns in 2-, 6-, and 10-month-olds illustrates the processes by which emotional traits self-organize in the context of adult–child interaction.

Like functionalist and discrete state theory, systems approaches maintain that emotional reactions serve adaptive functions for the organism and its social environs. However, some systems theorists suggest that the functions of emotional reactions are emergent products of activity within a context rather than definitive properties of emotions per se. For example, Dickson et al. suggest that different types of smiles may serve different functions in the context of different social interactions in the first year of life. Recall that Dickson et al. observed that, after 9 months of age, basic smiles tended to co-occur with comment laughter, whereas Duchenne smiles occurred more often with rhythmic laughter. The investigators speculated that, similar to adult practices, the production of basic smiles in the context of comment laughter may function to indicate interest in the ongoing interaction. In contrast, the co-occurrence of Duchenne smiles with rhythmic laughter suggests that such smiles may function to signal intense enjoyment. Thus, the differential functions of smiling can be seen as emergent products of the ways in which emotional elements coalesce within varied social contexts.

Mascolo and Griffin also suggest ways in which emotional functions may emerge in development and in particular social contexts and relationships. They suggest that appraisals involved in anger experiences undergo developmental transformation from "want violations" toward increasingly sophisticated "ought violations." As such, anger episodes may serve different functions at different points in development. For example, whereas anger might function to remove obstacles to one's sensorimotor goals in infancy (i.e., the violation of a want), with development, anger may function to preserve increasingly internalized social and moral standards (i.e., the violation of an ought). Furthermore, with development, anger may serve different functions in the context of different types of appraised ought violations. Anger episodes may function to direct a partner's attention to the status of one's relationship in the context of relational violations, to personal boundaries in personal violations, or to social rules and conventions in sociomoral violations. Indeed, variants on all three functions may occur simultaneously within any given anger scenario. Furthermore, to the extent that the participation of ought violations in anger are gender-related, anger may function differently as a function of gender. Still further, as anger becomes increasingly mediated by social and moral standards with development, it can function to maintain, extend, and define the sociomoral orders of one's local community. Thus, different functions of anger can emerge throughout development and within different interpersonal contexts.

Cognitive and Sociocultural Origins of Emotional Experiences

Contributors differed in their view of whether emotional experiences undergo developmental change. Whereas proponents of biological or discrete emotions theory argue for the invariance of emotional experience in onto-genesis, others argue that the subjective experience of emotion undergoes change as the processes that produce and evaluate experience change and develop (Frijda & Mesquita; Michael Lewis; Mascolo & Harkins; Mascolo & Griffin; Mancuso & Sarbin). Of these views, Michael Lewis and Mancuso and Sarbin have advanced two very different approaches to the development and experience of emotion.

Michael Lewis's Analysis of the Structure of Emotional States and Experiences

Michael Lewis's approach to emotion is comprehensive and spans several of the organizational categories developed in this chapter. Lewis proposes that emotions are structured in terms of five separable components, including emotional *elicitors, receptors, states, expressions,* and *experiences.* From his view, an emotional *state* is defined as the activation of emotional *receptors* by emotional *elicitors.* Emotional receptors can consist of either innate neuro-logical pathways or general, nonspecific arousal. Emotional elicitors can be either internal or external, automatic or learned. An important aspect of Lewis's approach is the separability of the five components. Like discrete emotions theorists, Lewis suggests that emotional states reflect the activation of specific central nervous system pathways. However, Lewis also suggests that existing work has not yet convincingly demonstrated that different emotional receptors underlie the production of different emotional states; as such, Lewis entertains the idea that nonspecific arousal may function as an emotional receptor system. Also, like differential emotions theorists, Lewis proposes that emotional expressions and experiences accompany emotional states. Although both Lewis and differential emotions theorists maintain that with age, children become increasingly able to dissociate their facial expressions from their inner experiences, Lewis argues for a greater separability of expression and internal state than do differential emotions theorists. For example, Lewis cites the relative scarcity of pure emotion-typical facial expressions in infancy (but see Ackerman et al. for a different view). In addition, Lewis questions the extent to which emotion-typical facial expressions in very young infants are reflective of their underlying emotional states.

Lewis is particularly explicit in his discrimination of emotional experiences from emotional states. Whereas emotional states consist of the activation of the emotional receptors by emotional elicitors, the experience of emotion "involves turning attention on the self in order to interpret and evaluate perceived emotional states and expressions. Emotional experiences require that individuals attend to emotional states and expressions. The attending refers to the turning of one's consciousness toward the self as a referent. It is not automatic" (p. 41). Lewis suggests further that "the development of experiences may occur long after the emergence of emotional states. Therefore, although newborns may show an emotional state of pain when pricked with a pin, it would not necessarily follow that they have an emotional experience of pain" (p. 44). In viewing emotional experiences as products of cognitive interpretation, Lewis's view of emotional experience departs significantly from that of differential emotions theorists, who maintain that emotional feelings can register directly in consciousness without cognitive participation (Izard, 1977). Again, it is possible that some of the distance between Izard's and Lewis's position can be diminished if we differentiate between the notions of subjective *feeling* on the one hand and emotional *experience* on the other. For example, one might suggest that the activation of emotional states produces *feeling tone* that at least becomes available to consciousness. With cognitive development and changes in the capacity for self-awareness, more articulated and encompassing emotional *experiences* would arise as children gain the capacity to focus on their emotional feelings and connect them to other aspects of their emotional states (see also Lewis, 1991).

As a product of cognitive interpretation of emotional states, emotional experience must await the development of self and abilities to locate and interpret internal changes within a bodily source that one calls "me." The capacities to experience self in terms of different emotions must await cognitive development and emerges in the context of social interaction. The development of emotional experiences is in part dependent on the ways in which others respond to a child's emotional state. Verbal and nonverbal reactions from others provide the interpretive contexts in which children develop ways to interpret and evaluate, and thus experience, their emotional states. As such, "infants become, in part, what others think them to be" (p. 45). Lewis suggests that with the onset of self-recognition, beginning around 15 months of age, children begin to be able to experience their emotional states as anger, sadness, and fear. Furthermore, the capacity to experience emotions "changes the nature of the earlier emotional states, but, more importantly, acts to create new emotional states and experiences" (p. 46), including secondary emotions such as pride, shame, and guilt. In arguing that changes in experience change the very nature of emotional states, Lewis advances a strong definition of development as structural transformation. Specifically, he states that the basic distinction between change and development is that "in the former, the structure remains but is subsumed by another process, whereas in the latter, the structure changes" (p. 30). Thus, Lewis postulates that emotion is composed of multiple interacting elements that develop along their own pathways through different mechanisms of change. Among these, "it is the development of experience that is likely to exert the most powerful force in the development of emotional life" (p. 47).

The Social Construction of Emotional Experiences

Constructivist and social constructionist approaches to emotion proceed from the premise that the events that persons call "emotional" are products of constructive processes that occur within and between individuals. In their approach to emotion, Mancuso and Sarbin explicitly reject the notion of discrete emotions as independent physiological or psychological entities. Rather, they suggest that mismatches between incoming sensory input and one's anticipatory constructions prompt mobilization reactions (preparations for effort) to reduce such mismatches to a subjectively optimal level. Sensory changes from such preparations for effortful action are labeled "feelings," and individuals come to attribute the source of their subsequent actions to these so-called "feelings." Mancuso and Sarbin hold, however, that the physiological changes that form a basis for reports of felt activity are but adjuncts rather than causes of an individual's emotional behavior. When laypersons or scholars speak of emotions as feelings that precipitate action, they engage in an unrecognized use of *metonymy*—the linguistic practice of referring to a whole in terms of some salient feature or associated part. In the case of the concept of emotion, persons invoke metonymy when they define an emotion as an independent feeling state rather than as a construed aspect of persons' ongoing activity in the world.

From this view, the very concept of emotion qua independent entity is a social construction. As such, it is a mistake to assume that the socially constructed concept of emotion reflects a real entity or process. As such, "questions about 'true emotions' are futile" (Mancuso & Sarbin, p. 297). It is better to ask questions about the origins and development of the processes by which persons construct understandings of their own and other's activities as "emotional," and how such constructions affect their activities and relationships. Thus, rather than attempting to define and specify the properties of real or specific emotions, researchers should conceptualize their work in terms of the metaphor of *emotional life*. In so doing, theorists and researchers would direct their research toward "actors involved in multipersoned plots that are identified as anger, fear, pride, envy, joy, and so on" (p. 298). Conceived in this way, persons *construct* their emotional life in terms of socially created narrative structures. The experience of emotion is a product of construing mobilization input in terms of emotional-life narratives that have their origins in interactions with social and cultural agents.

Mancuso and Sarbin also propose that emotional experiences undergo developmental transformation in ontogenesis. Like Michael Lewis, they locate the source of experiential change in cognitive and social development. Unlike Lewis, however, Mancuso and Sarbin do not postulate the existence of underlying emotional states. Rather, they suggest that bodily meanings are embedded in social meanings: Socially constructed narratives provide the primary organizational structures that create the experience of bodily change as emotion. As such, the experience of emotion undergoes developmental transformation from protonarrative to increasingly complex narrative structures that have their origins in social interaction, language, and cultural meaning systems. Thus, the transformation from protonarrative to increasingly complex narrative structures implies that emotional life undergoes qualitative and not just quantitative change in ontogenesis.

Within Mancuso and Sarbin's version of social constructionism, the mobilization changes that provide the bodily basis of constructions such as "feeling" or "emotion" serve the function of preparing the organism for effort of reducing the mismatch between events and failed anticipatory constructions. However, because Mancuso and Sarbin do not regard such bodily changes as emotions, questions about the functions of emotions give way to questions about the function of socially constructed ways of structuring one's experience into emotional-life narratives. For Mancuso and Sarbin, such narratives not only provide individuals with ways of making sense of their inner lives, but they also provide the sociomoral rule systems through which individuals enact their emotional lives in interactions with others. Furthermore, as a historical construction, the prevailing experience of emotional life in terms of "stirrings from within" is open to change. Mancuso and Sarbin suggest that full adoption of a narrative approach by experiencing individuals could transform emotional experience from a sense of "stirrings from within" to an awareness of one's construings of one's own bodily changes in contexts involving effortful activity in the world.

THINKING ABOUT EMOTIONAL DEVELOPMENT: CONTROVERSY AND CONSENSUS

There is considerable diversity in the approaches to emotional development advanced by contributors to this volume. Despite this diversity, several common themes runs through many of the approaches that have been advanced. These themes suggest some emerging points of consensus and pave the way for future exploration of the shapes of emotional development.

Modularity and Systems Metaphors in Models of Emotion

The subtitle of the Ackerman et al. chapter on discrete emotions theory calls for a need to be "mindful of modularity." The subtitle is timely, as most contributors to this volume advanced models of emotion that embraced some version of a modularity thesis. Indeed, three theorists (Ackerman et al; Lewis & Douglas; Panksepp et al.) explicitly argued that emotions themselves consist of modular systems that are independent of other psychological systems. Other theorists, while rejecting the modularity of emotions per se, nonetheless embraced the idea that emotional processes are composed of ensembles of multiple modular processes (e.g., cognitive, motivational, central nervous system, autonomic nervous system, behavioral, experiential, expressive; see contributions by Barrett; Dickson et al.; Frijda & Mesquita; Michael Lewis; Mascolo & Harkins). Alternatively, another group of theorists suggested the possibility that many or all emotional experiences may be based upon generalized rather than modular arousal or mobilization reactions (Kozak & Brown; Frijda & Mesquita; Michael Lewis; Mancuso & Sarbin). However, even among these theorists, Michael Lewis nonetheless argues for the separability of emotional states, expressions, and experiences, and does not rule out the possibility of modular receptor systems that produce different emotional states. Frijda and Mesquita, although skeptical of the existence of discrete patterns of physiological arousal, nevertheless treat emotions as coordinations of separable, culturally penetrable component processes.

A second and related theme concerns the increasing use of systems metaphors in models of emotion. According to systems theory, an integral system refers to a series of elements that are dependent upon each other and function as a unit. Although individual systems function according to their own principles, they also interact with and are modified by other such integral systems. In so doing, interacting systems mutually influence each other and self-organize into forms that are not specified in individual systems alone. The basic appeal of a systems account is the idea that individual systems have integrity even as they become modified through their interactions with other such systems. Because of this appeal, systems metaphors have attracted the attention of a variety of theorists and researchers, including those who do not refer to themselves as systems theorists. For example, Ackerman et al. explicitly make use of systems concepts in their discussion of the formation of emotion–cognitive structures. They maintain that "the emotions and cognitive systems are highly interactive and show reciprocal causality but also a degree of independent functioning, which is greatest in early childhood" (p. 93). They suggest further that

> treating emotions as a system *qua* system focuses attention on emergent properties and patterns that are not predicted by or reducible to the discrete elements alone. Order and complexity emerge out of elements and subsystems and form the basis of complex behavior.... Modularity focuses attention on intersystem connections and communication as proximal zones of development. (p. 93)

To be sure, different theorists use systems ideas in different ways. Ackerman et al. use the concept of systems to accentuate the modularity of emotion as a separable integral system. Dickson et al. use systems metaphors to describe ways in which emotional phenomena are derived from the inherent connectivity among multiple-component systems. Lewis and Douglas work to bridge the gap between models between independent and derivative views of emotions by focusing on the ways in which separable cognitive and emotional systems self-organize within any given context.

But even here, systems metaphors can help to orient research in ways that can test contradictory hypotheses. Thinking in systems terms, theorists and researchers would attempt to specify the nature of the modular systems that are relevant to the production of emotion and describe how those systems interact to produce various observed emotional phenomena. What constitutes a modular system? How will we know one when we see it? Once defined, how encapsulated is the system in question? How interconnected or dependent is the system with other such systems? How does the activity of any single modular system affect the activity of other such systems? In asking these questions, theory and research conducted from different theoretical perspectives can serve different scientific functions. Researchers sympathetic to Ackerman et al.'s admonition to be "mindful of modularity" will work to define the boundaries of modular emotion systems; functionalist and dynamic systems theorists will work to establish the permeability of interacting systems, however defined. Thus, tensions among competing perspectives can be useful in attempts to establish the boundaries and relations among emotion-relevant systems.

Intersystemic Transformations in Emotional Development

Analysis of emotional development requires not only a focus on the concept of emotion, but also clarification of what it means to speak of development. One can approach the concept of development in many ways. For example, one might define development in terms of age-related change or growth. From this view, any psychological change that covaries with age would qualify as a developmental change, including regression and quantitative change. Alternatively, one can adopt a strong definition of development as structural transformation—directed, qualitative changes in the organization of a psychological process. Werner's (Werner, 1948; Werner & Kaplan, 1963/1984) orthogenetic principle, for example, maintains that development involves movement from a global and undifferentiated state to states of increased differentiation and hierarchical integration. In adopting an orthogenetic view of development, one might ask whether and how emotions undergo developmental transformation in terms of differentiation and integration over the course of ontogenesis (Sroufe, 1979, 1996).

Different positions on whether emotions undergo developmental change are informed by different definitions of emotion and development. Biological and differential emotions theorists, who define emotion narrowly in terms of encapsulated physiological states, maintain that emotions do not undergo structural change subsequent to their emergence. Findings that basic emotional expressions emerge early in infancy and show stability thereafter are inconsistent with the concept of orthogenesis, which would predict increased differentiation of emotions from earlier global states of distress or excitement (as in Bridges, 1932). Functionalist and systems theorists, who define emotion in terms of broader ensembles of component processes, are more inclined to endorse the view that emotions undergo developmental change. Whereas functionalists appear to focus on continuity of changes in emotionality, systems theorists attempt to identify transformations in the organization of emotional elements as they develop in relation to each other. In so doing, however, none of the functionalist or systems models represented in this volume endorsed a strong differentiation model of emotional development (e.g., Bridges, 1932); instead, various emotional systems (e.g., which we label with terms such as anger, joy, etc.) are seen as differentiated from early infancy, but thereupon undergo further differentiation and integration throughout ontogenesis. Finally, those who view emotion as a derived social construction have argued that because "real" emotions do not exist, they cannot undergo developmental change. However, the socially constructed meaning systems from which experiences of emotion are derived undergo qualitative change.

Thus, there is much that develops in *emotional development*, even though not all theorists or researchers agree that *emotions* are what develops. However, cutting across theoretical orientation, and consistent with the themes of modularity of organismic systems, there is broad consensus that emotional development involves transformations in the ways in which organismic subsystems interact to produce more complex emotional wholes. In fact, in their characterization of what develops in emotional development, most contributors to this volume have proposed hypothetical constructs defined by some form of intersystemic interaction, regardless of whether a distinct emotional system is postulated. These include affective–cognitive structures (Ackerman et al.), emotional interpretations or emotional attractors (Lewis & Douglas), emotional families or processes (Barrett; Frijda & Mesquita), emotional experiences (Lewis; Mascolo & Harkins), emotional episodes (Lewis & Douglas; Mascolo & Harkins), and emotional-life narratives (Mancuso & Sarbin).

In examining developmental changes in such structures, the analyses reported in this volume do not support any attempt to map out broad states in the development of intersystemic emotional linkages or of emotional families. Instead, the research reported in this volume focuses on how emotion-relevant components develop along separable pathways and combine with each other in different ways as a function of individual, emotional domain, context, culture, and other variables. What is needed is the elaboration of more precise methods of measuring the organization of individual emotion-relevant systems as they develop in relation to each other within particular social and cultural contexts. For example, we need to find ways to make precise assessments of changes in brain systems, appraisal processes, bodily reactions, action-tendencies, experiences, expressions, and so forth, and examine how such changes influence each other throughout the course of ontogenesis. Only by charting transformations in relations among multiple emotion-relevant systems will we be able to exploit the richness of a developmental analysis of emotion.

The Multifunctionality of Emotion Processes

Despite the diversity in approaches to emotional development represented in this volume, a general consensus emerged among contributors about the functionality and even multifunctionality of emotional processes. Although disagreements occurred over whether specific emotions can be defined in terms of particular functions, virtually all contributors agreed that emotional states or processes served multiple adaptive functions for the individual and his or her social community. The view that emotions are functional phenomena stands in contrast to previous characterizations that emotions consist of disruptive processes. Barrett's distinction between *emotion processes* and *emotion-impacted processes* is quite useful in understanding the functionality of emotion. For Barrett, a psychological process is emotional to the extent that it serves functions relative to a significant relationship between the organism and its environs. As such, a particular emotional process may serve functions relative to a given organism–environment relation, but not for other presumably less significant ongoing relations. Thus, although emotional processes are always functional, they may disrupt behaviors that are unrelated to salient concerns and motives (e.g., an experience of fear induced by seeing a police officer in one's rearview mirror may function to reduce one's speed but may also disrupt one's conversation with a fellow passenger).

CONCLUSION

The concept of emotion has had a long and turbulent history in psychology and related disciplines (Calhoun & Solomon, 1984; Kleinginna & Kleinginna, 1981). Traditionally, theorists and researchers have been unable to reach consensus about the meaning of the concept of emotion or about the nature of emotional development. As is evidenced by the present volume, despite some emerging points of commonality among emotion researchers, a consensual approach to the study of emotional development has not yet been achieved. Some might argue that the lack of consensus among emotion researchers is a cause for dismay. How can we approach the study of a psychological domain if we cannot reach consensus on the nature of that domain? Although the absence of a shared understanding about emotion may seem initially unsettling, it is not necessarily a problem. The current state of the field is animated by multiple approaches that define the problems of emotion differently and thus produce disparate bodies of evidence. In this context, much can be gained by sharpening rather than smoothing distinctions among competing approaches to emotion, a goal that we hope to achieve in the present volume. As different researchers proceed with their research agendas, conflicting models and research findings may lead toward either a consensus model or the formation of a more precise system of theoretical constructs and supporting evidence that can account for the differences between competing approaches.

REFERENCES

Barrett, K. C., & Campos, J. J. (1987). Perspectives on emotional development II: A functional approach to emotions. In J. D. Osofsky (Ed.), *Handbook of infant development* (2nd ed., pp. 555–578). New York: Wiley.

Bridges, K. M. B. (1932). Emotional development in early infancy. *Child Development, 3*, 324–341.

Calhoun, C., & Solomon, R. C. (1984). *What is an emotion?* New York: Oxford University Press.

Izard, C. E. (1977). *Human emotions.* New York: Plenum Press.

Izard, C. E., Fantuauzzo, C. A., Castle, J. M., Haynes, O. M., Rayias, M. F., & Putnam, P. H. (1995). The ontogeny and significance of infants' facial expressions in the first nine months of life. *Developmental Psychology, 31*, 997–1013.

Izard, C. E., & Malatesta, C. Z. (1987). Perspectives on emotional development I: Differential emotions theory of early emotional development. In J. D. Osofsky (Ed.), *Handbook of infant development* (2nd ed., pp. 495–554). New York: Wiley.

Kleinginna, P. R., & Kleinginna, A. M. (1981). A categorized list of emotion definitions, with suggestions for a consensual definition. *Motivation and Emotion, 5*, 345–379.

Lewis, M. (1991). Ways of knowing: Objective self-awareness or consciousness. *Developmental Review, 11*, 231–243.

Sroufe, L. A. (1979). Socioemotional development. In J. D. Osofsky (Ed.), *Handbook of infant development* (1st ed., pp. 462–516). New York: Wiley.

Sroufe, L. A. (1996). *Emotional development: The organization of emotional life in the early years.* New York: Cambridge University Press.
Werner, H. (1948). *Comparative psychology of mental development* (2nd ed.). New York: Science Editions.
Werner, H., & Kaplan, B. (1984). *Symbol formation.* Hillsdale, NJ: Erlbaum. (Original published 1963)

Index

An "*f*" or "*t*" suffix indicates that a term appears in a figure or table.